Progress in Respiratory Research

Vol. 38

Series Editor

Chris T. Bolliger Cape Town

Paediatric Bronchoscopy

Volume Editors

Kostas N. Priftis Athens
Michael B. Anthracopoulos Patras
Ernst Eber Graz
Anastassios C. Koumbourlis Washington, D.C.
Robert E. Wood Cincinnati, Ohio

136 figures, 86 in color, 37 tables, and online supplementary material, 2010

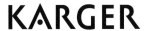

Basel · Freiburg · Paris · London · New York · Bangalore ·
Bangkok · Shanghai · Singapore · Tokyo · Sydney

Prof. Dr. Kostas N. Priftis
Allergy-Pneumonology Department
Penteli Children's Hospital
GR-152 36 P. Penteli, Athens (Greece)

Prof. Dr. Michael B. Anthracopoulos
Respiratory Unit, Department of Paediatrics
University of Patras
GR-265 04 Rio, Patras (Greece)

Prof. Dr. Ernst Eber
Klinische Abteilung für Pulmonologie/Allergologie
Universitätsklinik für Kinder- und Jugendheilkunde
Medizinische Universität Graz
Auenbruggerplatz 34
A-8036 Graz (Austria)

Prof. Dr. Anastassios C. Koumbourlis
Division of Allergy, Pulmonary and Sleep Medicine
Children's National Medical Center
George Washington University
Suite 1030, 111 Michigan Avenue, N.W.
Washington, DC 20010-2970 (USA)

Prof. Dr. Robert E. Wood
Pediatric Bronchology, Divison of Pulmonary Medicine
Cincinnati Children's Hospital Medical Center
University of Cincinnati College of Medicine
3333 Burnet Avenue MLC 2021
Cincinnati, OH 45229-3039 (USA)

Library of Congress Cataloging-in-Publication Data

Paediatric bronchoscopy / volume editors, Kostas N. Priftis ... [et al.].
      p. ; cm. -- (Progress in respiratory research ; v. 38)
  Includes bibliographical references and indexes.
  ISBN 978-3-8055-9310-6 (hard cover : alk. paper)
  1. Bronchoscopy. 2. Pediatric respiratory diseases--Diagnosis. I.
Priftis, Kostas N. II. Series: Progress in respiratory research ; v. 38.
  [DNLM: 1. Bronchoscopy--methods. 2. Child. 3. Lung--pathology. 4. Lung
Diseases--pathology. W1 PR681DM v.38 2010 / WF 500 P126 2010]
  RJ431.P34 2010
  616.2'3--dc22
                                          2010010546

Bibliographic Indices. This publication is listed in bibliographic services, including Current Contents®.

© Copyright 2010 by S. Karger AG, P.O. Box, CH–4009 Basel (Switzerland)
www.karger.com
Printed in Switzerland on acid-free and non-aging paper (ISO 9706) by Reinhardt Druck, Basel
ISSN 1422–2140
ISBN 978–3–8055–9310–6
e-ISBN 978–3–8055–9311–3

Contents

Flexible Bronchoscopy in Specific Clinical Conditions

Epilogue

▶ideo **Online supplementary material, www.karger.com/PRR038_suppl**

Foreword

Ten years ago, Praveen Mathur, Indianapolis, USA, and myself co-edited the book *Interventional Bronchoscopy* which was volume 30 in the series *Progress in Respiratory Research*. When we first presented the book at the European Respiratory Society congress in Madrid, we were overwhelmed by its success, and relatively soon the book was sold out and had to be reprinted. We thus realized that the topic had much broader appeal than we originally thought. Some time ago, I was approached by Kostas Priftis from Athens, Greece, who asked whether there might be interest for a similar book in paediatrics. I immediately showed my enthusiasm, and we quickly found a group of 5 eminent paediatric bronchoscopists who undertook to co-edit the now 38th volume of *Progress in Respiratory Research* entitled *Paediatric Bronchoscopy*. They are Michael Anthracopoulos, Patras, Greece; Ernst Eber, Graz, Austria; Anastassios Koumbourlis, Washington, D.C., USA, and Rob Wood, Cincinnati, Ohio, USA. Between them they could get the help of some of the most eminent paediatric bronchoscopists from all over the world to cover every aspect pertaining to bronchoscopy in children. Thanks to the never failing commitment of the volume editors under the leadership of Kostas Priftis, all chapters came in on time and were carefully reviewed by the editors.

As any book on endoscopy needs illustrations, we encouraged chapter authors to supply as much material as possible, including their best educational videos. A careful selection took place to choose the best pictures for the print version of this volume; the best videos, on the other hand, can all be found in an online repository and can be downloaded for free by the purchaser of the book. We are happy to announce another feature 'the electronic book' version of *Paediatric Bronchoscopy*, which was first tested in the most recent volume 37 of the series, *Clinical Chest Ultrasound*, and generated a lot of interest. This virtual book gives the reader the option to read the whole text on the screen and read it by actually turning the pages, or directly jump to a certain chapter or illustration. Quite a revolution, which – I am sure – will appeal to many readers!

True to the spirit of the series, Paediatric Bronchoscopy is not just another textbook but has its emphasis on the most modern technical developments in and approaches to the art of bronchoscopy in children. Among other things this is reflected in all chapters having the latest references available incorporated.

Finally a big thank you to the production team at Karger, led by Thomas Nold, Linda Haas and Stefan Sessler, who have supported authors, editors and myself to bring out another state-of-the-art book in *Progress in Respiratory Research*. Enjoy it in print or on your screen!

C.T. Bolliger, Cape Town

Preface

Bronchoscopy has come a long way since the times of Gustav Killian, who in 1897 used a rigid hollow tube and with the help of a headlight inspected the airways of cadavers. It has also markedly advanced from the times of Chevalier Jackson, who introduced both the illuminated endoscope and the practice of interventional endoscopy by removing foreign bodies from the oesophagus and the airway (although it has been rather difficult to surpass his reported success rate of 98% and the reduction of mortality from 24 to 2%). It has also been a long way since 1967 when the flexible fibre-optic bronchoscope was introduced in adult pulmonary medicine. At the time, nobody thought that the technique would ever be applicable to children because in addition to the lack of appropriate equipment there were no paediatric pulmonologists who would demand it and perform the procedure.

In this respect, the history of flexible bronchoscopy in children mirrors the development of paediatric pulmonology itself. The introduction, in 1980, of a flexible fibre-optic bronchoscope small enough to allow the inspection of the airways of small infants and children by Robert E. Wood (then at Case Western Reserve University and later at the University of North Carolina, Chapel Hill) provided not only a new diagnostic tool, but also helped define the new subspecialty of paediatric pulmonology. Almost 30 years later, flexible bronchoscopy has become one of the core components of paediatric pulmonary training around the world and an indispensable tool of clinical practice and research.

The aim of the current volume in the series *Progress in Respiratory Research* is to provide the interested reader with a comprehensive review and insight into paediatric bronchoscopy. Although it is the first on this subject in the English literature, it is not intended to be a classical 'textbook' but rather a 'state-of-the-art review' on specific clinical and research topics on the subject. Both the introductory and closing chapters emphasize a view of what is anticipated for the future regarding the application of this technique.

The book is divided into three sections. The first section covers a wide spectrum of technical issues regarding the preparation for and the performance of flexible bronchoscopy, ranging from common applications such as bronchoalveolar lavage to the less common such as bronchial biopsy, interventional bronchoscopy and total-lung lavage. Separate chapters also present an in-depth review of the two major alternatives to flexible bronchoscopy, i.e. rigid bronchoscopy and 'virtual' bronchoscopy.

The second section of the book is devoted to the bronchoscopic appearance of the normal upper and lower airways as well as congenital and acquired abnormalities.

The third section deals with the application of paediatric bronchoscopy in specific clinical conditions including asthma, atelectasis and plastic bronchitis, cystic fibrosis and other chronic suppurative lung diseases, endobronchial tuberculosis, chronic cough, lung transplantation and immunosuppression.

An innovation of the book series – born out of the belief that 'if a picture is worth a thousand words, a video speaks volumes' – is to include videos that can be seen online. Thus, 48 online original videos covering a large spectrum of airway pathology have been contributed by the authors of the book and greatly enhance the understanding of paediatric bronchoscopy (see online supplementary material, www.karger.com/PRR038_suppl).

Selecting the contributors among the many qualified candidates was a special challenge for the editors. In the end, it was felt that since the book is intended for an international audience, it was best to be written by an international panel

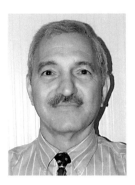
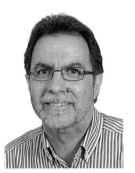
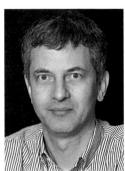
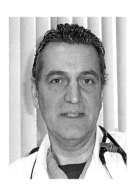
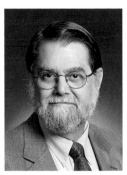

Kostas N. Priftis   Michael B.   Ernst Eber   Anastassios C.   Robert E. Wood
Anthracopoulos   Koumbourlis

of experts, thus providing multiple points of view and not just the ways of one institution or one country. We are grateful to all the authors for their effort, time and efficiency in this endeavour.

We are also indebted to the publisher, S. Karger AG, Switzerland, for adopting and supporting this project. Special thanks and gratitude go to the Series Editor, Prof. Chris Bolliger, for his 'tough love' and open-minded leadership that kept us in line throughout the process. Last but not least, we are grateful to the unsung heroes of every publication in the series, Mr. Thomas Nold and Mr. Stefan Sessler, for their technical advice, and Ms. Linda Haas, for her diligence, efficiency and incredible patience throughout this project.

With a great sigh of relief for reaching the end and satisfaction for the finished product,

Kostas N. Priftis, Michael B. Anthracopoulos, Ernst Eber,
Anastassios C. Koumbourlis, Robert E. Wood

Introduction

Priftis KN, Anthracopoulos MB, Eber E, Koumbourlis AC, Wood RE (eds): Paediatric Bronchoscopy.
Prog Respir Res. Basel, Karger 2010, vol 38, pp 2–10

Introduction

Andrew Bush

Paediatric Respirology, Imperial School of Medicine at National Heart and Lung Institute, and Department of Paediatric
Respiratory Medicine, Royal Brompton Hospital, London, UK

Sutton was an American bank robber, who, when asked why he robbed banks, replied 'because that is where the money is'. He thus gave us 'Sutton's law', and ever since then wise doctors have targeted their investigations in accord with that law, to go where the money is to be found. Since a large number of common diseases affect the airways, bronchoscopy is the tool which above all enables us to find out what is going on in airway disease, and the use of the procedure is ever increasing. The purpose of this introductory chapter is to give an overview of the scope of bronchoscopy; the details will be fleshed out in subsequent chapters.

The Key Requirements

The Bronchoscopist

Training in bronchoscopy continues all one's professional life; learning never ceases. Before setting up in independent practice, the bronchoscopist needs to acquire a thorough 3-dimensional knowledge of normal anatomy, from the tip of the nose to the lobar and segmental bronchi, together with the common normal variants (fig. 1). Furthermore, the bronchoscopist must have acquired the manual dexterity to manipulate the bronchoscope rapidly and safely along the course of the airway, and perform at least bronchoalveolar lavage (BAL), but also any other procedures being contemplated. Most bronchoscopists learn these skills on airway phantoms, animals, adult patients and finally while being carefully supervised during paediatric bronchoscopy. There is no real evidence as to how many procedures need to be performed before the individual can be considered competent; assessment on an individual basis is important. Mean times to perform procedures have been published (fig. 2) [1] and can serve as a valuable audit tool.

Finally, the bronchoscopist must have the humility to realize that discretion may be the better part of value. It is better to withdraw from the procedure and repeat it subsequently with a colleague (for example, a rigid bronchoscopist) than to get a diagnosis at the expense of serious destabilization of the child. For example, an endobronchial tumour may look tempting to biopsy (fig. 3), but severe bleeding may make control of the airway difficult unless a rigid bronchoscope is used.

The Bronchoscopy Team

Depending on what samples are being taken, the bronchoscopist will need at least one assistant and often more. These should be experienced people, who know in advance what is expected of them, and can respond rapidly to requests for equipment and process samples appropriately. Whether the team consists of nurses, technicians or respiratory therapists will depend on local practice. The main requirement is experience and competence.

The Anaesthetic Team

Increasingly, fibre-optic bronchoscopy is performed under general anaesthesia rather than sedation. If sedation is to be used, guidelines mandate that the standard of monitoring is at least as good as for an anaesthetized patient, which includes the presence of senior personnel whose role is solely the monitoring of the child [2]. General anaesthesia is my preferred option. Modern anaesthetic agents allow speedy induction of anaesthesia, complete amnesia and rapid recovery. The procedure needs to be discussed in detail with the anaesthetic team in advance – there is no point in trying to assess airway dynamics in an intubated, paralysed child. The anaesthetist needs to be very experienced. The fibre-optic bronchoscope will obstruct a large portion of the airway

[3–5], the child may be critically unstable, and a light anaesthetic allowing the child to breathe spontaneously may be required. We have no particular anaesthetic protocol, and in particular whether induction of anaesthesia is by inhalation or intravenous injection is left to the anaesthetist. It is important to stress to the family that, although the child should be encouraged to express preferences, the final word on how best to anaesthetize the child belongs not with the bronchoscopist, child or family, but is the sole prerogative of the anaesthetic team. The anaesthetist is also solely responsible for the safety of the child during the procedure and has the absolute authority to halt the procedure if the child is compromised. The bronchoscopist, no matter how senior, cannot be trusted simultaneously to perform the procedure and monitor the child's condition, because of the phenomenon of 'bronchoscopists's hypnosis' [6]. The one exception to the rule that the anaesthetist is always in charge is that a local anaesthetic should not be applied to the vocal cords before they are inspected if laryngomalacia is a possible diagnosis, because lignocaine can exaggerate the severity of this condition [7].

The Key Question: Why?

There are numerous ways of performing a bronchoscopy, and the most appropriate technique will depend upon the question being asked. The procedure should be discussed in detail with the anaesthetic team; for example, a child with stridor will need to be breathing spontaneously, and the bronchoscope will have to be passed through the nose to traverse the whole length of the respiratory tract (fig. 4). On the other hand, the immunocompromised, febrile child may be better served by being intubated for a swift diagnostic BAL. The child being bronchoscoped for haemoptysis should first have the lower airway inspected through a laryngeal mask, and only when this has been done, and a BAL performed, is the laryngeal airway mask removed and the upper airway inspected. This routine is to prevent lower airway contamination from iatrogenic upper airway bleeding.

When the procedure has been planned in detail, it is also important to return to the question of risk, which should not merely include the risk of doing the procedure, but the risks of *not* doing it. If the information is important, and can only be obtained by bronchoscopy, then the benefits justify the risks. Chevalier Jackson, the father figure of bronchoscopy, once famously but fatuously remarked that if doubt existed whether a bronchoscopy should be performed, then

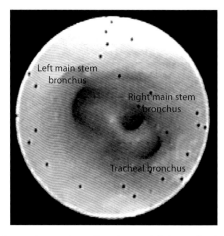

Fig. 1. Trifurcation of the trachea at the carina, due to a 'pig bronchus'. This is a normal variant usually of no clinical consequence.

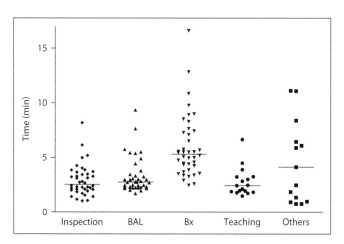

Fig. 2. Range of times spent performing different bronchoscopic procedures, reproduced with permission from Pediatr Pulmonol 2009;44:76–79. Bx = Endobronchial biopsy.

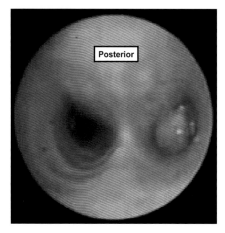

Fig. 3. There is a large endobronchial tumour protruding into the left main bronchus. Biopsy was performed with a rigid bronchoscope, which enabled safe control of the ensuing brisk haemorrhage.

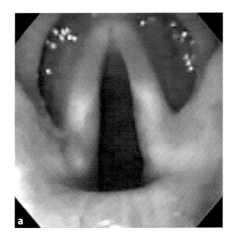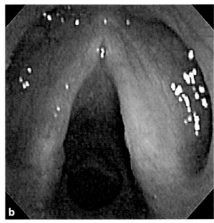

Fig. 4. a Normal true and false cords seen from above (the top is posterior). **b** There is severe subglottic stenosis secondary to previous intubation, viewed through a fibre-optic bronchoscope from above (the top is anterior). It is important not to try to advance the bronchoscope beyond the obstruction because of the risk of secondary haemorrhage and oedema causing complete airway obstruction.

a bronchoscopy ought to be performed. There have been frequent occasions when I have been in doubt about the performance of bronchoscopy, and subsequent events have made me glad that the doubts won the day.

The Specimens: Preplanning

Specimens obtained from bronchoscopy potentially include bronchial washings, BAL fluid, brush biopsy, endobronchial biopsy and transbronchial biopsy. Merely obtaining the samples is not an end in itself; there is no benefit in the most carefully obtained samples if they are not adequately processed. It is essential that all samples are rapidly transferred to the laboratory; there are no prizes for leaving precious samples in an out tray over the weekend. Some tests need to be discussed with the microbiology laboratory in advance so that the appropriate tests can be carried out at a time when the laboratory can receive the specimens.

Biopsy material may be used in multiple ways, and this should be discussed in advance. Material may need to be cultured if endobronchial tuberculosis or *Aspergillus fumigatus* is suspected. Different histological techniques may require biopsies to be snap-frozen, put in glutaraldehyde or sent fresh to the laboratory; putting the material in formalin and routinely transporting it to the laboratory is not appropriate. This is another area where preplanning is essential.

The Procedure: Having a Good Look

Inspection of the airways is routine, but other imaging procedures may be considered. The equipment used by adult pulmonologists for endobronchial ultrasound is too bulky at the moment to be used in children, but undoubtedly advances in technology will soon result in miniaturized devices, which should allow us to assess lymphadenopathy or confirm the presence of complete cartilage rings. Bronchography to diagnose bronchiectasis has passed into history, but the use of very low volumes of water-soluble contrast medium permits dynamic airway imaging (fig. 5) [8, 9]. However, it is likely that dynamic CT and MRI scanning and 'virtual bronchoscopy' may increasingly be used if imaging the airway is the only point of the procedure. Bronchoscopy will of course still be needed if specimen collection is to form part of the procedure.

The Procedure: Taking the Specimens

This is discussed in much more detail in specific chapters, but some general principles are given here. BAL is usually the first investigation to be performed, to avoid contamination from bleeding after brushing or biopsy. However, residual airway fluid may make endobronchial biopsy more difficult. It is worth considering therefore doing the lavage and the other procedures on opposite sides, if this is compatible with clinical needs.

Although pneumothorax is virtually unheard of after airway brushing or endobronchial biopsy, it is wise in my view to use only one side and never to do bilateral invasive procedures. This is most certainly true for transbronchial biopsy if it is to be performed. Since all 3 invasive procedures (airway brushing, endobronchial and transbronchial biopsy) can cause bleeding which may compromise further sampling, the order should be prioritized on an individual basis. For example, if endobronchial tuberculosis or another infection is suspected (fig. 6), my practice is to do a brush biopsy first

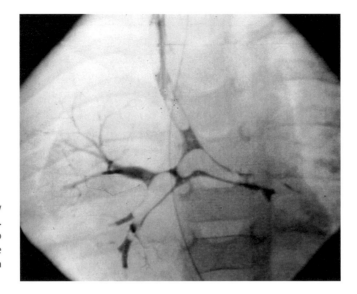

Fig. 5. Bronchogram performed with a low volume of water-soluble contrast medium. There is narrowing of the trachea due to complete cartilage rings. Contrast the tracheal diameter with that of the main bronchi.

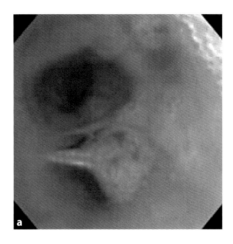
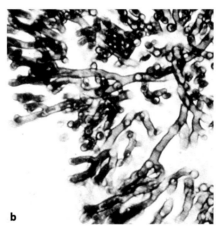

Fig. 6. a There is a thick purulent exudate adhering to the airway in this immunocompromised child. **b** Brush biopsy from the same child. There are the typical branching hyphae of *A. fumigatus*. The diagnosis was invasive aspergillosis.

and then endobronchial biopsy. If these are research procedures, then priority depends on the protocol.

The Procedure: Treatment as Well as Diagnosis

Increasing numbers of diagnoses in the fields of congenital and acquired airway disease are made bronchoscopically, but probably the main growth area in the next few years will be therapeutic bronchoscopy. Perhaps the commonest is endobronchial toilet, with removal of mucus plugs under direct vision. On occasion, they may be so large that the whole bronchoscope needs to be removed with the plug hanging off the end. Suction may be supplemented by instillation of recombinant human deoxyribonuclease under direct vision [10, 11]. Other treatments include airway stenting, endobronchial laser therapy and foreign-body removal. It is intriguing to speculate how advances in technology including 3-dimensional image guidance may allow precisely targeted, endobronchial therapy.

The Procedure: Worth Doing Anything Else?

As a general principle, it is worth considering whether there is any other procedure which does not of itself merit an anaesthetic, but is sufficiently disagreeable that it should be performed if the child has been anaesthetized for a bronchoscopy. Examples would include passing a pH probe, nasal brush biopsy for ciliary studies and intramuscular injection

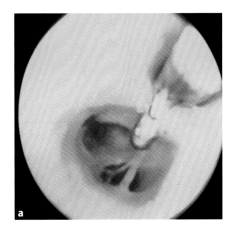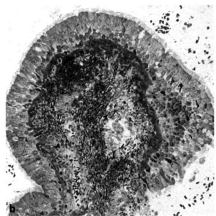

Fig. 7. Performance of endobronchial biopsy. **a** The biopsy forceps are grasping a subcarina. **b** Typical pinch biopsy obtained (2-mm biopsy channel).

of triamcinolone in severe asthma [12]. Conversely, if a child with an airway problem is being anesthetized for another procedure, it is worth considering whether a bronchoscopy should be performed under the same anaesthetic. Trying to maximize the information obtained when something invasive is being done to a child is a good principle under all circumstances.

The Procedure: Research Implications?

The principles of research in children are very clear [13]. Any procedure of more than minimal risk cannot be carried out purely for research purposes in a child. Bronchoscopy is clearly of more than minimal risk and thus can only be carried out if the individual child will derive benefit from the procedure; even if a parent or carer wishes the child to have a purely research bronchoscopy, this is not permissible. This is quite different from the situation in adults, where paying volunteers to be bronchoscoped is completely acceptable. However, what is not only permissible but actively desirable is to maximize the opportunities offered by bronchoscopy to obtain specimens for research [14]. The protocols must have been deemed scientifically valid by independent peer review, and have received approval from the ethics committee, the consent of parent and carers, and age-appropriate assent of the child. The samples should also be obtained by the most experienced bronchoscopist; this is not an appropriate training exercise. The anaesthetist should act as the guarantor of the integrity of the investigations and should stop the research component of the procedure if there is any risk due to unanticipated instability of the child.

What samples can legitimately be taken as a research procedure? Firstly, few would argue against the use for research of material that is left over after clinical tests have been performed, provided the conditions above have been met. In adult practice, BAL, endobronchial biopsy and bronchial brush biopsy are all considered low-risk procedures and are routinely performed for research. Although there has been controversy in particular about endobronchial biopsy [15–18] (fig. 7), most would think these procedures are legitimate for research in children, in the course of a clinically indicated bronchoscopy. The complication rate of transbronchial biopsy is not trivial [19], and I do not believe it is ever legitimate to undertake this procedure purely for research, during a bronchoscopy in which the procedure would not have been undertaken for clinical reasons.

The Procedure: Special Situations

Neonatal and Paediatric Intensive-Care Units
The added risks of bronchoscopy in intensive-care units have been summarized. The performance of a bronchoscopy in an already intubated child is deceptively easy but by definition these children are critically ill and may be easy to destabilize [20–22]. Depending on the patient group, important diagnoses were made in 44–90% of the patients [22, 23], and bronchoscopy represents an opportunity for therapy (as indicated above). However, if samples to rule out infection are all that is required, a blind BAL may be a safer, no less adequate technique.

There is one circumstance when bronchoscopy in the intensive-care unit is not indicated, and that is to assess the airway at the time of planned extubation 'while we take out the tube'. No useful purpose will be served by trying to inspect the airway as a vigorous child is making energetic

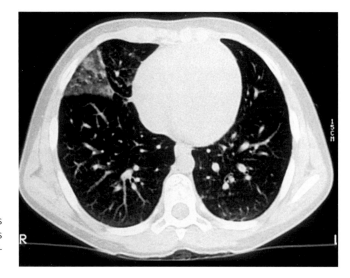

Fig. 8. CT scan appearances several hours after a BAL. There is atelectasis of the lateral segment of the right middle lobe, which is an area of disordered gas exchange which can contribute to hypoxaemia for up to 24 h.

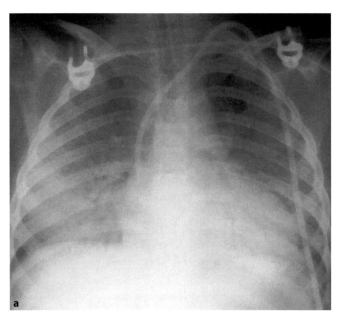

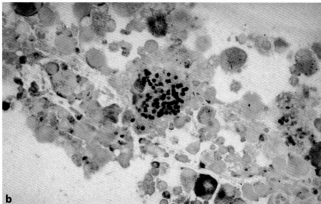

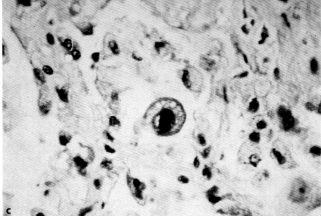

Fig. 9. a The chest radiograph in this immunocompromised child shows diffuse ground glass shadowing. The appearances are non-specific, and the differential diagnosis includes opportunistic infection and pulmonary drug toxicity. **b** Same case, silver stain of BAL. The diagnosis is *Pneumocystis jiroveci* pneumonia. **c** BAL in another immunocompromised child shows the owl's eye cells of cytomegalovirus pneumonitis.

respiratory efforts. The requirements of the intensivist and bronchoscopist are totally different; the former needs an active, non-sedated child, the latter an unhurried opportunity to assess the airway. It is much better to anaesthetize the child, have the anaesthetist remove the endotracheal tube while the airway is inspected, and then, if conditions for extubation look favourable, the child is either allowed to wake up extubated or is re-intubated, returned to the

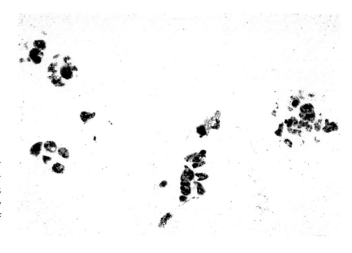

Fig. 10. Perls' stain of BAL. There are hae-mosiderin-laden macrophages due to previous pulmonary haemorrhage. These findings cannot distinguish idiopathic pulmonary haemosiderosis from secondary causes of pulmonary haemorrhage.

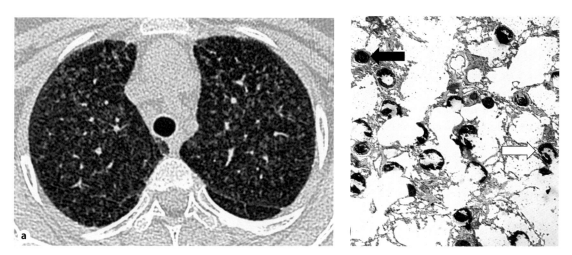

Fig. 11. **a** The CT scan in a child with ILD shows widespread nodular shadowing. **b** The transbronchial biopsy is diagnostic of alveolar microlithiasis. There are abundant calcospherites (black arrow) lying both within alveolar spaces and the interstitium. Many of them have fractured during cutting due to their hard nature (white arrow).

intensive-care unit and extubated when the effects of the anaesthetic have worn off.

Interstitial Lung Disease
In childhood interstitial lung disease (ILD), the role of bronchoscopy is much less clear than in adult ILD. If opportunistic infection is thought likely, flexible bronchoscopy and BAL constitute the next choice investigation [24] (fig. 9). A few specific diagnoses may be made on BAL (fig. 10). There are far fewer paediatric data to allow other ILDs to be diagnosed on BAL cytology, unlike in adults. Transbronchial biopsy has only a limited role because the samples obtained are very small. It may be diagnostic if the suspected ILD has very specific and focal features, which are uniformly distributed within the lung (fig. 11). Bronchoscopy is only likely to

be diagnostic in a very small number of children with ILD, and most would use open lung biopsy for the diagnosis. For research purposes, flexible bronchoscopy and BAL should be performed under the same anaesthetic to compare cytology with biopsy, with the hope that eventually we will be able to reduce the number of surgical biopsies that need to be performed.

And Afterwards?

Excellent postprocedure care is mandatory and just as important as the excitement of performing the procedure. Straightforward cases are able to be sent home on the day of the procedure. Even these children need careful monitoring of level of consciousness, oxygenation and blood pressure at the very least until they are fully awake. Admission of the patient for observation to an intensive-care unit should be considered in cases with a high probability of postoperative complications, e.g. infants with severe stridor and immunosuppressed children with rapidly evolving hypoxaemia. Postprocedure care should be planned just as carefully as the procedure itself.

Bronchoscopy: The Future

Modern medicine has reached a degree of sophistication that could not have been dreamed of years ago. With this have come novel iatrogenic problems, side effects of medications (such as the dramatic cytokine storm with the anti-CD28 monoclonal antibody TGN1412 [25]) and the complications of sophisticated procedures. Thus, the bronchoscopist must be alert to detect new airway diseases. An example is the complete tracheal infarction complicating unifocalization (an operation in which a pulmonary arterial trunk is created by stripping off and anastomosing bronchial arteries from the airway in children with complex congenital heart disease (fig. 12) [26].

Modern technology is becoming more sophisticated. Adult bronchoscopists are treating emphysema by inserting endobronchial valves and diagnosing the causes of lymphadenopathy by endobronchial-ultrasound-directed fine-needle aspiration. It is only a matter of time before these and other procedures become available for small children. The challenge will be to use them wisely; *the feasibil-*

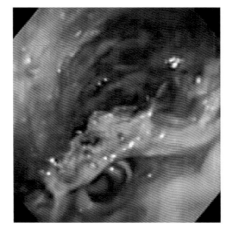

Fig. 12. Tracheal wall necrosis from infarction.

ity of a procedure is not necessarily the best indication for its performance.

Bronchoscopy: Summary and Conclusions

It is likely that the bronchoscope will become ever more versatile in terms of diagnostic and therapeutic interventions. However, the key principles of careful planning and discussion beforehand, meticulous execution during the procedure, and skilled aftercare of the child and analysis of the samples will remain important. Of these, careful thought and planning are the most important; *time spent in reconnaissance is seldom wasted.*

References

1 Regamey N, Balfour-Lynn I, Rosenthal M, Hogg C, Bush A, Davies JC: Time required to obtain endobronchial biopsies in children during fiberoptic bronchoscopy. Pediatr Pulmonol 2009;44:76–79.

2 Midulla F, de Blic J, Barbato A, Bush A, Eber E, Kotecha S, Haxby E, Moretti C, Pohunek P, Ratjen F. Flexible endoscopy of paediatric airways. Eur Respir J 2003;22:698–708.

3 Linnane B, Hafen GM, Ranganathan SC: Diameter of paediatric sized flexible bronchoscopes: when size matters. Pediatr Pulmonol 2006;41:787–789.

4 Hsia D, Di Blasi RM, Richardson P, Crotwell D, Debley J, Carter E: The effects of flexible bronchoscopy on mechanical ventilation in a pediatric lung model. Chest 2009;135:33–40.

5 Bush A: Primum non nocere: how to cause chaos with a bronchoscope in the ICU. Chest 2009;135:2–4.

6 Wood RE: Pitfalls in the use of the flexible bronchoscope in pediatric patients. Chest 1990;97:199–203.

7 Nielson DW, Ku PL, Egger M: Topical lidocaine exaggerates laryngomalacia during flexible bronchoscopy. Am J Respir Crit Care Med 2000;161:147–151.

8 MacIntyre P, Peacock C, Gordon I, Mok Q: Use of tracheobronchography as a diagnostic tool in ventilator-dependent infants. Crit Care Med 1998;26:755–759.

9 Burden RJ, Shann F, Butt W, Ditchfield M: Tracheobronchial malacia and stenosis in children in intensive care: bronchograms help to predict outcome. Thorax 1999;54:511–517.

10 Shah PL, Scott S, Hodson ME: Lobar atelectasis in cystic fibrosis and treatment with recombinant human DNase 1. Respir Med 1994;88:313–315.

11 Slattery DM, Waltz DA, Denham B. O'Mahoney M, Greally P: Bronchoscopically administered human DNase for lobar atelectasis in cystic fibrosis. Pediatr Pulmonol 2001;31:383–388.

12 Fleming L, Wilson N, Bush A: Difficult to control asthma in children. Curr Opin Allergy Clin Immunol 2007;7:190–195.

13 McIntosh N, Bates P, Brykczynska G, Dunstan G, Goldman A, Harvey D, Larcher V, McCrae D, McKinnon A, Patton M, Saunders J, Shelley P: Guidelines for the ethical conduct of medical research involving children. Royal College of Paediatrics, Child Health: Ethics Advisory Committee. Arch Dis Child 2000;82:177–182.

14 Bush A: Guidelines for the ethical conduct of medical research involving children. Arch Dis Child 2000;83:370.

15 Mallory GB Jr: Pitfalls in non-therapeutic research in children. Pediatr Pulmonol 2006;41:1014–1016.

16 Bush A, Davies JC: Rebuttal: you are wrong, Dr. Mallory... Pediatr Pulmonol 2006;41:1017–1020.

17 Mallory GB Jr: Re: pitfalls in non-therapeutic research in children. Pediatr Pulmonol 2007;42:656–657.

18 Bush A, Davies JC: Response to Mallory: you are civilized, but still wrong, Dr. Mallory. Pediatr Pulmonol 2007;42:658.

19 Whitehead B, Scott JP, Helms P, Malone M, Macrae D, Higenbottam TW, Smyth RL, Wallwork J, Elliott M, de Leval M: Technique and use of transbronchial biopsy in children and adolescents. Pediatr Pulmonol 1992;12:240–246.

20 Bush A: Bronchoscopy in paediatric intensive care. Paediatr Respir Rev 2003;4:67–73.

21 Schelhase DE, Graham LM, Fix EJ, Sparks LM, Fan LL: Diagnosis of tracheal injury in mechanically ventilated premature infants by flexible bronchoscopy. Chest 1990;98:1219–1225.

22 Manna SS, Durward A, Moganasundram S, Tibby SM, Murdoch IA: Retrospective evaluation of a paediatric intensivist-led flexible bronchoscopy service. Intensive Care Med 2006;32:2026–2033.

23 Bar-Zohar D, Sivan Y: The yield of flexible fiberoptic bronchoscopy in pediatric intensive care patients. Chest 2004;126:1353–1359.

24 Riedler J, Grigg J, Robertson CF: Role of bronchoalveolar lavage in children with lung disease. Eur Respir J 1995;8:1725–1730.

25 Suntharalingam G, Perry MR, Ward S, Brett SJ, Castello-Cortes A, Brunner MD, Panoskaltsis N: Cytokine storm in a phase 1 trial of the anti-CD28 monoclonal antibody TGN1412. N Engl J Med 2006;355:1018–1028.

26 Schulze-Neick I, Ho SY, Bush A, Rosenthal M, Franklin RC, Redington AN, Penny DJ: Severe airflow limitation after the unifocalization procedure: clinical and morphological correlates. Circulation 2000;102(suppl 3):III142–147.

Prof. Andrew Bush, MBBS (Hons), MA, MD, FRCP, FRCPCH
Department of Paediatric Respiratory Medicine, Royal Brompton Hospital
Sydney Street
London SW3 6NP (UK)
Tel. +44 207 351 8232, Fax +44 207 351 8763, E-Mail a.bush@rbh.nthames.nhs.uk

Techniques and Technical Issues

Priftis KN, Anthracopoulos MB, Eber E, Koumbourlis AC, Wood RE (eds): Paediatric Bronchoscopy.
Prog Respir Res. Basel, Karger 2010, vol 38, pp 12–21

Bronchoscopic Equipment

Ian M. Balfour-Lynn[a] · Jonny Harcourt[b]

[a]Department of Paediatric Respiratory Medicine, Royal Brompton Hospital, and [b]Department of Paediatric Otolaryngology, Chelsea and Westminster and Royal Brompton Hospitals, London, UK

Abstract

Bronchoscopic equipment is expensive and must be properly maintained. Sufficient initial outlay is required to provide adequate back-up equipment. Modern hybrid bronchofibrevideoscopes combine digital technology with fibre-optic glass rods to produce an instrument that is small enough for use in children. These provide extremely clear images which can be digitally recorded and reproduced. A workstation is required to hold the ancillary equipment – flat-screen monitor, light source and video processor. Extra equipment is required for cleaning and disinfecting the bronchoscopes and their removable parts, and a proper storage space is necessary.

Any hospital planning to set up a bronchoscopy service must be aware that this will require a significant start-up financial outlay. There will also be routine maintenance costs (e.g. cleaning, replacement of disposable parts) as well as occasional repair costs, which can be expensive if a bronchoscope is broken.

Flexible Bronchoscopes

It is important to have sufficient bronchoscopes to ensure that logistical problems are not encountered whilst servicing or repairs are being carried out. Occasionally a bronchoscope (or more usually its suction channel) malfunctions during a procedure itself, hence the need for a standby bronchoscope. Unfortunately some units may have difficulty with this due to the prohibitive price of bronchoscopes, which cost in the range of GBP 20,000.

There are several types of bronchoscopes available for paediatric use. Clearly the size of the bronchoscope used is dependent on the size of the airways (and hence the size of the child). In younger children, the smallest bronchoscope available should be used, in order to reduce blockage of the airway and minimize local trauma. The exception is if an endobronchial biopsy is to be performed, in which case it is better to use an instrument with the biggest available biopsy channel, provided that it is safe for the child [1]. The manufacturers usually describe the bronchoscope by the diameter of the distal tip; however, this is not always the maximum diameter of the bronchoscope. A small study has shown a discrepancy between the stated external diameter (of the tip) and the maximum diameter of the insertion tube that ranged from 0.19 to 0.66 mm, with a mean of 0.41 mm [2]. This is only likely to be relevant when a bronchoscope is used down an endotracheal tube (ETT) in a small child when the size is critical. In general, the larger the bronchoscope, the better the image obtained but even the smaller ones allow remarkably good views, with a 120-degree field of view. The image from the standard bronchofibrescopes is never as clear as that obtained by rigid bronchoscopes with their Hopkins rod lens telescopes. These are invariably the images found in textbooks, which can mislead trainees who need to be able to perform a bronchoscopy with suboptimal views. Since the advent of the hybrid bronchofibrevideoscopes and bronchovideoscopes however, pictures can be as clear as those obtained with rigid bronchoscopes.

If the bronchoscope is being inserted down an ETT for general anaesthesia with assisted breathing, its size is critical as it partially blocks the ETT. This means a relatively smaller bronchoscope may need to be used for the size of the child, compared to inserting it via a laryngeal mask or down the nose via a facemask (table 1). The proportion of the cross-sectional area that the bronchoscope blocks can be

Table 1. Sizes of flexible bronchoscopes that can be passed safely down differently sized ETTs, along with typical ages of relevant patients

Bronchoscope external diameter	ETT internal diameter	Size of patient
2.2 mm	3.0 – 3.5 mm	premature neonate
2.8 mm	4.0 mm	term neonate
3.6 mm	5.0 mm	small child (3–4 years)
4.0 mm	5.5 mm	child 4–8 years
4.9 mm	6.0 mm	child over 8 years

Table 2. Bronchofibrescopes

Manufacturer's code	External diameter mm	Size of patient	Suction/instrument channel mm	Biopsy	Brushings
Olympus bronchofibrescopes					
BF-N20	2.2	neonate	no	no	no
BF-XP60	2.8	neonate – infant	1.2	just	yes
BF-3C40	3.6	infant, small child	1.2	just	yes
BF-MP60	4.0	small child	2.0	yes	yes
BF-P60	4.9	big child (>7–8 years)	2.2	yes	yes
BF-IT60	6.0	adult	3.0	yes	yes
BF-XT40	6.2	adult	3.2	yes	yes
Pentax bronchofibrescopes					
FB-8V	2.7	neonate – infant	1.2	just	yes
FB-10V	3.4	infant, small child	1.2	just	yes
FB-15V	4.9	big child (>7–8 years)	2.2	yes	yes
FB-18V	5.9	adult	2.8	yes	yes
FB-19TV	6.2	adult	3.2	yes	yes

calculated from this formula: [1 – (bronchoscope radius^2/ ETT radius^2) × 100]. Hence a 3.6-mm bronchoscope down a 5-mm ETT blocks 48% of the potential space for airflow. Generally the ETT internal diameter needs to be at least 1 mm greater than the external diameter of the bronchoscope [3; chapter 5, this vol., pp. 54–63].

The smallest (Olympus) neonatal 2.2-mm bronchoscope has no suction channel, and its use has been limited since the advent of the 2.8-mm bronchoscope (with a 1.2-mm suction channel). Nevertheless, it may be used in a ventilated neonate with a 3-mm ETT in whom visualization of the airways is essential. The neonatal bronchoscope can only be used for a visual inspection, as lavage cannot be performed, but this can be hampered if mucus settles on the lens and obscures vision as it can usually not be cleared unless the whole scope is removed and wiped. In addition, the 2.2-mm bronchoscope is fragile and breaks easily.

The 1.2-mm suction/instrument channel is usually adequate for lavage and suction, the exception being when the secretions and mucus are excessively thick or sticky, as is typically found in children with more advanced cystic fibrosis lung disease. The larger 2-mm channel is also more useful when trying to suction up mucus plugs that have been blocking an airway. Excellent-quality biopsies can be obtained with 2-mm forceps that fit down the 2-mm working channel; reasonable biopsies can also be obtained from the smaller 1-mm forceps that fit the 1.2-mm channel but the procedure is more difficult and the biopsies are really quite small, hence often of poorer quality [4]. Lasers can be used in bronchoscopes with suction/instrument channels of 2 mm and above, and ultrasonic probes in the 2.8-mm channel and above. These technologies are not usually employed in children [chapter 4, this vol., pp. 42–53].

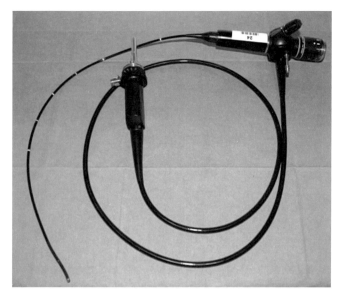

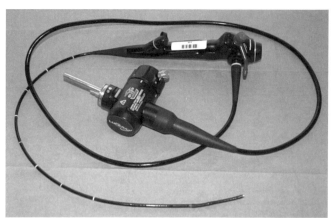

Fig. 2. Hybrid bronchofibrevideoscope with 4.0-mm outside diameter.

Fig. 1. Bronchofibrescope with 3.6-mm outside diameter.

Table 3. Hybrid bronchofibrevideoscopes manufactured by Olympus

Manufacturer's code	External diameter mm	Size of patient	Suction/instrument channel mm	Biopsy	Brushings
BF-XP260F	2.8	neonate – infant	1.2	just	yes
BF-P260F	4.0	small child	2.0	yes	yes

The principal manufacturers of paediatric broncho-scopes are Olympus and Pentax, and details of their available equipment are best seen on their respective websites (www. keymed.co.uk or www.olympusamerica.com; www.pentax. co.uk or www.pentaxmedical.com). Product information is accurate at the time of writing this chapter.

Bronchofibrescope
This is the classic fibre-optic bronchoscope (table 2, fig. 1) in which light and hence the image travels along extremely fine glass fibres (also known as image guide fibres or fibre-optic rods).

Hybrid Bronchofibrevideoscope
This has a built-in charge-coupled device in the control section and thus combines video and fibre-optic technol-ogy (table 3, fig. 2). This allows use of video technology in a smaller bronchoscope. The newer technology produces larger, clearer and brighter images, and there is an automatic focus and light adjustment. These scopes are also much lighter in weight and hence easier to handle.

Bronchovideoscope
These are generally larger bronchoscopes (table 4) as the charge-coupled device is incorporated into the distal end of the instrument ('chip in the tip'); they do not contain glass fibre rods.

Battery-Powered Bronchoscopes
Pentax make portable 'bedside' fibre-optic bronchoscopes (FB series) that run off a self-contained battery-powered light source. They can also be attached to a standard light source (table 5).

Intubation Bronchoscopes
Finally, Pentax make a series of fibre-optic intubation endo-scopes for anaesthetists (FI series). The smallest is 2.4 mm but has no suction channel.

Table 4. Bronchovideoscopes

Manufacturer's code	External diameter mm	Size of patient	Suction/instrument channel mm	Biopsy	Brushings
Olympus bronchovideoscopes					
BF-260	4.9	big child (>7–8 years)	2.0	yes	yes
BF-1T260	5.9	adult	2.8	yes	yes
Pentax bronchovideoscopes					
EB-1170K	3.8	infant, small child	1.2	yes	yes
EB-1570K	5.5	teenager/adult	2.0	yes	yes
EB-1970K	6.3	adult	2.8	yes	yes

Table 5. Battery-powered bronchoscopes manufactured by Pentax

Manufacturer's code	External diameter mm	Size of patient	Suction/instrument channel mm	Biopsy	Brushings
FB-15BS/ FB-15RBS	4.8	big child (>7–8 years)	2.0	yes	yes
FB-18BS/ FB-18RBS	5.9	adult	2.6	yes	yes

Hence to take advantage of the better images obtained by digital video technology, paediatricians will need to use the Olympus hybrid 2.8- and 4.0-mm bronchoscopes, or the Pentax 3.7- and 5.1-mm bronchoscopes.

Bronchoscope Components

The bronchoscope attaches to the light source and video processor from a fixed lead that comes off the control section (proximal part of bronchoscope). The eyepiece (on bronchofibrescopes) is at the tip of this part, and when attached to a TV monitor an attachment locks onto the eyepiece with a bayonet mount. A manual focus button is on this attachment as well as remote control buttons that can be used to control video recording and still pictures. Hybrid and videoscopes do not require this attachment, and the buttons to control recording are just distal to the suction valve; focus is automatic, so there is no separate control button.

The suction valve is sited on the control section (convenient for the index finger) but can be taken off to be autoclaved. Stand-alone suction pumps (or wall suction) connect to the valve with disposable suction tubing.

Lower down this section is the biopsy port, through which lavage fluid, biopsy forceps and brushes are inserted.

The control section also has the lever (convenient for the thumb) which controls the distal tip of the bronchoscope; this allows a bending angle upwards of 180° and downwards of 130°. The Pentax K series (3.7 and 5.1 mm) bronchoscopes have an extended upward angulation of 210°.

On the distal tip of the bronchoscope there are the objective lens, light guide (2 of these in larger instruments) and instrument/suction channel (fig. 3). In the adult large videoscopes, the charge-coupled device is located on the tip as well.

Bronchoscopy 'Tower'

The workstation holds all the ancillary electronic equipment, which is specific to the manufacturer of the bronchoscope (fig. 4).

A bright light source is essential (unless using the battery-operated Pentax bronchoscopes).

A video system centre (a multifunction processor) is available for use with hybrid and videoscopes. A keyboard is attached to put in patient details etc.

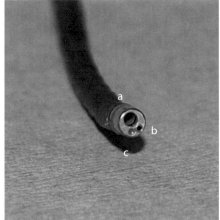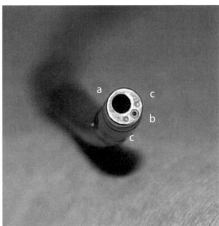

Fig. 3. Distal tips of hybrid bronchofibrevideoscopes. On the left is the tip of a 2.8-mm bronchoscope with suction/instrument channel (a), objective lens (b) and light guide (c). On the right is the tip of a 4.0-mm bronchoscope which has 2 light guides (c).

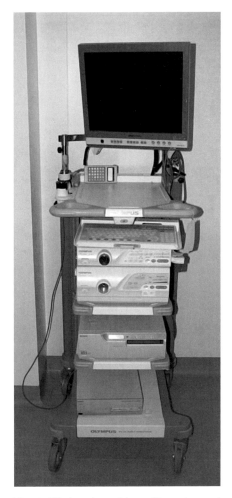

Fig. 4. Workstation with ancillary electronic equipment. From the top down are shown: the flat-screen LCD monitor, the keyboard for data entry, light source, video processor and photo printer.

There is a colour video monitor or high-definition flat-screen LCD monitor. With the standard bronchofibrescopes, the bronchoscopy can be performed with the operator using the eyepiece, which gives a surprisingly clear (albeit small) picture. However, with hybrid and videoscopes, a high-definition monitor is needed to see the images. This has the advantage of allowing others to watch the procedure at the same time, and a large clear image is helpful for the bronchoscopist.

An adaptor is available so that the older bronchofibrescopes can be attached to the newer video monitoring system (backward compatibility); this locks over the eyepiece with a bayonet mount. This is useful when changing over to the newer system as older bronchoscopes can still be used, although it makes them somewhat top heavy and unbalanced.

Recording equipment is essential to be able to record all procedures. This allows review with colleagues (useful if the findings are complex or for discussion with surgeons), review if the procedure is being repeated at a later date, use in teaching sessions and as an aid for potential medicolegal issues. It can also be helpful for demonstrating findings to parents and patients when necessary. The videoscopes record onto CD-ROMs, but the older systems utilize a digital tape recorder or standard video tape recorder. The CD-ROMs are particularly useful as bronchoscopy clips can be stored on a hard drive and are easily inserted into presentation software for teaching purposes.

Colour video printers are also available to produce instant colour images, which can be helpful for explaining findings to parents and are also useful for recording results in notes and for sending to referring centres.

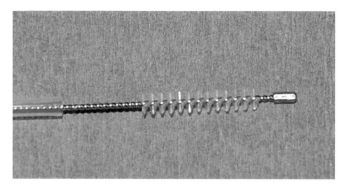

Fig. 5. Tip of cytology brush, shown outside its sheath.

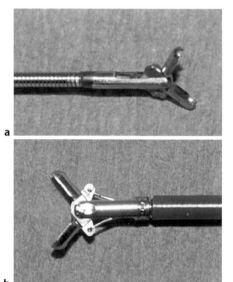

a

b

Fig. 6. Ends of endobronchial biopsy forceps. **a** Reusable cupped forceps that fit down a 1.2-mm instrument channel. **b** Disposable swing jaw forceps that fit down a 2-mm channel.

a single-use unsheathed brush is available [chapter 4, this vol., pp. 42–53].

Biopsy forceps can be used for endobronchial mucosal biopsies under direct vision and transbronchial biopsies under radiological image intensifier control. There are a number of types including single-use disposable or reusable ones. Although disposable forceps are more expensive, the reusable ones become blunt with time and hence less efficient; the reusable forceps must also be autoclaved. There are a number of tips available, including smooth oval cup forceps (with or without a needle), alligator jaw forceps and rat tooth forceps; the smallest size (for the 1.2-mm channel) only come as reusable ones (fig. 6). The tip of the forceps is visible at a minimum distance of 5 mm from the distal end of the scope and 3 mm in smaller scopes. The 2-mm forceps come in a low-friction sheath that makes them easier to pass down the instrument channel, especially when there is an acute bend at the distal end of the scope [chapter 4, this vol., pp. 42–53].

In adult bronchoscopy, aspiration needles, grasping forceps (for foreign bodies), balloon catheters, electrosurgical and laser attachments, and ultrasonic probes are also available. In paediatric practice, use of endobronchial ultrasound has been described [5]. There is a 1.2-mm diameter 20-MHz endobronchial ultrasound probe (UM-S20–17S, Olympus, Tokyo, Japan) which is placed inside a 1.7-mm plastic guide sheath. This can then be passed down a 2-mm instrument channel (for relevantly sized bronchoscopes, see tables 2 and 4) to perform radial probe endobronchial ultrasound in order to localize peripheral lung lesions. Use of linear probe endobronchial ultrasound to sample hilar and mediastinal lymph nodes requires a specific bronchoscope (Olympus BF-UC160F-OL8) which has a 6.9-mm external maximum diameter, so this is limited to older children who are large enough (usually weighing >50 kg) for an 8-mm ETT.

Equipment for Procedures

Equipment for bronchoalveolar lavage is simple but must all be sterile. It includes a bag of 0.9% normal saline, a jug/container for the saline, syringes (10 or 20 ml) and sputum traps that connect to the suction valve [chapter 3, this vol., pp. 30–41].

Cytology brushes (fig. 5) are disposable, and for the larger bronchoscopes with 2-mm channels, brushes can be used that have a sheath to withdraw the brush into during insertion and removal of the brush from the instrument channel. For the bronchoscope with a 1.2-mm working channel,

The Trolley

A trolley is useful for the accessory equipment needed. Ours is set up to contain: jug with room temperature 0.9% (normal) saline, which is used to fill the syringes for lavage and also to suction up through the bronchoscope at the end of the procedure to clear the suction channel prior to full cleaning; 10- or 20-ml syringes for inserting saline lavage fluid; sputum traps for the lavage; sterile gauze swabs; lubricant jelly for the distal end of the bronchoscope; alcohol wipe for the tip of the scope; brushes and forceps; containers for brushings/biopsies; sterile gloves.

We also keep percutaneoulsy inserted central catheters (long lines) and an assortment of blood bottles as we take advantage of the general anaesthesia to perform venepuncture and insert a long line if the child needs intravenous antibiotics following the procedure.

Bronchoscopic Logs

It is important to carefully record the results from the procedure, including normal findings, in addition to whether lavage and biopsies were performed, as well as any complications that might have occurred. Whilst this would be best done electronically, we still record this by hand on a paper proforma that is in duplicate (Appendix). Ideally a department will also keep an electronic database of all bronchoscopies performed.

Consent Form

This is obviously mandatory and it is best to use procedure-specific forms for parents and/or the patient to sign. This should outline the procedure itself (detailing what happens before, during and after the bronchoscopy), as well as benefits, complications and risks. Consent should also include bronchoalveolar lavage as well as biopsy and brushings. There should be a separate section for any research use that may be made from surplus material (lavage fluid, biopsies), including whether material will be stored for future use. Finally it should be made clear that an electronic recording of the procedure is made that may be used for training (once anonymized). Consequently, our consent form is 7 pages long.

Models for Training

It is useful for any department involved in training to have a model that trainees can practise on. Models of the whole head/neck and lungs exist, as do latex casts of the airways. Some anatomical models are available from Adam Rouilly Ltd. (www.adam-rouilly.co.uk). Bronchoscopic simulator training models can also be useful [6].

Cleaning Equipment

Detailed information on cleaning and disinfecting equipment should be obtained from the manufacturer of the bronchoscopes that a department owns. Adherence to recommendations is critical to avoid cross-infection and contamination of lavage samples that could lead to false-positive microbiological results [7]. Equipment will include brushes (e.g. channel-cleaning and port-cleaning), detergents, disinfectants and 70% ethyl or isopropyl alcohol to assist drying. A leakage testing device is also used, and if the test is not satisfactory, the bronchoscope should not be immersed in the cleaning fluids but must be sent back to the manufacturer [4]. Bronchoscopes are best stored hanging in a purpose-built ventilated cupboard and should not be kept in their carrying cases as the foam fillings in the cases can harbour bacteria.

Instructions on cleaning flexible bronchoscopes issued by KeyMed (Medical & Industrial Equipment) Ltd. takes the form of 10 steps:

1 Take a secure hold of the endoscope and wipe down the insertion tube with a neutral detergent solution using a soft cloth or gauze square
2 Depress the suction valve and with the tip of the bronchoscope immersed, suck up some of the detergent solution through its channel
3 Remove all valves and adaptors for separate cleaning; disconnect the bronchoscope from the light source, video processor (if applicable) and suction pump
4 Perform a leakage test on the bronchoscope; in the case of videoscopes, the waterproof cap must be attached prior to full immersion
5 Immerse the bronchoscope fully in a neutral detergent solution and use the port cleaning brush (MH-507) to clean the biopsy port opening, suction port opening and also to carefully clean the distal end of the bronchoscope
6 Pass the channel cleaning brush through (a) the biopsy port and down the insertion tube, (b) the suction port and down the insertion tube, (c) through the suction connector and control body (if applicable); it is important to clean the brush head each time it emerges from the endoscope
7 Immerse endoscope and irrigate channels with (a) detergent, (b) disinfectant, (c) water; it is important to ensure adequate irrigation/contact times
8 Dry the external surface of the endoscope; the use of an alcohol wipe is recommended to assist in the drying process
9 Remove residual fluid from the channel; the use of a little 70% ethyl or isopropyl alcohol is recommended to assist in the drying process
10 Hang the bronchoscope in a ventilated cupboard

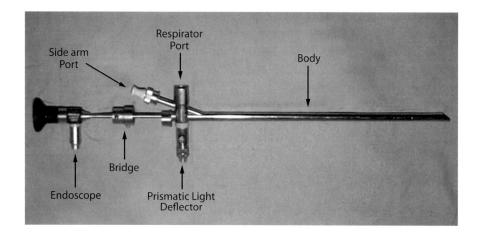

Fig. 7. Rigid paediatric bronchoscope.

Table 6. Suitable sizes of Storz bronchoscopes by age of child with normal-sized airways

Age of child	Tracheal diameter, mm	Storz bronchoscope	
		size	outer diameter, mm
Preterm to 1 month	5	2.5	4.2
1–6 months	5–6	3	5.0
6–18 months	6–7	3.5	5.7
18 months to 3 years	7–8	4	6.7
3–6 years	8–9	4.5	7.3
6–9 years	9–10	5	7.8
9–12 years	10–13	6	8.2
12–14 years	13	6	8.2

Rigid Bronchoscopes

The most widely available range of paediatric broncho-scopes is manufactured by Karl Storz (www.karlstorz.com). The appropriate size of bronchoscope depends on the child's age (table 6), but if a subglottic (or tracheal) stenosis is suspected, the size of the bronchoscope may be reduced by 1 or 2 sizes [chapter 8, this vol., pp. 83–94].

The bronchoscope has 6 main parts (fig. 7):
- *Body:* age-appropriate size (and length); may have side ports for improved ventilation but these may not be appropriate in the presence of a tracheal stenosis or inflammatory disorder as the edge of the side ports may traumatize the trachea; bronchoscopes without side ports are available or the side ports may be covered in tape
- *Side arm:* for suction tubing and instrumentation (microforceps)

- *Prismatic light deflector:* for illumination if naked eye and lens are used to main port; otherwise put at position 1 (the first stop on the port) to seal
- *Bridge:* to stabilize the endoscope and seal the bronchoscope
- *Endoscope:* usually attached to camera and monitor allowing others to observe the procedure
- *Respirator port:* to attach to anaesthetic circuit

For safety, a full set of laryngoscopes and bronchoscopes should be available, to adapt to any circumstances encountered during the case.

Apart from a full range of bronchoscopes, the following should also be available:
- Optical forceps to remove any foreign bodies; these are a separate grasping instrument passed down the bronchoscope, with their own intrinsic 0-degree

endoscope, giving an excellent view of the entrapment and withdrawal of the foreign body

- Biopsy forceps
- Bronchoscope-size-appropriate 0- and 30-degree endoscopes to give a range of views of the airway

Conflict of Interest

The paediatric respiratory department at Royal Brompton Hospital runs a paediatric flexible bronchoscopy course on alternate years. Key Med (Medical & Industrial Equipment) Ltd. is the UK sales outlet for Olympus bronchoscopes and has been involved with this course since its inception in 1998.

Appendix

Proforma for recording results of bronchoscopy

Royal Brompton & Harefield NHS
NHS Trust

Hospital number:

Indications -

Surname:

Forenames:

DOB:

Ward: Rose / PICU

Consultant:

Date: BRONCHOSCOPY REPORT

Bronchoscopist: Anaesthetist:

Bronchoscope: 2.8 / 3.6 / 4.0 / 4.9   Facemask / LMA / ETT / tracheostomy

FINDINGS -

Right   *Left*

BAL	Lobe(s) -	Vol. IN -	Ciliary brushings
Endobronchial biopsy	Lobe(s) -	Number -	pH probe
Brushings	Lobe(s) -	Number -	Bloods
			PICC line
			IM triamcinolone
			Other

Complications:

Recommendations: Signed:
                                             Print name:

DOB = Date of birth; PICU = paediatric intensive-care unit; LMA = laryngeal mask airway; BAL = bronchoalveolar lavage; PICC = peripherally inserted central catheter; IM = intramuscular.

References

1 Midulla F, de Blic J, Barbato A, Bush A, Eber E, Kotecha S, Haxby E, Moretti C, Pohunek P, Ratjen F, ERS Task Force: Flexible endoscopy of paediatric airways. Eur Respir J 2003;22:698–708.

2 Linnane B, Hafen GM, Ranganathan SC: Diameter of paediatric sized flexible bronchoscopes: when size matters. Pediatr Pulmonol 2006;41:787–789.

3 Jaggar SI, Haxby E: Sedation, anaesthesia and monitoring for bronchoscopy. Paediatr Respir Rev 2002;3:321–327.

4 Regamey N, Hilliard TN, Saglani S, Zhu J, Scallan M, Balfour-Lynn IM, Rosenthal M, Jeffery PK, Alton EW, Bush A, Davies JC: Quality, size, and composition of pediatric endobronchial biopsies in cystic fibrosis. Chest 2007;131:1710–1717.

5 Steinfort DP, Wurzel D, Irving LB, Ranganathan SC: Endobronchial ultrasound in pediatric pulmonology. Pediatr Pulmonol 2009;44:303–308.

6 Davoudi M, Colt HG: Bronchoscopy simulation: a brief review. Adv Health Sci Educ Theory Pract 2009;14:287–296.

7 British Thoracic Society Bronchoscopy Guidelines Committee, a Subcommittee of Standards of Care Committee of BTS: BTS guidelines on diagnostic flexible bronchoscopy. Thorax 2001;56(suppl 1):i1–i21. www.brit-thoracic.org.uk.

Dr. I.M. Balfour-Lynn
Department of Paediatric Respiratory Medicine, Royal Brompton Hospital
Sydney Street
London SW3 6NP (UK)
Tel. +44 0 207 351 8509, Fax +44 0 207 349 7754, E-Mail i.balfourlynn@ic.ac.uk

Priftis KN, Anthracopoulos MB, Eber E, Koumbourlis AC, Wood RE (eds): Paediatric Bronchoscopy.
Prog Respir Res. Basel, Karger 2010, vol 38, pp 22–29

Sedation and Anaesthesia for Bronchoscopy

Jacques de Blic[a] · Caroline Telion[b]

[a]Paediatric Pulmonology Unit and [b]Department of Anaesthesiology, Hôpital Necker-Enfants Malades, and Université Paris Descartes, Paris, France

Abstract

Appropriate sedation is important for a well-tolerated broncho-scopic procedure. Pre-assessment of the child is essential in order to anticipate potential difficulties and complications. The available techniques include conscious and deep sedation. Various protocols may be used during flexible bronchoscopy that entail the administration of a single oral or intravenous drug or drug combination (e.g. midazolam, meperidine, propofol, ketamine, remifentanyl), or inhalational agents (premixed nitrous oxide, sevoflurane). Whichever the choice of sedation and the technique of oxygen delivery (nasal prongs, face mask, laryngeal mask, endotracheal intubation), it is essential to maintain and preserve spontaneous ventilation. Controlled ventilation is often used during rigid bronchoscopy for foreign-body removal. The most frequent complication of sedation is hypoxaemia, either as an isolated problem or in association with laryngospasm and/or bronchospasm. Transcutaneous oxygen de-saturation can be secondary to partial or total airway obstruction by the bronchoscope and/or depression due to sedation. Pre-operative detection of high-risk patients, administration of appropriate anaesthesia and monitoring of patients are essential for a successful procedure and help to minimize potential complications.

Bronchoscopy has become an indispensable tool for the diagnosis and treatment of infants and children with respiratory disease. Since its introduction in the mid-70s, an increasing number of flexible bronchoscopies (FBs) are being performed each year. The diagnostic value of FB is now widely accepted: it can be used to visualize the lower airways directly and to take samples, particularly of bronchoalveolar lavage fluid by performing bronchoalveolar lavage during the procedure [1; chapter 3, this vol., pp. 30–41]. Its indications are hardly limited to exploring stridor, persistent atelectasis or recurrent pneumonia in ambulatory patients; more severely ill children, who are in an unstable respiratory status, may also require bronchoscopy [2], sometimes under mechanical ventilation, in neonatal or paediatric intensive-care units [chapter 5, this vol., pp. 54–63]. Performing a safe and successful examination and sampling of the airways depend on the experience and skill of the operator and on how well the child tolerates the procedure. This chapter discusses sedation in FB and, briefly, in rigid bronchoscopy (RB). The process of sedation includes various parts, which are intricate and interdependent. These may be artificially separated in 3 phases: (a) the prebronchoscopic procedures; (b) the sedation/anaesthesia period that involves the procedure itself, and (c) the postbronchoscopic period, i.e. the time during and after the awakening of the patient.

Prebronchoscopic Procedures

FB can be performed in a day care or an inpatient setting. Both the bronchoscopist and the anaesthetist should obtain a detailed history and perform a complete physical examination. Pre-operative assessment of the child is essential, including current respiratory status, medications and associated diseases. The ASA numerical scale, described by the American Society of Anaesthesiologists, is predictive of the peri-operative adverse events [3]. A written, fully informed consent should be obtained. The family and child (when age appropriate) should be offered detailed information on the procedure prior to admission. This should include the risks of the procedure and the likelihood that a particularly high-risk child may require postbronchoscopic care in an intensive or a high-dependency care unit. The anticipated anaesthesia or sedation of the patient and the need for intravenous access should also be discussed [1].

Fasting prior to the procedure is usually 4–6 h for milk and solids and 2 h for water. The need for premedication is at the discretion of the anaesthetist. In general, if adequate explanation is provided, it is unnecessary to administer sedative premedication as this may delay postprocedural recovery. However, if the child is distressed or unable to cooperate, premedication is advisable. Oral atropine (0.01–0.02 mg/kg) minimizes bradycardia induced by vasovagal stimulation and also decreases airway secretions [4]. Systemic administration of atropine is not usually required with sevoflurane, but it maintains cardiac output in the presence of high inspired concentrations of halothane.

Topical anaesthesia is of particular importance when conscious sedation is used. Lidocaine 2–5% is applied in the nose and larynx and 0.5–1% below the larynx. Lidocaine may be instilled directly, sprayed or nebulized (3–5 ml of 2–4% lidocaine). The total dose should not exceed 5–7 mg/kg [5], but the exact amount applied is difficult to assess as most of the lidocaine administered is removed by suction, spitting or swallowing. Insufficient topical anaesthesia will result in pain, cough, laryngospasm and/or bronchospasm due to vagal stimulation. A further consideration is the possible effect of local anaesthetic agents on the larynx. In a study of 156 infant FBs, in whom sedation with midazolam and nalbuphine was administered, topical lidocaine inadvertently resulted in worsening of laryngomalacia (arytenoidal collapse and epiglottal folding). The authors concluded that during FB the larynx should be inspected before topical anaesthesia is applied [6].

Sedation and Anaesthesia

Bronchoscopy, like any invasive technique, may induce anxiety, fear, pain and unpleasant memory of the experience. Paediatric patients should almost always be sedated for bronchoscopy. The available techniques are conscious sedation and deep sedation (i.e. general anaesthesia).

Conscious sedation and analgesia describe the state that allows the patients to tolerate 'unpleasant' procedures while maintaining adequate cardiorespiratory function and the ability to respond purposefully to verbal commands and tactile stimulation. A child in a state of conscious sedation should be comfortable, not anxious, responsive to verbal and other sensory input but indifferent to that input. The Joint Commission on Accreditation of Healthcare Organizations has mandated that children undergoing sedation for various procedures must receive the same standard of care as those who undergo general anaesthesia [7].

Deep sedation (synonym for general anaesthesia) with complete loss of consciousness is defined as the failure to respond to verbal commands or tactile stimulation. It is achieved by drugs administered by a trained anaesthesiologist [7].

Sedation is contraindicated in patients who are at risk for airway obstruction, respiratory depression or intubated. Young infants may not require sedation if transnasal laryngoscopy is performed, but attention should be paid to their comfort.

As no single agent adequately provides anxiolysis, analgesia and amnesia, a combination of drugs is most often used, especially if conscious sedation is instituted [8].

Conscious Sedation in FB

There is no unique protocol for inducing conscious sedation. It appears that combinations of agents are more effective than single agents. However, published data suggest that drug combinations may increase the likelihood of adverse outcomes. Anxiolysis and analgesia may also be achieved with nitrous oxide via a face mask with a mixture of 50% nitrous oxide and oxygen. Sedation should be given in small incremental doses until the desired effect is obtained.

Table 1 lists the main agents which are usually used to induce conscious sedation; these are briefly discussed below:

- Midazolam is a water-soluble benzodiazepine. Its advantages are that it reduces anxiety and causes amnesia of the procedure. Midazolam has a short onset of action (15–30 min when administered orally), and its duration of action is approximately 90 min (peaks at 30 min). Its effects are additive to those of narcotics. Flumazenil is used as an antagonist. Midazolam is not intended for use as a sole agent in paediatric sedation but should be administered in association with a narcotic or nitrous oxide via a face mask. It may also be useful as an oral agent for presedation.
- Meperidine is a synthetic opiate that produces both sedation and analgesia; it has the advantage of rapid onset of action and easy reversibility by its antagonist, naloxone. Meperidine is preferably administered intravenously by fractional doses in order to achieve the desired effect with the minimum drug dose. The use of a benzodiazepine reduces the required dose of meperidine. Known adverse effects are: respiratory depression that may last longer than its other clinical effects, transient urticaria due to release of histamine, transient hypotension, nausea and vomiting.
- Inhalation of premixed 50% nitrous oxide and oxygen provides both anxiolysis and analgesia. In a prospective double-blind study, Fauroux et al. [9] compared the

Table 1. Main drugs used for sedation in paediatric FB

Drug	Actions	Dose	Onset of action, min	Duration of action, min	Antagonist
Midazolam	anxiolysis, amnesia	intravenous (bolus): 75–300 µg/kg	1–5	90	flumazenil 0.01 mg/kg
Meperidine	analgesia	intravenous (bolus): 0.5–2 mg/kg	5	180–240	naloxone 0.01 mg/kg
Ketamine	analgesia, anaesthesia, amnesia	intravenous (intermittent bolus): 0.25–0.5 mg/kg	2–4	10–20	–
Propofol	anaesthesia	intravenous (intermittent bolus): 0.5–1 mg/kg intravenous (continuous infusion): 100 µg/kg/min	<1	30	–
Remifentanyl	anaesthesia, analgesia	intravenous (continuous infusion): 0.05 µg/kg/min	2–5	2–3	–

effect of this fixed inhalational mixture with a control gas mixture (premixed 50% nitrogen and oxygen). One hundred and five children, aged 1 month to 18 years, were studied. Inhalations were performed through a face mask following intrarectal midazolam and topical anaesthesia with lidocaine. The primary outcome was the number of treatment failures and the need to switch to an open inhalation treatment if the child felt pain or discomfort at any time. The failure rate was significantly lower in the nitrous oxide group: 11 versus 43% (p < 0.00003). The efficacy of nitrous oxide was also confirmed by a higher satisfaction score, a lower Children's Hospital of Eastern Ontario Pain Scale rating, better visual analogue scale rating and improved behaviour scores.

In a 1997 survey of 51 European bronchoscopic centres [10], midazolam was by far the most frequently used sedative (50%), followed by meperidine.

Deep Sedation in FB

Deep sedation may be achieved either by an intravenous drug (propofol, ketamine, sulfentanyl, remifentanyl) or a volatile agent (halothane, sevoflurane), which can be used alone or in combination (table 1). The use of appropriate equipment and the presence of a trained anaesthesiologist are dictated by the type of sedation. The required equipment includes pulse oximeter, blood-pressure-measuring device, electrocardiograph, capnograph (when a tracheal tube or laryngeal mask is used) and if possible a temperature monitor.

- Propofol is an intravenous sedative hypnotic agent administered at a dose of 2–5 mg/kg. It has a rapid onset and a short duration of action. The level of sedation and that of respiratory depression are dose dependent. Pain at the injection site is common, but it cannot be completely eliminated by lidocaine. To date, propofol has not been approved for neonates.
- The use of ketamine as an anaesthetic agent is less common in children. Ketamine has been associated with laryngospasm and bronchospasm. It should be used in combination with atropine because it may increase bronchial mucus secretion via stimulation of the central cholinergic receptors. Ketamine can be used successfully but requires attention to topical anaesthesia of the airway in order to reduce the risk of laryngospasm; the addition of a benzodiazepine is also recommended to prevent the emergence of hallucinations. Berkenbosch et al. [11] have reported their experience of 59 procedures in 55 infants (mean age 6.1 ± 3.1 months). Sedation was achieved either with a combination of ketamine and midazolam or a combination of ketamine, midazolam and fentanyl. The mean dose of intravenous fentanyl was 3.1 ± 1.7 mg/kg. Only 1 infant could not be adequately sedated. There were no major complications, while the incidence of minor complications was 23.7%, most commonly mild hypoxaemia.
- Inhalational agents are commonly used to induce anaesthesia in children. Inhalational induction is

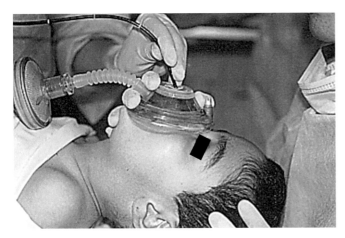

Fig. 1. Face mask used for FB. The bronchoscope is passed through a port on the mask while the anaesthetic gas or a mixture of 50% nitrous oxide and oxygen is delivered.

generally rapid, painless and well tolerated, particularly when sevoflurane is used [12]. Indeed, sevoflurane has a rapid onset of action, its effects quickly resolve after discontinuing drug administration, it does not cause pain, has minimal cardiovascular and no bronchoconstrictive effects, and allows deep sedation with preservation of spontaneous ventilation. Halothane can also be used for induction. It is a direct myocardial depressant but its use numbers decades of experience. It is not irritating to the airways, depresses airway reflexes and may cause some bronchial dilatation. When using inhalational agents, the preferred technique for administration is usually by face mask with the bronchoscope passed through a port on the mask, while the anaesthetic gas is delivered (fig. 1). An alternative technique is the use of a laryngeal mask.

- Remifentanyl is a synthetic opioid agent which is a strong analgesic. It is preferred to fentanyl or sufentanyl due to its pharmacological properties. When compared to fentanyl, it has a short duration of action. It has a short half-life (1–2 min), which essentially eliminates the risk of a cumulative effect. Its adverse effects include respiratory depression, nausea and rigid chest syndrome, which is characterized by markedly decreased compliance of the chest wall when the drug is given as a rapid bolus [13]. It is rarely used in anaesthesia for FB, but it is used in rigid endoscopy.

Currently, when deep sedation is used, the usual techniques employed are sevoflurane alone, propofol alone or the combination of the two.

Conscious or Deep Sedation?

The technique of sedation used depends on many factors: respiratory status, psychological and emotional status of the patient, underlying disease, drugs available, availability of an anaesthetist and type(s) of procedure(s) to be performed. Deep sedation is unequivocally preferred for children with chronic disease, those who undergo numerous procedures, and for very anxious and disruptive patients. In the past, most FBs were performed under conscious sedation but currently most units have moved to general anaesthesia, which appears to be more comfortable for both the child and the medical team. In the future, improvements in gas- and/or drug-induced anaesthesia will eventually result in short deep sedation, followed by quick recovery after the termination of the procedure.

Techniques to Ensure Adequate Ventilation during FB

Whichever the combination of drugs and the technique utilized to deliver oxygen, it is essential to maintain and preserve spontaneous ventilation. The procedure is far more demanding in a child who is not breathing spontaneously. This is applicable particularly to young infants who, if heavily sedated, are prone to apnoeas after the procedure. The techniques available include nasal prongs, face mask, laryngeal mask and endotracheal intubation [12].

- Nasopharyngeal prongs are easy to pass down through one nostril, while the bronchoscope is passed through the other. They allow inspection of most of the upper airway and assessment of the airway dynamics, and do not limit the size of the bronchoscope that can be used.
- A face mask allows the inspection of the entire airway and the assessment of its dynamics [14]. The bronchoscope is passed through an adaptor on the face mask. This method permits the application of positive end-expiratory pressure [15]. Problems may arise if a complication occurs as the airway is shared during the entire process between the bronchoscopist and the anaesthesiologist.
- The use of a laryngeal mask allows for a larger bronchoscope to be introduced, avoids tracheal intubation and is well tolerated [16, 17]. Airway control is better achieved than with the use of a face mask. Disadvantages are that the upper airways and vocal cord movement cannot be assessed. Size No. 1 is recommended for children weighing less than 6.5 kg and size No. 2 for children weighing 6.5–25 kg [18]. In a retrospective analysis of 2,836 paediatric FBs during a period of 21 years, the laryngeal mask was the most common route for the procedure in patients 2 years

of age and older [19]. The use of a laryngeal mask was associated with a lower rate of complications (1.9%) as compared to the nasal route (3.5%) or endotracheal intubation (3.3%).

- Lastly, endotracheal intubation allows to repass the bronchoscope easily and quickly when necessary. Disadvantages are that upper airway anatomy, vocal cord movement and airway dynamics cannot be assessed and that the size of the bronchoscope is limited by the size of the endotracheal tube.

Sedation and Anaesthesia in RB
RB should always be performed under deep sedation. Induction of anaesthesia is similar to that of FB, i.e. by using an intravenous drug or an inhalational agent (halothane/sevoflurane) alone or in combination. Inhalational anaesthesia and oxygen delivery are maintained through a T piece connected to the side arm of the rigid bronchoscope. Two modes of ventilation are routinely used: spontaneous ventilation or (preferably) positive-pressure-controlled ventilation [20]; the use of jet ventilation has also been reported. The use of a muscle relaxant (e.g. suxamethonium 1.5 mg/kg) has been proposed for cases when interventional endoscopy is performed; however, it appears to be less useful in children than in adults.

Recovery and Postprocedural Care

Upon completion of the procedure, the child should be awakened while still being fully monitored. Monitoring of transcutaneous oxygen saturation should continue during the recovery period. An intravenous line should be left in situ until the child is completely awake and tolerating oral fluids. Late complications are rare but may include progressive stridor necessitating intubation. The sedated child should not be left unobserved and may require the same recovery facilities that are formally implemented after general anaesthesia, including complete monitoring and resuscitation facilities. Sedative drugs may exert a hangover effect that lasts for several hours, during which time the patient should continue to be monitored. The child must remain in the recovery area until cardiovascular and respiratory stability have been assured, and is awake and orientated. If local anaesthetic agents have been applied to the airway, the laryngeal reflexes may be depressed for up to 1 h after the procedure. Children should not drink during this period because there is increased risk of aspiration.

Complications

Complications of FB
Induction of sedation or general anaesthesia has been associated with increased morbidity [10]. Few paediatric fatalities have been reported [21, 22]. The complications during FB can be divided into physiological, mechanical, infectious and anaesthetic.

Physiological Complications
These represent the most frequent complications and include: hypoxaemia with or without hypercapnia, laryngospasm and bronchospasm, and cardiac arrhythmia and bradycardia. Respiratory depression is the most concerning adverse effect of sedation. Partial or total airway obstruction by the bronchoscope and depression of respiratory drive due to sedation are the most frequent causes of transcutaneous oxygen desaturation during FB in children and may worsen pre-existing hypoxaemia [23]. Oxygen desaturation may also be a consequence of laryngospasm or bronchospasm. In children undergoing bronchoscopy, when the airway is compromised by both the underlying condition and the procedure itself, any depressant effect of sedation is likely to be poorly tolerated. Oxygen supplementation may delay detection of reduced ventilation but this should be sought by close observation of the child and capnography when appropriate. If desaturation episodes are moderate and transient (no decrease in oxygen saturation below 90%, episodes lasting less than 1 min), they do not preclude completion of the procedure. However, if the transcutaneous oxygen saturation falls to below 90%, intervention is required and, on occasion, the procedure needs to be terminated.

Laryngospasm may be mild and transient, or severe causing hypoxaemia. Such episodes can be limited by careful topical anaesthesia of the vocal cords. Bronchospasm occurs more frequently in children with bronchial hyperreactivity and should be prevented by inhalation of a β-agonist prior to the bronchoscopy. Cardiac arrhythmia and bradycardia may be favoured by vagal stimulation and/or inadequate sedation or topical anaesthesia [24].

Mechanical Complications
Epistaxis is probably the most common complication of FB; it is usually mild and can be prevented by a topical vasoconstrictor. Haemoptysis occurs if coagulopathy or a platelet count of less than $20,000/mm^3$ is present. It is more frequently observed after transbronchial rather than bronchial biopsy. Pneumothorax is rare and often occurs secondarily to transbronchial biopsy. Finally, postbronchoscopic subglottic

Table 2. Complications during 1,328 FBs (adapted from de Blic et al. [25])

	Conscious sedation	General anaesthesia	Total
Patients	1,233	95	1,328
At least 1 complication	84 (6.8)	7 (7.3)	91 (6.9)
Minor complications	63 (5.1)	6 (6.3)	69 (5.2)
Isolated excessive coughing	22 (1.8)	0	22 (1.7)
Excessive nausea reflex with coughing	20 (1.6)	0	20 (1.5)
Isolated desaturation (SpO$_2$ ≥90%)	9 (0.7)	6 (6.3)*	15 (1.1)
Epistaxis	6 (0.5)	0	6 (0.5)
Transient laryngospasm	6 (0.5)	0	6 (0.5)
Major complications	21 (1.7)	1 (1)	22 (1.7)
Desaturation with SpO$_2$ <90%	20 (1.6)	1 (1)	21 (1.6)
Isolated	9 (0.7)	1 (1)	10 (0.8)
Associated	11 (0.9)	0	11 (0.9)
Pneumothorax	1 (0.1)	0	1 (0.1)

Results are expressed as numbers of cases, with percentages in parentheses; SpO$_2$ = transcutaneous oxygen saturation measured by pulse oximetry; * p < 0.001, conscious versus deep sedation.

oedema is rare when performing FB but constitutes the most common complication of RB.

Bacteriological Complications

These are rare and are related to inefficient cleaning of the bronchoscope rather than sedation itself. Spread of infections by the bronchoscope is most likely a very rare complication [1].

Anaesthetic Complications

Most life-threatening adverse events during FB involve drug overdose, inadequate monitoring or inappropriate sedation.

FB is considered to be an invasive procedure. Many studies have focused on its clinical value but relatively few have dealt with the safety and the side effects of FB in children. Many of these studies are now outdated, and most have included small clinical series. In the European survey [10], the majority of the bronchoscopy centres reported adverse effects in less than 5% of their procedures with the flexible instrument. The main complications were bleeding, bronchospasm, laryngospasm and reactions to the medication. Two centres reported bronchospasm in over 10% of procedures; one of these centres also reported reactions to drugs, and the other also reported laryngospasm in over 10% of

cases. The frequency of side effects after FB was evenly distributed among centres that performed either more or fewer than 100 procedures per year.

In our hospital, complications of FB were prospectively evaluated between 1997 and 2001 in 1,328 diagnostic procedures in children, excluding those that were performed in intensive-care units [25]. Only 7.2% of the procedures were performed under deep sedation, while the rest were performed under conscious sedation. Supplementary oxygen was provided in approximately 80% of cases via a face mask (n = 783) or nasal prongs (n = 290). At least 1 complication was recorded in 91 cases (6.9%; table 2). Minor complications were observed in 5.2% of cases and included: transient moderate episodes of desaturation, isolated excessive coughing, excessive nausea reflex with coughing, transient laryngospasm and epistaxis. Major complications occurred in 1.7% of cases and included: oxygen desaturation to below 90% that was either isolated or associated with other untoward events (laryngospasm, excessive coughing, bronchospasm) and pneumothorax. The overall frequency of complications was similar in patients under conscious (6.7%) and those under deep (7.3%) sedation. However, the frequency of transient transcutaneous oxygen desaturation was significantly higher in children undergoing FB under deep sedation (p < 0.001).

Major complications involving oxygen desaturation were associated with age under 2 years and laryngotracheal abnormalities. These results are in agreement with those of others who have found oxygen desaturation to be more frequent in younger infants [16]. Episodes of oxygen desaturation are common particularly whilst the bronchoscope is in the mid-trachea and can occur despite oxygen supplementation. However, the frequency and severity of hypoxaemia decreases when oxygen is administered during procedures performed under sedation. In children under 10 kg, hypoxaemia was common even when oxygen was being administered; thus, an increase in the fraction of inspired oxygen was necessary [23].

Upper airway pathology, persistent radiographic changes, oxygen dependency, weight <10 kg and age below 2 or 3 years are significantly associated with an increased risk of adverse events [8, 12, 25, 26].

The pre-operative detection of high-risk patients by carefully evaluating the indication for bronchoscopy and the clinical status of each patient, in association with appropriate anaesthesia and monitoring during the examination, essentially ensure a successful procedure with the minimum of complications.

Complications of RB

The complications associated with RB include: coughing and bucking, pneumothorax, mediastinal and subcutaneous emphysema, laryngospasm, laryngeal oedema, cardiac arrhythmia, cardiac arrest, convulsions and death. Local anaesthesia of the larynx and carina is of great importance in order to prevent most of these complications.

In a series of 36 children who underwent RB to remove airway foreign body, Soodan et al. [27] compared the patients' tolerance to controlled and spontaneous ventilation techniques. In this study, all spontaneously ventilated children had to be converted to assisted ventilation because of desaturation or inadequate depth of anaesthesia. Ventilatory arrhythmia was observed in 4/36, laryngospasm in 4/36 and postoperative laryngeal oedema in 9/36 children.

In another series, 287 children with suspected tracheobronchial foreign-body aspiration were evaluated. RB was performed under general anaesthesia with sevoflurane/halothane and muscle relaxation. Adverse events secondary to anaesthesia were manifested in 0.7% of cases (2 cases of laryngospasm at extubation), and peri-interventional complications in 7.6% (4 cases of desaturation, 11 cases of stridor after extubation, 4 cases of postinterventional bronchospasm, 3 cases of severe laryngeal oedema and 7 cases of prolonged mechanical ventilation) [28].

References

1 Midulla F, de Blic J, Barbato A, Bush A, Eber E, Kotecha S, Haxby E, Moretti C, Pohunek P, Ratjen F: Flexible endoscopy of paediatric airways. Eur Respir J 2003;22:698–708.

2 Payne D, McKenzie SA, Stacey S, Misra D, Haxby E, Bush A: Safety and ethics of bronchoscopy and endobronchial biopsy in difficult asthma. Arch Dis Child 2001;84:423–426.

3 American Society of Anesthesiologists: Classification of Physical Status. Manual for Anesthesia Department Organisation and Management. Park Ridge, American Society of Anesthesiologists, 2001, pp 6–16.

4 Shaw CA, Kelleher AA, Gill CP, Murdoch LJ, Stables RH, Black AE: Comparison of the incidence of complications at induction and emergence in infants receiving oral atropine vs no premedication. Br J Anaesth 2000;84:174–178.

5 Amitai Y, Zylber-Katz E, Avital A, Zangen D, Noviski N: Serum lidocaine concentrations in children during bronchoscopy with topical anesthesia. Chest 1990;98:1370–1373.

6 Nielson DW, Ku PL, Egger M: Topical lidocaine exaggerates laryngomalacia during flexible bronchoscopy. Am J Respir Crit Care Med 2000;161:147–151.

7 Committee on Drugs, Section on Anesthesiology: Guidelines for the elective use of conscious sedation, deep sedation, and general anesthesia in pediatric patients. Pediatrics 1985;76:317–321.

8 Slonim AD, Ognibene FP: Amnestic agents in pediatric bronchoscopy. Chest 1999;116:1802–1808.

9 Fauroux B, Onody P, Gall O, Tourniaire B, Koscielny S, Clement A: The efficacy of premixed nitrous oxide and oxygen for fiberoptic bronchoscopy in pediatric patients: a randomized, double-blind, controlled study. Chest 2004;125:315–321.

10 Barbato A, Magarotto M, Crivellaro M, Novello A Jr, Cracco A, de Blic J, Scheinmann P, Warner JO, Zach M: Use of the paediatric bronchoscope, flexible and rigid, in 51 European centres. Eur Respir J 1997;10:1761–1766.

11 Berkenbosch JW, Graff GR, Stark JM: Safety and efficacy of ketamine sedation for infant flexible fiberoptic bronchoscopy. Chest 2004;125:1132–1137.

12 Jaggar SI, Haxby E: Sedation, anaesthesia and monitoring for bronchoscopy. Paediatr Respir Rev 2002;3:321–327.

13 Reyle-Hahn M, Niggemann B, Max M, Streich R, Rossaint R: Remifentanil and propofol for sedation in children and young adolescents undergoing diagnostic flexible bronchoscopy. Paediatr Anaesth 2000;10:59–63.

14 Erb T, Hammer J, Rutishauser M, Frei FJ: Fibreoptic bronchoscopy in sedated infants facilitated by an airway endoscopic mask. Paediatr Anaesth 1999;9:47–52.

15 Antonelli M, Conti G, Riccioni L, Meduri GU: Noninvasive positive-pressure ventilation via face mask during bronchoscopy with BAL in high-risk hypoxemic patients. Chest 1996;110:724–728.

16 Naguib ML, Streetman DS, Clifton S, Nasr SZ: Use of laryngeal mask airway in flexible bronchoscopy in infants and children. Pediatr Pulmonol 2005;39:56–63.

17 Nussbaum E, Zagnoev M: Pediatric fiberoptic bronchoscopy with a laryngeal mask airway. Chest 2001;120:614–616.

18 Mason DG, Bingham RM: The laryngeal mask airway in children. Anaesthesia 1990;45:760–763.

19 Nussbaum E: Pediatric fiberoptic bronchoscopy: clinical experience with 2,836 bronchoscopies. Pediatr Crit Care Med 2002;3:171–176.

20 Farrell PT: Rigid bronchoscopy for foreign body removal: anaesthesia and ventilation. Paediatr Anaesth 2004;14:84–89.

21 Picard E, Schlesinger Y, Goldberg S, Schwartz S, Kerem E: Fatal pneumococcal sepsis following flexible bronchoscopy in an immunocompromised infant. Pediatr Pulmonol 1998;25:390–392.

22 Wagener JS: Fatality following fiberoptic bronchoscopy in a two-year-old child. Pediatr Pulmonol 1987;3:197–199.

23 Schnapf BM: Oxygen desaturation during fiberoptic bronchoscopy in pediatric patients. Chest 1991;99:591–594.

24 Katz AS, Michelson EL, Stawicki J, Holford FD: Cardiac arrhythmias: frequency during fiberoptic bronchoscopy and correlation with hypoxemia. Arch Intern Med 1981;141:603–606.

25 De Blic J, Marchac V, Scheinmann P: Complications of flexible bronchoscopy in children: prospective study of 1,328 procedures. Eur Respir J 2002;20:1271–1276.

26 Malviya S, Voepel-Lewis T, Tait AR: Adverse events and risk factors associated with the sedation of children by nonanesthesiologists. Anesth Analg 1997;85:1207–1213.

27 Soodan A, Pawar D, Subramanium R: Anesthesia for removal of inhaled foreign bodies in children. Paediatr Anaesth 2004;14:947–52.

28 Tomaske M, Gerber AC, Weiss M: Anesthesia and periinterventional morbidity of rigid bronchoscopy for tracheobronchial foreign body diagnosis and removal. Paediatr Anaesth 2006;16:123–129.

Jacques de Blic
Paediatric Pulmonology Unit
149, rue de Sevres
FR–75015 Paris (France)
Tel. +33 1 4449 4838, Fax +33 1 4438 1740, E-Mail j.deblic@nck.aphp.fr

Priftis KN, Anthracopoulos MB, Eber E, Koumbourlis AC, Wood RE (eds): Paediatric Bronchoscopy.
Prog Respir Res. Basel, Karger 2010, vol 38, pp 30–41

Bronchoalveolar Lavage: Indications and Applications

Fabio Midulla · Raffaella Nenna

Department of Paediatrics, 'Sapienza' University of Rome, Rome, Italy

Abstract

Bronchoalveolar lavage (BAL) is a diagnostic procedure used to recover cellular and non-cellular components of the epithelial lining fluid from the alveolar and bronchial airspaces. Two types of the procedure have been described: bronchoscopic and non-bronchoscopic BAL. The preferred site for bronchoscopic BAL is the middle lobe or the lingula. Gentle manual or mechanical aspiration is applied in order to collect the lavage specimen in the collection trap, while the tip of the flexible bronchoscope is maintained wedged in the bronchus of the selected lavage site. The parameters measured in BAL fluid (BALF) include the percentage of the instilled normal saline that is recovered as well as various BALF cellular and non-cellular components. BAL is performed for diagnostic, therapeutic and research purposes. The most common indication for BAL is the investigation of lower respiratory tract infection. In chronic interstitial lung disease, BAL may have an important role in reaching a specific diagnosis, characterizing alveolitis, and monitoring patients during treatment and follow-up. BAL is still considered the gold standard for diagnosing chronic pulmonary aspiration. In general, BAL is a well-tolerated and safe procedure; however, on occasion, cough, transient wheezing and pulmonary infiltrates have been observed, which usually resolve within 24 h.   Copyright © 2010 S. Karger AG, Basel

Bronchoalveolar lavage (BAL) is a diagnostic procedure used for recovering cellular and non-cellular components of the epithelial lining fluid (ELF) of the alveolar and bronchial airspaces. The procedure usually entails the instillation and immediate withdrawal of prewarmed sterile 0.9% (normal) saline solution (NSS) through the working channel of a flexible bronchoscope, which has been wedged into a bronchus with a matching diameter.

The first reports on BAL derive from its use in adults [1]. In the year 2000, a European Respiratory Society Task Force published their results on BAL in children [2]. The major childhood application of BAL is the diagnosis of infection, particularly in immunocompromised children. The worldwide increase in the use of this procedure in children has established the role of BAL in the diagnosis and follow-up of several childhood lung diseases and has revealed its potential usefulness in paediatric research.

Bronchoalveolar Lavage Techniques

Current clinical practice utilizes two techniques: non-bronchoscopic and bronchoscopic BAL. Non-bronchoscopic BAL involves the insertion of simple catheters or balloon-type devices (size 4–8 Fr) through an endotracheal tube [3]. Unfortunately, this method does not allow visualization of the lavage site, although the turning of the child's head to the left predictably directs the catheter into the right lung [3].

Bronchoscopic BAL is performed by injecting NSS via a syringe into the working channel of a paediatric flexible bronchoscope; the paediatric instruments have external diameters of 2.8, 3.5 or 3.7 mm with a working channel of 1.2 mm in children younger than 9 years, and external diameters of 4.6–4.9 mm with a working channel of 2.2 mm in children older than 9 years [2; chapter 1, this vol., pp. 12–21]. In neonates it is possible to use the 2.8-mm bronchoscope with a 1.2-mm working channel.

Bronchoalveolar Lavage Site

The preferred site for BAL in diffuse lung diseases is the middle lobe or the lingula [chapter 10, this vol., pp. 114–119] because, being the smallest lobe of each lung, it offers better fluid recovery. When lung disease is localized, BAL must target the radiologically or endoscopically identified involved lobe. In patients with cystic fibrosis (CF), samples from multiple sites should be obtained in order to avoid underestimation of the extent of infection [4]. To avoid contamination, BAL must precede any other planned bronchoscopic procedure.

Amount of Fluid

Three optional methods are currently used for calculating the amount of sterile NSS for lavage and the number of aliquots required to obtain samples that are representative of the alveolar compartment [5]. Some authors base their recommendations on adult protocols and choose to use 2–4 aliquots of equal volume (10 ml per aliquot for children less than 6 years, and 20 ml per aliquot for children over 6 years of age), irrespective of the patient's body weight [6]. Others suggest the use of 3 aliquots, each consisting of 1 ml/kg body weight for children weighing up to 20 kg, and three 20-ml aliquots for heavier children. Lastly, de Blic et al. [7] have recommended that the amount of instilled NSS be adjusted up to a maximum volume of 10% of the child's functional residual capacity, i.e. 5- to 20-ml aliquots depending on the child's size. The saline utilized for BAL is prewarmed to body temperature (37°C) in order to prevent the cough reflex. Flow from the distal tip of the bronchoscope is observed during injection. After each instillation, enough air must be injected in order to empty the dead space of the working channel.

Fluid Recovery

While maintaining the tip of the bronchoscope wedged into the selected site, gentle manual or mechanical suction (3.33–13.3 kPa, i.e. 25–100 mm Hg) is applied in order to obtain the lavage specimen in the dedicated collection trap. At higher suction pressures, distal airways may collapse. In such cases, suction pressures should be reduced or suctioning should be applied intermittently with the use of a syringe. Manual suctioning may be preferable to mechanical aspiration into a collection trap because it is easier to perform, the suction pressure can be easily manipulated, and the procedure is less costly.

In general, BAL is considered technically acceptable if more than 40% of the total NSS instilled is recovered, and the lavage fluid (except for the first sample) contains few epithelial cells. A portion of the instilled volume is absorbed by the lymphatics. BAL fluid (BALF) is often recovered in

Table 1. Variables measured in BALF

Percent of BALF recovered
Cellular components
Number of cells per millilitre of BALF recovered
Differential cell count
Lymphocyte subsets
Morphological features
Specific inclusions
Proliferation assay
Non-cellular components
Microbiological studies

smaller amounts in children with obstructive lung disease as compared to those with diffuse parenchymal lung disease.

Throughout the procedure, patients should undergo routine monitoring using pulse oximetry and electrocardiography with intermittent checks of blood pressure. Oxygen supplementation is recommended during the lavage. After the end of the procedure, children should be observed and monitored for at least 1 h [chapter 2, this vol., pp. 22–29].

Processing Bronchoalveolar Lavage Fluid

Similarly to adult patients, BALF specimens should be processed as soon as possible. To optimize cell viability, BALF must be kept at 4°C until analysed. The variables measured in the BALF include the percentage of fluid recovered (as compared to the amount of NSS instilled) as well as various cellular and non-cellular components (table 1). The first unfiltered BALF aliquot is usually processed separately for microbiological studies. The rest of the aliquots are filtered through sterile gauze to remove mucus; then they are pooled and submitted for cytological studies and analysis of the BALF solutes.

Data on the cellular components suggest that, in healthy children as well as those with lung disease, the first BALF sample differs from subsequent ones, possibly because small-volume lavage recovers BALF from proximal airways (bronchial and oral cells), whereas increased lavage volumes recover material from the more distal airways and the alveoli [8]. Another important difference is that the initially obtained aliquots usually contain more neutrophils and fewer lymphocytes than the subsequent ones. For these reasons, at least 3 aliquots should be obtained during a BAL procedure.

BALF can be prepared in 2 ways: (a) by obtaining cytospin preparations of the whole BALF and (b) by resuspension of

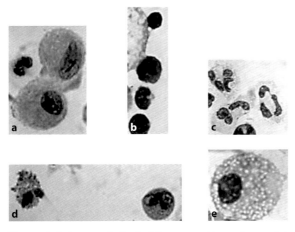

Fig. 1. Cellular morphological features. **a** Macrophages. **b** Lymphocytes. **c** Neutrophils. **d** Eosinophils. **e** Foamy macrophage. May-Grünwald Giemsa stain. ×100.

the specimen in a small amount of medium which is then centrifuged. At least 4 slides should be prepared for each patient, and we recommend storing 1 or 2 slides for research purposes. The number of cells per millilitre in the recovered BALF is counted with a cytometre on whole BALF specimens stained with trypan blue, or with a cytoscan. Alternatively, slides can be stained with May-Grünwald, Giemsa or Diff-Quick stains for the evaluation of differential cell counts and cellular morphological features (fig. 1). Macrophages are large cells with an abundant pale cytoplasm surrounding 1 or more uniform oval nuclei, which may also present with diverse shapes (e.g. round, oval, indented, folded or bean shaped). The presence of foamy macrophages indicates interstitial lung disease [9]. Lymphocytes have a large, dark-stained nucleus with little or no basophilic cytoplasm. In healthy children, the coarse dense nucleus of a lymphocyte is approximately the size of a red blood cell (approx. 7 μm in diameter). Eosinophils are cells with bilobed nuclei, which are normally transparent but after eosin staining by the Romanowsky method they appear brick-red.

In particular clinical settings, slides can also be prepared with specific stains, e.g. oil red O stain to detect lipid-laden macrophages (LLMs), iron stain to identify iron-positive macrophages in patients with alveolar haemorrhage, and periodic acid-Schiff to identify glycogen. Immunocytochemical staining of lymphocyte surface markers is used to differentiate lymphocyte subsets in specific clinical settings such as diffuse parenchymal lung disease.

Materials for the evaluation of non-cellular components must be obtained from the supernatant after centrifugation. The composition of BALF can be influenced by several technical factors, including site of lavage, fluid pH, temperature and volume of instilled NSS, number of aliquots, size of bronchoscope, dwell time and suctioning pressure. Two further important points in the interpretation of BALF findings are that its removal may preferentially select, activate or injure particular cells, and that the composition of the ELF may change during the BAL process.

The identification of an elevated erythrocyte count is an early sign of alveolar haemorrhage, while the presence of phagocytosed erythrocytes indicates that the alveolar haemorrhage has occurred within 48 h. The presence of haemosiderin-laden macrophages in the BALF implies that the alveolar haemorrhage has occurred prior to 48 h.

Reference Values

Several papers have reported on the normal values of BALF in children [10–15]. Such data are difficult to be collected from a healthy population that, for evident ethical reasons, cannot be studied by using an invasive procedure. Hence, the data available come in part from children undergoing bronchoscopy for a variety of clinical indications such as stridor [10, 12], chronic cough, evaluation of stenosis of a main bronchus and follow-up after foreign-body removal [13, 14], and in part from children without pulmonary illness, under general anaesthesia for minor surgery [11, 15].

Table 2 shows BALF differential cell counts of healthy children. The mean BALF total cell count ranges from 10.3 to 59.9×10^4 cells/ml, with a mean of 81.2–90% for macrophages, 8.7–16.2% for lymphocytes, 1.2–5.5% for neutrophils and 0.2–0.4% for eosinophils (fig. 1). The predominant cells, regardless of the child's age, are macrophages, followed by lymphocytes. The BALF neutrophil percentage appears to be higher in children younger than 12 months as compared to children aged 13–36 months.

An increased total number of BALF cell counts (more than 150×10^6/l) is a common characteristic of many lung diseases. Positive BALF cultures are associated with abnormally increased cell counts and abnormal differential counts; in the event of a positive culture, such an increase supports the diagnosis of lung infection as opposed to bacterial contamination from the upper respiratory tract [12].

Normal values of BALF lymphocyte subsets in children (table 3) resemble those found in healthy adults, except for the CD4/CD8 ratio, which is often lower in children, possibly because children frequently suffer from viral infections [11, 12].

Table 2. Total and differential cell counts in BALF from control children

	Clement et al. [10]	Ratjen et al. [11]	Riedler et al. [12]	Midulla et al. [13]	Tessier et al. [14]
Number of patients	11	48	18	16	16
Age range	1–15 years	3–16 years	3 months to 10 years	2–32 months	2 months to 8 years
Sedation	LA	GA	GA	LA	LA
Number of aliquots	6	3	3	2	6
Lavage saline volume	10% FRC	3 ml/kg	3 ml/kg	20 ml	10% FRC
BALF recovered, %					
Mean ± SD	NR	58±15	NR	43.1±12.2	69.7±9.6
Median	NR	NR	62.5	42.5	68
Range	NR	NR	42.5–71.5[1]	20–65	52–87
Cell count, $\times 10^4$ cells/ml					
Mean ± SD	25.5±4.1	10.3±11.1	NR	59.9±8.2	35.1±18.4
Median	24	7.3	15.5	51	30.5
Range	7–50	0.5–57.1	7.5–25.8[1]	20–130	9–68
AM, %					
Mean ± SD	89.7±5.2	81.2±12.7	NR	86±7.8	89.9±5.5
Median	89	84	91	87	92.5
Range	82–99	34.6–94	84–94[1]	71–98	77–98
Lymphocytes, %					
Mean ± SD	8.7±4.6	16.2±12.4	NR	8.7±5.8	8.9±5.6
Median	10	12.5	7.5	7	8
Range	1–17	2–61	4.7–12.8[1]	2–22	2–22
Neutrophils, %					
Mean ± SD	1.3±0.9	1.9±2.9	NR	5.5±4.8	1.2±1.2
Median	1	0.9	1.7	3.5	1
Range	0–3	0–17	0.6–3.5[1]	0–17	0–3
Eosinophils, %					
Mean ± SD	NR	0.4±0.6	NR	0.2±0.3	NR
Median	NR	0.2	0.2	0	NR
Range	NR	0–3.6	0–0.3[1]	0–1	NR

Modified from de Blic et al. [2]. LA = Local anaesthesia; GA = general anaesthesia; FRC = functional residual capacity; NR = not reported; AM = alveolar macrophages.
[1] Second and third interquartiles.

Establishing reference values for non-cellular components is a complex task owing to the absence of valid BALF dilution markers [13, 16, 17]. The concentration of serum-derived proteins is higher in children than in adults, whereas locally produced mediators do not differ. Surfactant phospholipid concentrations are higher in 3- to 8-year-old than in older children, whereas surfactant protein concentrations are independent of the child's age (tables 4, 5). Many pulmonary diseases result in an increase in the content of total protein and of serum-derived proteins of the BALF, probably reflecting the increased permeability associated with inflammation. Studies designed to investigate non-cellular BALF components have few clinical indications and are more important in the research setting.

Table 3. Lymphocyte subsets in BALF from control children

	Ratjen et al. [15]	Riedler et al. [12]
Number of patients	28	10 (5)
Age range	3–16 years	3 months to 10 years
CD3, %		
Mean ± SD	85.8±4.9	NR
Median	87	81
Range	72–92	75.5–88[1]
CD4, %		
Mean ± SD	33.1±12.8	NR
Median	34.5	27
Range	10–57	22–32[1]
CD8, %		
Mean ± SD	56.8±13.1	NR
Median	57	45
Range	30–84	33.8–57[1]
CD4/CD8 ratio		
Mean ± SD	0.7±0.4	NR
Median	0.6	0.6
Range	0.1–1.9	0.4–1[1]
CD19, %		
Mean ± SD	0.9±1.5	NR
Median	0.5	5
Range	0–7	4–9.5[1]
CD25, %		
Mean ± SD	1.9±1.3	NR
Median	2	(2)
Range	0–4	(0–3[1])
CD3/HLA-DR, %		
Mean ± SD	1.4±1.7	NR
Median	1	NR
Range	0–7	NR
CD56, %		
Mean ± SD	7.8±8.2	NR
Median	5	4
Range	0–40	1.5–7.5

Modified from de Blic et al. [2]. NR = Not reported; HLA-DR = human leucocyte antigen DR.
[1] Second and third interquartiles.

Because of the fluid exchange among the airspace, the vascular compartment and the interstitium, correction of the BALF solutes for the ELF volume would be highly desirable.

Unfortunately, the only two substances proposed, i.e. urea and albumin, have important limitations. Urea diffuses into BALF in a time-dependent manner and can be higher when there is an alteration of the capillary permeability. Moreover, albumin concentrations are modified during lung disease [2]. Therefore, BALF solutes are currently referenced to the BALF volume.

Microbiological Studies

Usually the first aliquot of BALF is used for microbiological studies. Samples must be processed as soon as possible, avoiding contamination and without use of filters that withhold cells or other diagnostic material. Another important precautionary measure is to keep the samples in anaerobic transport media that contain reducing agents in order to avoid air exposure that destroys anaerobic bacteria.

Bacteria, fungi, protozoa and viruses are detected by direct light microscopy after centrifugation or alternatively by smears. Special stains such as Gram, Papanicolaou, Gomori-Grocott or toluidine blue are used in air-dried preparations. In addition, the samples that are to be cultured for fungi, protozoa and viruses are first centrifuged, whereas those for bacterial cultures are processed without centrifugation.

Indications for Bronchoalveolar Lavage

BAL is performed for diagnostic, therapeutic and research applications, which require evaluation of microbiological and/or cellular components. Indications for BAL include non-specific chronic respiratory symptoms, non-specific radiological findings and clinical symptoms suggestive of interstitial lung disease.

Lower Respiratory Tract Infection
BAL is an important tool in the diagnosis of lung infection in both immunocompromised and immunocompetent patients because pathogens can be easily identified from small BALF samples.

BALF is diagnostic when pathogens not usually found in the lung are recovered, such as *Pneumocystis jiroveci*, *Toxoplasma gondii*, *Strongyloides stercoralis*, *Legionella pneumophila*, *Histoplasma capsulatum*, *Mycobacterium tuberculosis*, *Mycoplasma pneumoniae*, influenza virus and respiratory syncytial virus. Other infectious diseases, in which isolation of the infectious agent from BALF is not diagnostic but may

Table 4. Concentration (mg/l) of serum-derived proteins in BALF from control children

	Midulla et al. [13]	Ratjen and Kreuzfelder [16]		Braun et al. [17]	
		Children	Adults	Children	Adults
Number of patients	7	37 (30)	15 (8)	39	16
Age range	1–3 years	3–15 years	adults[1]	3–15 years	adults[2]
Total protein					
Mean ± SD	108±39	103±65	(62±10)	NR	NR
Median	67	92	(47)	NR	NR
Range	44–336	43–426	(29–115)	NR	NR
Albumin					
Mean ± SD	58±26	NR	NR	21±16	11±5.9
Median	29	NR	NR	16	9.7
Range	14–210	NR	NR	0.5–70	3.8–24
Immunoglobulin A					
Mean ± SD	NR	(3.6±1.4)	3.4±2	NR	NR
Median	NR	(3.2)	2.9	NR	NR
Range	NR	(0–7.7)	0–6.2	NR	NR
Immunoglobulin G					
Mean ± SD	NR	(9.1±7.4)	8.6±6.8	NR	NR
Median	NR	(6.4)	7.8	NR	NR
Range	NR	(2.8–3.7)	0–2.2	NR	NR
α_1-Antitrypsin					
Mean ± SD	NR	NR	NR	1.3±1.2	0.3±0.3
Median	NR	NR	NR	1.05	1.8
Range	NR	NR	NR	0.3–5.7	0.1–9.8
α_2-Macroglobulin					
Mean ± SD	NR	NR	NR	0.5±0.8	0
Median	NR	NR	NR	0.15	0
Range	NR	NR	NR	0–3.8	0
β_2-Microglobulin					
Mean ± SD	NR	(1.4±1.2)	0.8±0.5	NR	NR
Median	NR	(1)	0.7	NR	NR
Range	NR	(0–5)	0–2.2	NR	NR

Modified from Midulla and Ratjen [5]. NR = Not reported; figures in parentheses indicate parameters evaluated in number of patients in parentheses.
[1] Age range of patients: 22–54 years.
[2] Mean age of patients: 24.7 years.

contribute to their diagnosis and management, include herpes simplex virus, cytomegalovirus, *Aspergillus, Candida albicans, Cryptococcus* and atypical mycobacteria. Therefore, the presence of $\geq 10^4$ colony-forming units/ml in the BALF will identify patients with bacterial pneumonia with reasonable accuracy. Hence, when evaluating the microbiological results, the physician must take into account the underlying disease and the overall clinical picture.

In HIV-infected children, BAL can identify one or more infectious agents that alone or in combination cause interstitial pneumonitis. Similar findings are observed in children with primary immune deficiency, immunosuppression secondary

Table 5. Concentration (mg/l) of locally produced mediators in BALF from control children

	Midulla et al. [13]	Braun et al. [17]	
		Children	Adults
Number of patients	7	39	16
Age	1–3 years	3–15 years	adults[1]
Fibronectin			
Mean ± SD	172±83	240±120	89±52
Median	80	115	75
Range	25–640	10–370	10–200
Hyaluronic acid			
Mean ± SD	26±5	NR	NR
Median	18	NR	NR
Range	16–45	NR	NR
Myeloperoxidase			
Mean ± SD	NR	58±51	19±17
Median	NR	0	24
Range	NR	0–161	1–51
Lactoferrin			
Mean ± SD	NR	50±61	37±21
Median	NR	31	27
Range	NR	2–289	10–84
Elastase			
Mean ± SD	NR	1.4±1.2	0.8±0.5
Median	NR	0	2
Range	NR	0–21	1–14

Modified from Midulla and Ratjen [5]. NR = Not reported.
[1] Mean age of patients: 24.7 years.

to chemotherapy for malignancy, and bone marrow or non-lung organ transplantation. The role of BAL in lung and heart-lung transplantation patients is debated because, although helpful in diagnosing lung infection, it cannot replace transbronchial biopsy in the diagnosis of graft rejection [18]. Several efforts have been made to identify a marker of rejection in the BALF by analysing combinations of various cell counts and non-cellular components. Unfortunately, the results of these studies remain inconclusive. Nevertheless, BAL continues to play a role in the routine surveillance of lung transplant recipients [chapter 18, this vol., pp. 191–197].

The role of BAL in the diagnosis of lung infection in immunocompetent children is more controversial. This invasive procedure is hardly ever justified as a first step in the diagnosis of primary respiratory infection in otherwise healthy children but should be reserved for patients with atypical manifestations. BAL is a useful tool in patients with chronic pneumonia, tuberculosis and CF. In CF patients, BAL has an important role in detecting respiratory pathogens and inflammation, especially in young children who are unable to expectorate or in those who fail to improve after therapy [chapter 15, this vol., pp. 156–172]. In these patients, samples should be taken from more than one site so that the collected BALF is representative of the entire lung [4]. Moreover, flexible bronchoscopy can be used in these patients to remove obstruction leading to atelectasis by directly injecting DNAse into the airways.

Chronic Interstitial Lung Disease
Chronic interstitial lung disease (CILD) is a heterogeneous group of disorders characterized by typical radiological findings, restrictive lung disease and inflammation of the pulmonary interstitium [19]. In these patients, BAL may have an important role in reaching or confirming a specific diagnosis, in characterizing the alveolitis and in monitoring the patient during treatment and follow-up [20].

Fan et al. [21] published one of the first papers on the clinical application of BAL in children with CILD. They studied 29 patients with a clinical and radiological diagnosis of CILD and reported a positive BALF finding in 20 [22]. Unfortunately, BALF findings proved diagnostic of a primary disorder in only 5 patients (17%), while in another 15 they were consistent with a diagnosis; in 8 patients, BAL uncovered a secondary pulmonary disorder. In 2004, a study that was conducted as part of the European Respiratory Society Task Force on CILD in immunocompetent children provided an update on the current understanding of the pathophysiology of these diseases and the ongoing research directions [23].

In addition, BALF findings usually provide a specific diagnosis in children with alveolar proteinosis, pulmonary haemorrhage, pulmonary histiocytosis, chronic lipoid pneumonia and pulmonary microlithiasis.

In alveolar proteinosis, BAL can be diagnostic because the BALF recovered has a milky appearance due to the presence of periodic-acid-Schiff-positive material (fig. 2) and enlarged foamy alveolar macrophages (fig. 1) with the characteristic 'onion-like' cytoplasmic inclusions on electron microscopy [chapter 7, this vol., pp. 75–82].

When BALF has a bloody or orange pink colour in patients presenting with haemoptysis, infiltrates on chest X-ray and anaemia, the diagnosis of alveolar haemorrhage is confirmed. Usually in such cases, the fluid becomes increasingly haemorrhagic with each aliquot. However, the diagnosis is more difficult to reach when free red blood cells,

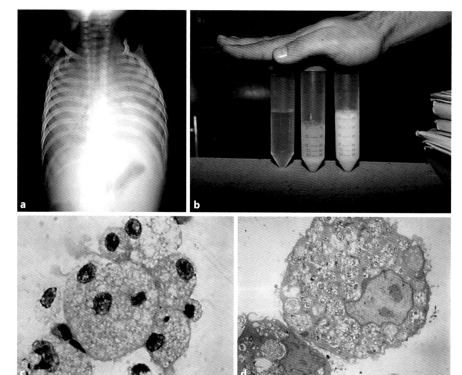

Fig. 2. Radiological and BALF findings in a patient with idiopathic alveolar proteinosis. **a** Chest X-ray showing diffuse ground-glass lesions. **b** BALF aliquots with milky appearance (first and second aliquots from the right), compared to normal-appearing BALF (third aliquot from the right) at the end of a therapeutic total lung lavage. **c** Foamy macrophages. May-Grünwald Giemsa stain. ×100. **d** Macrophages (electron microscopy) showing inclusion bodies specific for alveolar proteinosis.

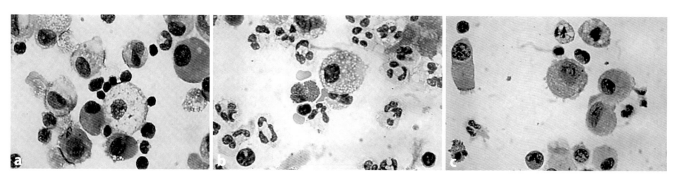

Fig. 3. BALF cytological features in various clinical conditions. **a** Lymphocytic alveolitis. **b** Neutrophilic alveolitis. **c** Eosinophilic alveolitis. May-Grünwald Giemsa stain. ×100.

red blood cells phagocytosed by alveolar macrophages or haemosiderin-laden alveolar macrophages become evident only at microscopy.

Detection of more than 5% CD1a-positive cells in the BALF is diagnostic of pulmonary histiocytosis [24].

Finally, in chronic lipoid pneumonia, BALF samples from alveolar structures usually contain lipoid material originating from external or internal sources [25].

In several types of CILD, BAL is a useful tool, even if not per se diagnostic of the disease. Lung biopsy is often indicated in order to reach a definitive diagnosis and decide on the appropriate therapy. However, lung biopsy should not be considered if the diagnosis can be reached by using less invasive techniques [22].

With BALF analysis, 3 different forms of alveolitis can be identified, lymphocytic, neutrophilic and eosinophilic (fig. 3):

(a) When patients present with clinical manifestations typical of sarcoidosis, a high percentage of lymphocytes (more than 30%) with predominating CD4 T cells in the BALF is strongly suggestive, although not definitively confirmatory, of the diagnosis [26]. Results obtained in recent years suggest that the CD4/CD8 T lymphocyte ratio in patients with sarcoidosis varies greatly from patient to patient [27]. BALF samples in which CD4 T lymphocytes predominate can also be found in children with Crohn disease.

Hypersensitivity pneumonitis typically causes lymphocytic alveolitis with the BALF containing predominantly CD8 T lymphocytes. Similarly, in children with histiocytosis X, or with interstitial lung disease related to collagen disease, or in cryptogenic organizing pneumonia (previously termed bronchiolitis obliterans and organising pneumonia) the predominant cells are CD8 T lymphocytes.

(b) Features of BALF reminiscent of neutrophilic alveolitis are usually found in idiopathic pulmonary fibrosis and in cryptogenic organizing pneumonia. The histological features are an accumulation of macrophages accompanied by mild chronic interstitial pneumonia and, at the very worst, mild interstitial fibrosis.

(c) Patients with eosinophilic alveolitis or interstitial lung disease always show a predominance of eosinophils in BALF with focal eosinophilic abscesses. The aetiology of this condition often remains elusive; a number of causes (e.g. drug reactions, fungi, parasites and vapour inhalation) have been described. There is a dramatic response to corticosteroid therapy.

Chronic Pulmonary Aspiration
BAL is still considered to be the gold standard for the diagnosis of chronic pulmonary aspiration (CPA), i.e. the repeated passage of food material, gastric refluxate or saliva into the subglottic airways causing chronic or recurrent respiratory symptoms [28]. Several predisposing factors (neurological disorders, underlying medical conditions such as prematurity, anatomical abnormalities of airways, vocal cord paralysis), when coinciding with other stressors (respiratory tract infection, gastro-oesophageal reflux), predispose to this condition. CPA arises from anatomical defects in the separation of the gastrointestinal from the respiratory tract, swallowing dysfunction and the inability to protect the airway from oral secretions and gastric refluxate. The typical presenting signs and symptoms are chronic cough, wheezing, recurrent pneumonia, failure to thrive, apnoea and choking on food or secretions; optimal management entails a multidisciplinary approach. Chest radiographs usually disclose diffuse air-trapping, subsegmental infiltrates and peribronchial thickening, which involve the basilar and superior segments of the lower lobes and posterior upper lobe segments. High-resolution computed tomography scans may show bronchiectasis, centrilobular opacities,

air-trapping and bronchial thickening [29]. Reflux aspiration is usually evaluated by pH and/or impedance monitoring [30] or by gastro-oesophageal scintigraphy.

Flexible bronchoscopy with BAL is a useful tool for assessing aspiration. This procedure helps to evaluate swallowing, allows direct assessment of airway anatomy and inflammatory changes in airway mucosa, and can detect evidence of gastro-oesophageal reflux. BAL remains the procedure of choice to diagnose CPA by determining the LLM index [31], by immunocytochemical staining for α-lactoalbumin and β-lactoglobulin [32], and by measuring gastric pepsin concentrations [33, 34].

The presence of LLM in BALF is a sensitive marker of aspiration in children. In CPA the lipids present in aspirated food are phagocytosed by alveolar macrophages. Theoretically, an increased prevalence of LLM in the lower airways suggests aspiration of food with swallowing or after gastro-oesophageal reflux.

The LLM index can be calculated by assigning each LLM a score that ranges from 0 to 4 according to the amount of cytoplasmic lipid (fig. 4) and scoring 100 consecutive alveolar macrophages; thus, the highest possible score (LLM index) is 400. An LLM index of more than 100 is considered positive for aspiration [31]. However, the LLM index has certain limitations such as the lack of reproducibility, the inability to differentiate between exogenous and endogenous lipids, and the false-positive results that it may yield in patients with lung disease unrelated to aspiration or even in healthy children [35, 36]. LLMs may also be observed in cases of fat embolism [37] and endogenous lipoid pneumonia [38]. Advantages of its use are: it is simple to perform, it remains elevated for several days after aspiration, and a specific cut-off increases its diagnostic specificity [35]. The LLM index remains a useful diagnostic tool in the evaluation of children with a history and clinical symptoms suggestive of aspiration. Therefore, such children should undergo diagnostic bronchoscopy.

Immunocytochemical staining for α-lactoalbumin and β-lactoglobulin proteins has also rendered interesting results in animal models of pulmonary aspiration [39]. Unfortunately, these findings have not been confirmed by studies in paediatric patients [32].

With respect to other potential biomarkers, tracheal pepsin has been used as a marker of reflux aspiration [33]. Pepsin is a proteolytic enzyme that is secreted by the gastric chief cells and mucus neck cells as inactive pepsinogen and then cleaved in the stomach at a pH of 5, thus forming active pepsin. Pepsin detection in the BALF has been shown to have high sensitivity and specificity values for reflux-related pulmonary aspiration [34]. Unfortunately, pepsin detection

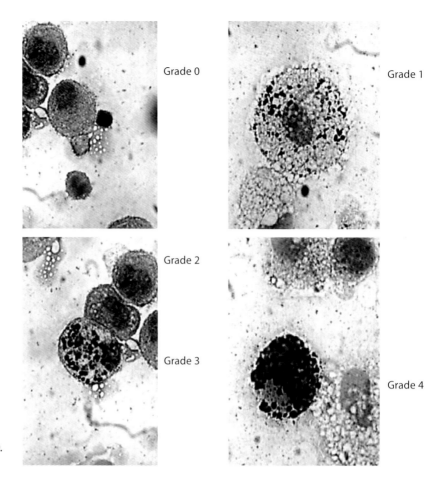

Fig. 4. Lipid index graded from 0 to 4. Oil red O. ×100.

is still a 'home-made' assay, and its use is limited strictly to the diagnosis of gastric reflux-related aspiration.

Therapeutic Applications

BAL has a major role in the therapy of certain lung diseases, in the form of total lung lavage [chapter 7, this vol., pp. 75–82] or mucus plug removal. In particular, children with persistent and massive atelectasis can successfully undergo selective lavage with DNAse [chapter 14, this vol., pp. 149–155].

Complications

In general, BAL is a well-tolerated and safe procedure. Sometimes cough, transitory wheeze and pulmonary infiltrates, which in most cases resolve within 24 h, are observed [40]. As far as minor complications are concerned, in approximately 10–30% of children a transient fever is reported after BAL, while bronchospasm is observed in approximately 1% of patients. Notwithstanding its good safety profile, BAL may cause hypoxaemia, hypercapnia or both as it increases

the duration of the bronchoscopic procedure [chapter 2, this vol., pp. 22–29].

Severe bleeding, bronchial perforation, mediastinal emphysema, pneumothorax and cardiac arrest are extremely rare. A large prospective study [41] showed that less than 2% of patients suffer a major complication, and, to date, no published report has described a lethal complication directly related to the BAL procedure. If necessary, BAL can also be undertaken in intubated patients who require mechanical ventilation. Contraindications to the procedure include: bleeding disorders, severe haemoptysis and severe hypoxaemia that persists despite oxygen treatment.

Research Applications

The worldwide increase in the use of paediatric BAL and the opportunity to study cellular as well as non-cellular components in the ELF have made this procedure useful in the investigation of the pathogenesis of lung disease. By direct evaluation of local response to therapy, BALF studies may contribute to improvements in the management of a number of lung diseases [42]. For example, the new multiplex PCR for *Streptococcus pneumoniae, Haemophilus influenzae, M. pneumoniae* and *Chlamydophila pneumoniae* appears to be a useful tool in the investigation of the aetiology of lower respiratory tract infection, particularly in patients previously treated with antibiotics [43].

Several attempts have been made to evaluate the balance between pro-inflammatory and anti-inflammatory mechanisms involved both in the early stages as well as during resolution of paediatric lung disease, including wheezing and asthma, bronchiolitis, CF, CILD and complications of lung transplantation. Thus, a method capable of valid measurement of cytokine expression during the course of various paediatric lung diseases may prove to be a powerful tool to assess disease activity, and will have important implications for the planning of therapy. Furthermore, the identification of the genes involved in disease pathogenesis will probably enhance our understanding of these conditions and provide new therapeutic targets [23].

Analysis of BALF in wheezing children [chapter 13, this vol., pp. 142–148] during relatively quiescent periods of their disease by Stevenson et al. [44] has suggested that the pathophysiological mechanisms underlying atopic asthma that is characterized by airway inflammation with recruitment of eosinophils and mast cells differ from those operating in viral wheeze. Despite these differences, children with viral wheeze, regardless of aetiology, were found to have elevated histamine levels, whereas eosinophil cationic protein was elevated only in children with atopy [45]. The investigation of the underlying inflammatory processes in wheezing children in an attempt to detect subjects at risk for subsequent asthma could prove to be an exciting path for BALF-related research in the near future. Airway neutrophilia observed in early childhood asthma and in severe asthma suggests that bacterial infection may be important in promoting airway inflammation [46]. In recent years, studies have provided evidence that corticosteroid therapy may actually induce airway inflammation [47].

In children with bronchiolitis BAL may prove helpful in evaluating processes within the peripheral airways by identifying markers that could help to explain the clinical presentation of the inflammatory process, the predisposition of wheezers to subsequent asthma, or both. Moreover, alveolar macrophages infected by respiratory syncytial virus may indeed have a role in the pulmonary response to infection [48].

In CF, research on BALF could prove to be helpful in the assessment of disease prognosis and the selection of the subjects who are fit to receive organ transplantation. BALF research may also help to elucidate the pathogenetic mechanism that links the abnormal CF transmembrane regulator function to lung inflammation. Several studies in young patients with CF suggest that infection is a fundamental driving force behind the inflammatory process [49; chapter 15, this vol., pp. 156–172]. Conversely, studies in children at 4 weeks of age have demonstrated that airways inflammation develops at a very early stage, thus suggesting that inflammation precedes infection [50].

Lastly, in patients scheduled for lung or heart-lung transplantation, BALF analysis, a procedure that has already proved to be helpful in the diagnosis of infections, may be used in the future to evaluate organ rejection, a task currently achievable only by performing transbronchial biopsy [chapter 18, this vol., pp. 191–197].

References

1 Klech H, Pohl W, European Society of Pneumology Task Group on BAL: Technical recommendations and guidelines for bronchoalveolar lavage (BAL). Eur Respir J 1989;2:561–285.

2 De Blic J, Midulla F, Barbato A, Clement A, Dab I, Eber E, Green C, Grigg J, Kotecha S, Kurland G, Pohunek P, Ratjen F, Rossi G: ERS Task Force on bronchoalveolar lavage in children. Eur Respir J 2000;15:217–231.

3 Heaney LG, Stevenson EC, Turner G, Cadden IS, Taylor R, Shields MD, Ennis M: Investigating paediatric airways by non-bronchoscopic lavage: normal cellular data. Clin Exp Allergy 1996;26:799–806.

4 Gutierrez JP, Grimwood K, Armstrong DS, Carlin JB, Carzino R, Olinsky A, Robertson CF, Phelan PD: Interlobar differences in bronchoalveolar lavage fluid from children with cystic fibrosis. Eur Respir J 2001;17:281–286.

5 Midulla F, Ratjen F: Special considerations for bronchoalveolar lavage in children. Eur Respir Rev 1999;9:38–42.

6 Ratjen F, Bruch J: Adjustment of bronchoalveolar lavage volume to body weight in children. Pediatr Pulmonol 1996;21:184–488.

7 De Blic J, McKelvie P, Le Bourgeois M, Blanche S, Benoist MR, Scheinmann P: Value of bronchoalveolar lavage in the management of severe acute pneumonia and interstitial pneumonitis in the immunocompromised child. Thorax 1987;42:759–765.

8 Pohunek P, Pokorna H, Striz I: Comparison of cell profiles in separately evaluated fractions of bronchoalveolar lavage (BAL) fluid in children. Thorax 1996;51:615–618.

9 Costabel U, Guzman J, Bonella F, Oshimo S: Bronchoalveolar lavage in other interstitial lung diseases. Semin Respir Crit Care Med 2007;28:514–524.

10 Clement A, Chadelat K, Massliah J, Housset B, Sardet A, Grimfeld A, Tournier G: A controlled study of oxygen metabolite release by alveolar macrophages from children with interstitial lung disease. Am Rev Respir Dis 1987;136:1424–1428.

11 Ratjen F, Bredendiek M, Bredel M, Meltzer J, Costabel U: Differential cytology of bronchoalveolar lavage fluid in normal children. Eur Respir J 1994;7:1865–1870.

12 Riedler J, Grigg J, Stone C, Tauro G, Robertson CF: Bronchoalveolar lavage cellularity in healthy children. Am J Respir Care Med 1995;152:163–168.

13 Midulla F, Villani A, Merolla R, Bjermer L, Sandstrom T, Ronchetti R: Bronchoalveolar lavage studies in children without parenchymal lung disease: cellular constituents and protein levels. Pediatr Pulmonol 1995;20:112–118.

14 Tessier V, Chadelat K, Baculard A, Housset B, Clement A: A controlled study of differential cytology and cytokine expression profiles by alveolar cells in pediatric sarcoidosis. Chest 1996;109:1430–1438.

15 Ratjen F, Bredendiek M, Zheng L, Brenel M, Costabel U: Lymphocyte subsets in bronchoalveolar lavage fluid of children without bronchopulmonary disease. Am J Respir Crit Care Med 1995;152:174–178.

16 Ratjen F, Kreuzfelder E: Immunoglobulin and beta2-microglobulin concentrations in bronchoalveolar lavage of children and adults. Lung 1996;174:383–391.

17 Braun J, Mehnert A, Dalhoff K, Wiessmann KJ, Ratjen F: Different protein composition of BALF in normal children and adults. Respiration 1997;64:350–357.

18 Riedler J, Grigg J, Robertson CF: Role of bronchoalveolar lavage in children with lung disease. Eur Respir J 1995;8:1725–1730.

19 Fan LL, Langston C: Chronic interstitial lung disease in children. Pediatr Pulmonol 1993;16:184–196.

20 Ronchetti R, Midulla F, Sandstrom T, Bjermer L, Zabrak J, Pawlik J, Villa MP, Villani A: Bronchoalveolar lavage in children with chronic diffuse parenchymal lung disease. Pediatr Pulmonol 1999;27:1–8.

21 Fan LL, Mullen AL, Brugman SM, Inscore SC, Parks DP, White CW: Clinical spectrum in chronic interstitial lung disease in children. J Pediatr 1992;121:867–872.

22 Fan LL, Lung MC, Wagener JS: The diagnostic value of bronchoalveolar lavage in immunocompetent children with chronic diffuse pulmonary infiltrates. Pediatr Pulmonol 1997;23:8–13.

23 Clement A, Allen J, Corrin B, Dinwiddie R, Ducou le Pointe H, Eber E, Laurent G, Marshall R, Midolla F, Nicholson AG, Pohunek P, Ratjen F, Spiteri M, de Blic J: Task force on chronic interstitial lung disease in immunocompetent children. Eur Respir J 2004;24:686–697.

24 Réfaber L, Rambaud C, Mamou-Mani T, Scheinmann P, de Blic J: CD1a-positive cells in bronchoalveolar lavage samples from children with Langerhans cell histiocytosis. J Pediatr 1996;129:913–915.

25 Midulla F, Strappini PM, Ascoli V, Villa MP, Indinnimeo L, Falasca C, Martella S, Ronchetti R: Bronchoalveolar lavage cell analysis in a child with chronic lipid pneumonia. Eur Respir J 1998;11:239–242.

26 Chadelat K, Baculard A, Grimfeld A, Tournier G, Boule M, Boccon-Gibod L, Clement A: Pulmonary sarcoidosis in children: serial evaluation of bronchoalveolar lavage cells during corticosteroid treatment. Pediatr Pulmonol 1993;16:41–47.

27 Kantrow SP, Meyer KC, Kidd P, Raghu G: The CD4/CD8 ratio in BAL fluid is highly variable in sarcoidosis. Eur Respir J 1997;10:2716–2721.

28 Boesch RP, Daines C, Willging JP, Kaul A, Cohen AP, Wood RE, Amin RS: Advances in the diagnosis and management of chronic pulmonary aspiration in children. Eur Respir J 2006;28:847–861.

29 Kuhn JP, Brody AS: High-resolution CT of pediatric lung disease. Radiol Clin North Am 2002;40:89–110.

30 Borrelli O, Battaglia M, Galos F, Aloi M, De Angelis D, Moretti C, Mancini V, Cucchiara S, Midulla F: Non-acid gastro-oesophageal reflux in children with suspected pulmonary aspiration. Dig Liver Dis 2009, E-pub ahead of print.

31 Corwin RW, Irwin RS: The lipid-laden alveolar macrophage as a marker of aspiration in parenchymal lung disease. Am Rev Respir Dis 1985;132:576–581.

32 Miller J, Colasurdo GN, Khan AM, Jajoo C, Patel TJ, Fan LL, Elidemir O: Immunocytochemical detection of milk proteins in tracheal aspirates of ventilated infants: a pilot study. Pediatr Pulmonol 2002;34:369–374.

33 Krishnan U, Mitchell JD, Messina I, Day AS, Bohane TD: Assay of tracheal pepsin as a marker of reflux aspiration. J Pediatr Gastroenterol Nutr 2002;35:303–308.

34 Farrell S, McMaster C, Gibson D, Shields MD, McCallion WA: Pepsin in bronchoalveolar lavage fluid: a specific and sensitive method of diagnosing gastro-oesophageal reflux-related pulmonary aspiration. J Pediatr Surg 2006;41:289–293.

35 Knauer-Fischer S, Ratjen F: Lipid-laden macrophages in bronchoalveolar lavage fluid as a marker for pulmonary aspiration. Pediatr Pulmonol 1999;27:419–422.

36 Ding Y, Simpson PM, Schellhase DE, Tryka AF, Ding L, Parham DM: Limited reliability of lipid-laden macrophage index restricts its use as a test for pulmonary aspiration: comparison with a simple semiquantitative assay. Pediatr Dev Pathol 2002;5:551–558.

37 Vichinsky E, Williams R, Das M, Earles AN, Lewis N, Adler A, McQuitty J: Pulmonary fat embolism: a distinct cause of severe acute chest syndrome in sickle cell anemia. Blood 1994;83:3107–3112.

38 McDonald JW, Roggli VL, Bradford WD: Coexisting endogenous and exogenous lipoid pneumonia and pulmonary alveolar proteinosis in a patient with neurodevelopmental disease. Pediatr Pathol 1994;14:505–511.

39 Elidemir O, Fan LL, Colasurdo GN: A novel diagnostic method for pulmonary aspiration in a murine model: immunocytochemical staining of milk proteins in alveolar macrophages. Am J Respir Crit Care Med 2000;161:622–626.

40 Klech H, Pohl W, Hutter C: Safety and side-effects of bronchoalveolar lavage. Eur Respir Rev 1992;2:57.

41 De Blic J, Marchac V, Scheinmann P: Complications of flexible bronchoscopy in children: prospective study of 1,328 procedures. Eur Respir J 2002;20:1271–1276.

42 Connett GJ: Bronchoalveolar lavage. Paediatr Respir Rev 2000;1:52–56.

43 Stralin K, Korsgaard J, Olcén P: Evaluation of a multiplex PCR for bacterial pathogens applied to bronchoalveolar lavage. Eur Respir J 2006;28:568–575.

44 Stevenson EC, Turner G, Heaney LG, Schock BC, Taylor R, Gallagher T, Ennis M, Shields MD: Bronchoalveolar lavage findings suggest two different forms of childhood asthma. Clin Exp Allergy 1997;27:1027–1035.

45 Ennis M, Turner G, Schock BC, Stevenson EC, Brown V, Fitch PS, Heaney LG, Taylor R, Shields MD: Inflammatory mediators in bronchoalveolar lavage samples from children with and without asthma. Clin Exp Allergy 1999;29:362–366.

46 Marguet C, Jouen-Boedes F, Dean TP, Warner JO: Bronchoalveolar cell profiles in children with asthma, infantile wheeze, chronic cough, or cystic fibrosis. Am J Respir Crit Care Med 1999;159:1533–1540.

47 Payne DN, Wilson NM, Hablas H, Agrafioti C, Bush A: Do oral corticosteroids cause sputum neutrophilia in children with severe asthma? Thorax 1999;54:A46.

48 Midulla F, Villani A, Panuska JR, Dab I, Kolls JK, Merolla R, Ronchetti R: Respiratory syncytial virus lung infection in infants: immunoregulatory role of infected alveolar macrophages. J Infect Dis 1993;168:1515–1519.

49 Amstrong DS, Grimwood K, Carlin JB, Carzino R, Olinsky A, Phelan PD: Bronchoalveolar lavage or oropharyngeal cultures to identify lower respiratory pathogens in infants with cystic fibrosis. Pediatr Pulmonol 1996;20:267–275.

50 Khan TZ, Wagener JS, Bost T, Martinez J, Acurso FJ, Riches DWH: Pulmonary inflammation in infants with cystic fibrosis. Am J Respir Crit Care Med 1995;151:1075–1082.

Dr. Fabio Midulla
Department of Paediatrics, 'Sapienza' University of Rome
Viale Regina Elena 324
IT–00165 Rome (Italy)
Tel. +39 06 4997 9363, Fax +39 06 4997 7412, E-Mail midulla@uniroma1.it

Priftis KN, Anthracopoulos MB, Eber E, Koumbourlis AC, Wood RE (eds): Paediatric Bronchoscopy.
Prog Respir Res. Basel, Karger 2010, vol 38, pp 42–53

Special Procedures

Andrew A. Colin[a] · David A. Waltz[b]

[a]Division of Pediatric Pulmonology, Miller School of Medicine, University of Miami, Miami, Fla., and [b]Harvard Medical School, Children's Hospital Boston, and Novartis Institutes for Biomedical Research, Boston, Mass., USA

Abstract

As paediatric flexible bronchoscopy has become more prevalent over the past 3 decades, procedures in which the primary aim is beyond visual inspection have similarly become more common. Interventional bronchoscopy procedures are performed less frequently in the paediatric compared to the adult population due to the relative lack of airway tumours as well as limitations of the size of the instrumentation in the former. However, the ability to perform these special procedures when indicated is nonetheless an important part of the armamentarium of the paediatric flexible bronchoscopist. Predominant among these procedures are endobronchial (EBB) and transbronchial biopsy (TBB), although segmental bronchography, assessment and therapy of airway bleeding, drug concentration measurement, assisted intubation and therapy of bronchitis obliterans have also been performed. This chapter reviews each of these indications, focusing in particular on the clinical, research and technical aspects of EBB and TBB. EBB in the paediatric population remains predominantly a research procedure, as evidence to support its use in clinical contexts is lacking. In contrast, TBB has an established role in clinical care, particularly following lung transplantation.

The use of flexible bronchoscopy became prevalent in paediatric practice in the 1980s and 1990s. In 1997, the first large survey was published on the practice of bronchoscopy (rigid and flexible) in Europe [1]. In this study, 51 European centres performed a total of 7,446 bronchoscopic procedures within the 12 months of the survey. There is no mention of special procedures and more specifically the performance of biopsies.

Interventional pulmonology has developed into a specialty field within adult pulmonology, and the range of procedures has recently been reviewed in an ERS/ATS statement [2]. The use of instrumentation and specifically biopsy via

forceps is routine for adult patients but infrequent in paediatric bronchoscopy, where inspection and bronchoalveolar lavage (BAL) are the mainstay. The cause of this discrepancy lies in the different sets of pathologies that drive adult bronchoscopy; predominant amongst these are airway malignancies that are rare in the paediatric airway. The technical limitations of obtaining usable samples via bronchoscopes with small working channels also reduce the use of the paediatric bronchoscopes for biopsy procedures. Where training programmes are formalized (e.g. in the USA), there are no specific requirements for training in brochoscopic bioptic techniques. We therefore do not know the extent to which training is given or proficiency obtained in these techniques around the world. It is likely, however, that in contrast to adult bronchoscopists, many paediatric pulmonologists are not trained to perform endobronchial (EBB) or transbronchial biopsies (TBB). In some countries, the training of paediatric bronchoscopists includes rigid bronchoscopy, thus enabling such specialists to be more flexible with invasive procedures. The focus of this chapter will be on flexible bronchoscopy; we will limit the discussion on rigid bronchoscopic procedures to occasional comparative comments between the two procedures.

Definitions

For the purpose of this chapter we will use the terminology EBB to indicate acquisition of histological samples by use of forceps, typically under direct visualization. Most commonly the sample is obtained from the bronchial mucosa and less frequently from masses invading the wall or ones occupying the bronchial lumen. A complimentary procedure to bronchial forceps that uses a brush in lieu of forceps is termed bronchial brush biopsy. It is limited to morphological and functional studies of bronchial epithelial cells and is optimized when the brush is protected by a sheath; such 'protected' brushes are limited to bronchoscopes with larger working channels. Some of the studies cited in this review include bronchial brush biopsy, and we have incorporated those data within the EBB segment.

TBB depicts acquisition of tissue samples from regions of the lung that are not directly visible through the bronchoscope. This typically includes alveolar samples obtained from the lung periphery, but can also encompass tissue samples obtained by a needle passed through the bronchial wall. The ERS Task Force recommends that TBB be preceded by a plain chest radiograph, a full blood count including platelet count, and a coagulation screen [3].

Technical details of EBB and TBB and assessment of quality of the samples are discussed below.

Endobronchial Biopsy

EBB in Clinical Practice

We reviewed the existing literature in an attempt to define the range of clinical conditions for which EBB is indicated. Specifically, we evaluated the indication(s) for a biopsy of the bronchial mucosa, normal or inflamed, that does not reveal an obvious lesion or a mass on the surface of the mucosa. We failed to find convincing evidence that such EBB is indicated for any clinical condition.

In a review on the role of brush and mucosal biopsies [4] and in the frame of clinical context, a retrospective analysis of 278 biopsies over 10 years is presented from the centre in Prague. While technical and safety data are offered, there is no analysis of the actual clinical yield from the procedures. The largest study to date stating clinical indications for the procedure [5] included 170 paediatric patients who underwent bronchoscopy with EBB for persistent respiratory problems. The study was published only to state the safety of the procedure but limited the diagnostic or therapeutic impact of the procedure to state that '…broad conclusions about the biopsy findings are not possible owing to the variability in the patients' symptoms and drug treatment regimens…'. Thus, this large study failed to report the effect of the intervention on guiding medical management or consequent health of the patients. The lack of reported relevant outcome data in this large and unique series of patients, and in particular the authors' suggestion to utilize EBB, presumably based on an unsupported conclusion on the relative diagnostic advantage of EBB over conventional BAL,

have been a cause of concern in a recent editorial on the role of EBB in childhood [6]. Saglani et al. [7] analysed the yield of a comprehensive set of investigations in 47 young children with severe recurrent wheeze. The investigations included bronchoscopy and EBB. In 44% of the patients, tissue eosinophilia was identified, and 28% had a thickened reticular basement membrane (RBM). The authors made no attempt to analyse the specific influence of these results on the clinical management of patients and appropriately presented the results as a hypothesis-generating work that could form the basis of future interventional studies.

The use of EBB for specific diagnoses, in contrast to exploratory biopsies from the mucosal surface, appears to be limited as well. The ERS Task Force on flexible endoscopy of paediatric airways [3] cites the procedure as a well-established clinical technique for obtaining ciliated cells for the diagnosis of primary ciliary dyskinesia. It is, however, the current practice of centres for ciliary disorders to use predominantly nasal brush biopsy, and therefore tissue samples obtained by bronchoscopy are unnecessary and consequently EBB is not indicated [8, 9].

While samples of bronchial mucosa do not appear to have proven evidence for clinical utility, histological sampling of lesions of the bronchial wall or intraluminal lesions or masses are likely to offer diagnostic advantages. There is little in the way of systematic reviews of such interventions in childhood, suggesting that the occurrence of such interventions in paediatrics is not common enough to generate meaningful data on its yield. Figure 1 is an example of bronchial lesions that were biopsied and led to the diagnosis of Wegener's granulomatosis. Figure 2 depicts an endobronchial carcinoid from our own practice in which a forceps biopsy failed to yield the diagnosis (which was subsequently made following lobectomy) but was complicated by airway bleeding.

The specific role of EBB in the diagnosis of tuberculosis, a common condition, is of particular interest. The ERS Task Force [3] states that EBB is a safe procedure for the diagnosis of tuberculosis and other infectious or granulomatous disorders. Similarly, a review on bronchial biopsy states that EBB (both forceps and brush) is a routine clinical procedure in bronchial tuberculosis in children [10]. Both reviews provide no references to these statements. In a review on the role of EBB in childhood, Bush and Pohunek [4] also specify tuberculosis as a condition in which EBB has an established diagnostic role, citing a study on 17 adult patients with endobronchial lesions in whom EBB was helpful in the diagnosis [11]. A careful review of the literature reveals, however, that the use of EBB is substantially more limited in paediatric tuberculosis. In a paper assessing the value of

Subglottic space   Trachea   Main carina

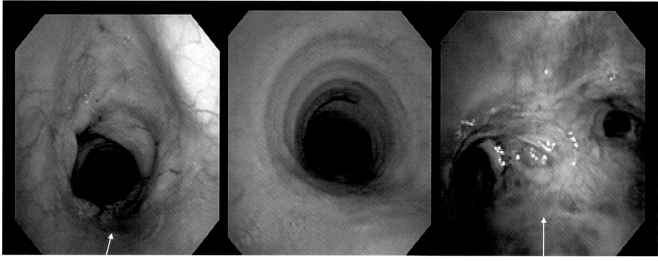

Acute inflammatory lesion   Acute and healed lesions

Fig. 1. Bronchoscopic images of an adolescent with haemosiderosis. EBBs of the skip lesions established the diagnosis of Wegener's granulomatosis with airway involvement. Courtesy of Eric Edell, MD, Mayo Clinic.

Fig. 2. a Endobronchial carcinoid. **b** Forceps biopsy via a flexible bronchoscope failed to yield the diagnosis and was complicated with airway bleeding.

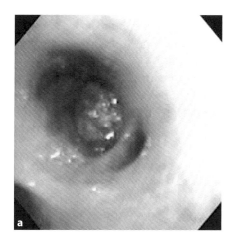

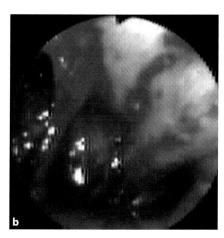

flexible bronchoscopy for childhood tuberculosis, de Blic et al. [12] state that bronchial brushings and transbronchial biopsy, which have been shown to be useful in increasing bacteriological yield in adults, cannot be performed with the smaller paediatric flexible bronchoscope due to the inadequate diameter of the operating channel. They do not comment on older children or use of larger bronchoscopes, and it should be noted that this report predated the description of alternative approaches, such as advancing a biopsy forceps through a separate catheter under direct fibre-optic visualization [13], or the subsequent development of biopsy forceps with a diameter small enough to be advanced through the working channel of a paediatric flexible fibre-optic bronchoscope. In a review of the role of bronchoscopy for pulmonary tuberculosis, Donato et al. [14] note that protected endobronchial brushing and biopsy of a granuloma with culture are sometimes useful but suggest caution in young children because of the risk of bleeding. Fine-needle TBB is deemed inappropriate in these age groups because of the risk of bleeding secondary to the proximity of the airway to the mediastinal great vessels. These authors view a biopsy of an endobronchial lesion as possibly providing a rapid diagnosis if the histological analysis reveals necrotic granulomas. None of these statements are, however, supported by literature or documented experience. A recent study [15] reviews 70 patients with tuberculosis who underwent 118 flexible bronchoscopies and of whom almost half had endobronchial tuberculosis, yet EBB was not obtained in any of the cases to substantiate or follow the diagnosis. It appears that EBB is not widely used for the diagnosis of tuberculosis, nor has it been proven to be superior to conventional diagnostic modalities. Beyond the impression that the technique may be useful, evidence to it is lacking. Thus, the role of EBB in the diagnosis of tuberculosis is overstated.

The ethics of EBB are beyond the scope of this chapter, but given the absence of convincing data supporting clinical utility for EBB, the statement that failure to perform EBB when the opportunity is given could be perceived as unethical, not best practice, and a wasted opportunity [4] is not substantiated by current evidence.

Use of EBB for Research
There are numerous publications on the paediatric use of EBB to evaluate tissue alterations in response to disease conditions, and some of these studies also used controls. These studies encompass predominantly paediatric asthma and to a lesser degree cystic fibrosis and other conditions. The totality of these studies has yielded invaluable information and insight into the underlying pathologies of these diseases and their natural history. Such detailed information and its inconsistent relationship to non-invasive parameters could not have been obtained by other, less invasive means [16], and as such EBB should be viewed as a valuable research tool. The following paragraphs are a concise summary of the scope of discoveries obtained by the use of EBB in infants and children.

A number of studies on asthmatic children have used EBB to examine eosinophilic infiltration and remodelling of airways in asthma. Remodelling is typically defined as an increase in the thickness of the RBM. Such changes were previously observed in adults, and many of the paediatric studies confirmed the presence of such changes in early asthma. Using EBB, thickening and hyalinization of the basement membrane, loss of cilia of epithelial cells, predominance of fibroblasts, degranulating mast cells and lymphocyte infiltration but rarely eosinophils were observed in the mucosa by Cokugras et al. [17] in moderately asthmatic children. Barbato et al. [18] demonstrated an increase in RBM thickness and in mucosal eosinophils in children with asthma compared to non-asthmatic controls. Similarly, early thickening of the RBM was found in children with difficult asthma, and was comparable to asthmatic adults [19]. This observation was independent of age, symptom duration, lung function

or concurrent eosinophilic airway inflammation. In a subsequent study [20], EBBs from children with difficult asthma following treatment with systemic corticosteroids were compared to non-asthmatic children. RBM thickness was greater in the asthmatic than in the control group, but no other significant tissue difference was seen. It was also noted that in such patients treated with systemic corticosteroids, persistent airflow limitation was associated with a greater density of CD4+ T lymphocytes in EBB specimens. In a study designed to investigate whether the increases in airway smooth muscle alterations observed in adults with asthma and cystic fibrosis (CF) occur in children, Regamey et al. [21] found that an increase in both number and size of airway smooth muscle cells occurs in children with chronic inflammatory lung diseases including asthma, CF and non-CF bronchiectasis. The ultrastructure of fibrils and matrix in the thickened RBM of infants, children and adults with asthma revealed no difference in comparison to the respective normal controls. These findings were different from the ones expected in fibrosis [22].

Studies on the natural history and subgroups of wheezing infants and children also revealed important information. Pohunek et al. [23] obtained repeated EBB in children with early respiratory symptoms before a clear clinical diagnosis of bronchial asthma could be made. Increased eosinophils in the bronchial mucosa and increased thickness of the subepithelial lamina reticularis were found in children who were subsequently diagnosed as having bronchial asthma, compared with the children who did not progress to asthma. Thus, markers of inflammation and tissue remodelling are present in children with early respiratory symptoms before a clear clinical diagnosis of bronchial asthma can be made.

EBB from wheezy infants at a median age of 12 months revealed that the RBM thickening and eosinophilic inflammation characteristic of asthma in older children and adults were not present in symptomatic infants who had reversible airflow obstruction, even in the presence of atopy [24]. In contrast, EBB from preschool children with confirmed wheezing revealed significant thickening of the RBM and increased subepithelial eosinophil density when compared to controls. These results suggest that the characteristic pathological features of asthma in adults and school-aged children develop in preschool children with confirmed wheeze between the ages of 1 and 3 years [25]. The presence of asthma-related pathological changes in children at a median age of 4–5 years was demonstrated when a set of pathologies assumed to be limited to atopic children was also found in non-atopic ones by Turato et al. [26]. Both atopic and non-atopic wheezing children had increased epithelial loss, thickened RBM, increased number of vessels and eosinophils, as well as an increase in cytokine expression (interleukins 4 and 5) when compared to normal controls.

A number of studies examined the relationship between clinical markers and the underlying asthma-related pathology. Payne et al. [27] examined the relationship between exhaled nitric oxide and eosinophilic inflammation in EBB from children with difficult asthma after 2 weeks of prednisolone, compared to non-asthmatic controls. Exhaled nitric oxide was associated with eosinophilic inflammation in children with difficult asthma following prednisolone and may serve as a marker for persistent airway eosinophilia. Cysteinyl leukotrienes in exhaled breath condensate, a non-invasive marker of inflammation in the airway, were found to be associated with RBM thickening in asthma [28]. The value of the high-resolution CT scan as a marker of airway remodelling in children with difficult asthma was studied by Saglani et al. [29]. The relationship between RBM thickness and bronchial wall thickening on high-resolution CT, which was found in adults with asthma, did not appear to hold true in children with difficult asthma.

While invasive studies for asthma go back to the 1990s, systematic studies using EBB for CF are more recent. Innovative research on CF using EBB in addition to BAL in patients aged 0.3–16.8 years was undertaken by Hilliard et al. [30]. Multiple inflammatory and matrix breakdown markers in BAL as well as RBM thickness were studied. The authors concluded that two types of changes were observed in these patients: some of the CF patients had indicators of matrix breakdown determined by high concentrations of glycosaminoglycans, elastin and collagen compared to control groups. These correlated positively with neutrophils and negatively with pulmonary function. Other patients had an increase in the median RBM thickness compared to controls. These correlated positively with levels of transforming growth factor β_1 but not with other inflammatory markers or pulmonary function. As cited above for asthma, Regamey et al. [21] demonstrated an increase in airway smooth muscle in children with chronic inflammatory lung diseases including CF.

Safety of EBB
There is now a large body of literature to support the safety of EBB and presumably also TBB, albeit no study specifically addressed the latter procedure in paediatric populations. The Prague centre reported 278 EBB over 10 years, predominantly using fibrescopes at a mean patient age of 11.6 years [4]. Trivial and superficial bleeding typically lasting less than 2 min was noted, oxygen saturation and EKG were monitored throughout the procedure and for 2 h after, and revealed no significant changes. No other complications were reported.

Asthma and Persistent Inflammation
The safety of bronchoscopy and EBB, via flexible and rigid bronchoscopy, in children with difficult asthma and matched normal controls at a mean age of 10.9 years was investigated in a 3-year prospective study [31]. The complications were few and included desaturation and bronchospasm. There were no cases of significant bleeding or pneumothorax. Curiously, the rate of complications was much higher in the control group (17/35 control children versus 1/38 of the asthma patients). At the same centre, the safety of bronchoscopy and EBB was studied in younger patients at a mean age of 31 months [32]. Comparisons were made between patients who underwent EBB versus an identical number of patients who had bronchoscopy without a biopsy. None of the complications in the respective groups were life threatening and between the two groups included fever, grunting, desaturation, stridor, treatment (other than paracetamol), antibiotics, oxygen, paediatric intensive-care unit observation and dexamethasone. Based on a statistical analysis of the comparison groups, the authors concluded that there was no significant difference in the complications. This was likely due to small sample size, since the absolute numbers of subjects experiencing at least one complication was almost double in the group that underwent biopsy: 13 of 33 patients compared to 7 of 33 in the bronchoscopy group alone. The largest study addressing the safety of EBB included a non-homogeneous group of 170 patients [5]. A single patient had a prolonged oxygen desaturation, none had laryngo- or bronchospasm, none of the patients required topical adrenaline to control bleeding. There were no episodes of pneumothorax, haemoptysis, pneumonia or significant fever. Of note, a single dose of intravenous ampicillin was administered to patients younger than 4 years of age. This study reported the average duration of flexible bronchoscopy and biopsy to be 12 min (range 6–27). Regamey et al. [33] evaluated the impact of performing EBB as a part of fibre-optic bronchoscopy on the length of the total procedure time. The median time to obtain 3 biopsies was 5.3 min (range 2.5–16.6) which the authors consider an acceptable increase in the duration of fibre-optic bronchoscopy for biopsy sampling. Of note, however, the median durations for the conventional elements of the procedure were 2.5 min (1.0–8.2) for airway inspection and 2.8 min (1.7–9.4) for BAL. Thus, EBB doubled the procedure time.

Cystic Fibrosis
There are few publications on EBB for CF and a single systematic review of the safety of the procedure in this population [34]. EBB was performed in 45 bronchoscopies for patients with CF at a mean age of 7 years and compared to controls with

EBB for other conditions. The complications were minor and infrequent, and there were no significant differences between disease groups in the number, type or severity of complications occurring during or in the first 12 h after the procedure.

In conclusion, it appears that neither significant bleeding nor pneumothorax are serious risks in EBB, and thus a routine chest radiograph is not deemed necessary following the procedure [3, 4]. The concerns over an increased risk of bleeding with EBB in CF have not materialized, but the number of procedures in patients with CF in comparison to asthma is relatively small. It appears that performance of EBB by expert practitioners with adequate anaesthesia support reduces complications to a minimum. The milder complications, oxygen desaturation of varying severity, bronchospasm and to a lesser degree laryngospasm, and postprocedure fever are very variable and may be underreported.

Transbronchial Biopsy

TBB in Clinical Practice
TBB has an established role in the paediatric lung or heart-lung transplant patient [35–38], in whom surveillance bronchoscopy with TBB is often performed on a scheduled basis for at least the first year after transplantation to evaluate for rejection and/or infection [39]. Detection of asymptomatic rejection of grade A2 or greater has been reported in 4% [39] to 24% [38] of cases. TBB is also performed when the clinical condition of the lung or heart-lung transplant patient changes, typically in the setting of a decline in pulmonary function or the development of cough, dyspnoea and/or fever in the presence of a radiographic infiltrate. When TBB is performed for clinical indications other than routine surveillance, a change in clinical management based on the results of TBB has been reported to occur in 64% of cases [40].

TBB has also been performed in other clinical settings in paediatric patients. In an early report, Fitzpatrick et al. [41] reported a specific diagnosis established by TBB in 6 of 12 patients with a persistently abnormal chest X-ray. Subsequent reports of the diagnostic yield of TBB in immunocompromised and immunocompetent patients, including those with chronic interstitial lung disease, range from 50 to 67% [36, 42–44], although the use of TBB in the non-transplant setting is termed 'controversial' by the ERS Task Force [3].

Safety of TBB
The most common serious complications following TBB in paediatric patients are bleeding and pneumothorax. Minor bleeding is relatively common. Clinically significant bleeding has been reported in up to 6% of cases [40]. The incidence of pneumothorax reported in the literature ranges up to 12% [45], although more recent publications generally report an incidence of 1–3% [38, 40]. Other complications of TBB include transient hypoxaemia, dyspnoea and pyrexia [3]. In general, however, TBB in paediatric patients under carefully controlled conditions is relatively safe.

Technical Aspects of Invasive Bronchoscopy

Sedation/Anaesthesia
A shift towards a more controlled environment for paediatric fibre-optic bronchoscopy, replacing the prevailing conscious sedation approach, emerged in the early 2000s [chapter 2, this vol., pp. 22–29]. Stacey et al. [46] note that in their large centre in the UK they have almost completely transitioned to the use of general anaesthesia with inhalational agents. In the same year, the largest study to date addressing the use of laryngeal mask airway for flexible bronchoscopy with general anaesthesia was published from the USA [47]. The following comments relate exclusively to anaesthesia used for airway biopsies. There appears to be wide agreement in the literature that EBB should be performed under general anaesthesia. The report by Payne et al. [31] was subsequently applied in the publications emanating from the Royal Brompton centre in the UK [32, 34, 48]. In these reports, the procedure was done in theatre under general anaesthesia, administered by a specialized anaesthetist. Nebulized albuterol (salbutamol) was given to asthmatic patients 30 min before induction of anaesthesia and when adequate, atropine or glycopyrrolate had been added. Intravenous access was secured in all subjects. Anaesthesia was induced with intravenous (propofol) or volatile (sevoflurane) agents, and maintained with volatile agents (isoflurane, sevoflurane or halothane) or intravenous propofol. Carrier gases were oxygen, oxygen/air mixture or oxygen/nitrous oxide mixture. The choice of muscle relaxant, if used, was between vecuronium, atracurium, rocuronium or mivacurium. Similarly Barbato et al. [18] used intravenous propofol (3 mg/kg) and atropine for premedication, with local anaesthesia of lidocaine 0.5% in the lower airway. Salva et al. [5] performed the procedures with an anaesthesiologist with either controlled or assisted breathing. A laryngeal mask airway was used in all instances. Induction with sevoflurane in oxygen and nitrous oxide was followed by peripheral intravenous catheter placement with propofol. Sevoflurane in 100% oxygen with or without intermittent intravenous propofol (0.5–1.0 mg/kg) was used for maintenance of anaesthesia.

Size of Bronchoscope

For optimal results of EBB and TBB, by both brush and forceps, the 4.9- or 5-mm bronchoscope with its 2.2-mm working channel should be preferentially used [3]. The 4.0-mm bronchoscope with a 2.0-mm working channel is an acceptable alternative. The larger-sized working channels allow the use of a protected brush and larger-size forceps. When the size of the patient dictates the use of the smaller flexible bronchoscopes with a working channel of 1.2 mm, brush biopsies can only be obtained with a non-protected brush with the risk of loss of the cellular material if the brush is retracted through the channel. In such cases, the brush can be pulled into the tip of the bronchoscope and the bronchoscope in its entirety is pulled out and the brush subsequently processed [3]. The use of the smaller bioptic forceps for EBB is reported by some authors to be associated with material that is uninterpretable. Thus, Salva et al. [5] report abandoning the use of the smaller forceps after a third failed attempt and limiting acquisition of biopsies to the larger-sized biopsy forceps. Remarkably, however, in a study of EBB in infants and preschool children below the age of 5 years, Saglani et al. [32] used the 2.7-mm bronchoscope for children aged up to 2 years and 3.6-mm instruments for those aged 2–5 years. Both these bronchoscope types have a 1.2-mm suction channel. Yet the authors report an excellent yield with suitable biopsies for assessment for 30 of the 33 patients studied. In a later study of EBB from the same centre [48] spanning a wider patient age (from 0.2 to 16.8 years) and including also patients with CF, they report a significantly lesser likelihood of success with the smaller-sized forceps. The probability of obtaining at least 1 evaluable biopsy specimen was found to be mainly dependent on the size of the forceps used: with a large forceps, a 93% success rate, and with the small forceps, a 57% success rate. This difference was statistically significant (p < 0.001). These results were independent of the diagnosis of the patient in this mixed population. It is likely albeit not clearly emerging from the analysis by Regamey et al. [48] that operator experience in EBB has an important impact on the quality of the bioptic specimen; this may be of more importance with the use of the smaller forceps. Our own experience with the use of the smaller forceps is closer to that reported in the latter study. In addition, because of frequent damage to the bioptic material, we stopped using the 'rat tooth jaw' forceps in favour of an oval cup forceps. Disposable forceps appear to be superior to reusable ones for EBB, as Payne et al. [31] note that each set of forceps was used on a maximum of 5 patients.

A technique that is commonly used by surgeons for EBB is punch biopsy via a rigid bronchoscope. This was reported as an alternative to the EBB via a flexible bronchoscope in one of the large paediatric studies from the UK [31] and as the primary approach in a study from Turkey using a circular cup biopsy forceps [17].

An adult flexible bronchoscope, allowing for the use of a larger forceps, is also preferred for TBB, although an alternative approach entails TBB being performed through a rigid bronchoscope [35, 36, 45]. However, the difference in yield appears less striking in TBB than in EBB. Visner et al. [44] reported a yield of adequate tissue in 97% of procedures performed with an adult bronchoscope and 85% of procedures performed with a paediatric bronchoscope. This yield is consistent with reports, predominantly in transplant patients, in which the yield of adequate tissue ranges from 84 to 92% although the sizes of the biopsy forceps and/or bronchoscope were unspecified [13, 37, 40].

Localization of Biopsy Site

The ERS Task Force recommends that EBBs be taken from segmental subcarinae, which are sharper and thus allow a better grip by the forceps [3]. There is no evidence in the literature that the anatomical origin of the biopsy results in a different sample quality. In various studies EBB are reported from the main carina [18, 31], in the majority of the research studies (mostly deriving from a single centre), a standardized approach used segmental subcarinae of the right lower lobe [31, 32, 34, 48]. The single study that stated clinical indications for a series of EBB also used the right bronchial tree at the level of the third branch in children less than 10 years old and at the third or fourth branch in the older children [5].

When a rigid bronchoscope was used for EBB, the samples were obtained from the main carina or the carina between the right middle and lower lobes [31] or the left main bronchus [17].

The technique of TBB generally involves obtaining a sample from a distal airway in the manner described by Whitehead et al. [26] and Midulla et al. [3]. In the absence of localized disease, 2 or more lobes are often sampled, although only one lung is sampled to avoid the potential for bilateral pneumothoraces. Commonly, the closed forceps are advanced gently until resistance is met, indicating that the forceps have been placed into an airway of approximately the same diameter. The forceps are then withdrawn 1–2 cm, the jaws opened and the forceps advanced again until resistance is met. Following closure of the jaws, the forceps are withdrawn firmly from the airway. The airway into which the TBB forceps were advanced is visualized for a few minutes to evaluate for bleeding. Minor bleeding is common, but generally resolves spontaneously. If significant bleeding occurs, the bronchoscope itself can be wedged in the airway and blood aspirated through the suction channel to prevent spillover into adjacent airways. Persistent significant bleeding can be addressed via instillation of topical vasoconstrictors such as 1:10,000 epinephrine.

TBB performed through a rigid bronchoscope is similar to that performed through a flexible bronchoscope [36].

The ERS Task Force views fluoroscopy as mandatory for TBB for the accurate positioning of the biopsy forceps [3]. The opening and closing of the forceps jaws can also be directly ascertained and the peripheral location of the forceps visualized. It should be recognized, however, that typical fluoroscopic visualization is 2-dimensional, and thus the proximity of the biopsy forceps to the pleural surface perpendicular to the plane of the image is difficult to judge.

Sample Quality and Processing
Jeffery et al. [10] provide a comprehensive review of the methods of EBB for research, including the quality and processing of samples in adults and children. The degree of detail provided is beyond the scope of this chapter, but it is important to bear in mind that the small size of paediatric instruments is a limiting factor to obtaining adequate samples. Suitable samples for analysis are those that include RBM preferably sized at least 1 mm, sufficient subepithelial stroma for the assessment of inflammation, areas of smooth muscle and submucosal glands [32].

Considerations regarding sample quality and processing are similar for TBB. For the diagnosis of rejection in the lung transplant population, an adequate sample is considered to contain 100 alveoli.

Number of Samples
Because of the limitations of instrument size in paediatrics, an adequate number of samples is needed to ascertain interpretable results. The number of EBB samples obtained for reliable analysis varies in the published literature. Barbato et al. [18] used a single biopsy from the trachea. A minimum of 3 biopsies and no more than 3 attempts were needed to obtain a macroscopically adequate sample by Salva et al. [5] and Bush and Pohunek [4], respectively. Studies from the UK reported up to 6 biopsies [31, 32] and up to 5 biopsies in a subsequent analysis [34]. Saglani et al. [32] analysed the number of biopsies taken relative to the overall biopsy quality concluding that there was no clear relation between these parameters. These authors therefore stated that their results suggest that no additional clinical information is obtained by taking more than 3 biopsies per subject.

When a rigid bronchoscope is uscd for EBB, up to 6 specimens were obtained in one study [31] and 2 samples in another [17].

At least 3 specimens are obtained with TBB [3, 36]. In our experience, 8–10 samples are generally required to provide an adequate sample with TBB; this is slightly more than the 4–7 specimens advocated by Kurland et al. [37].

Less Common Procedures Using Flexible Bronchoscopy

Segmental Bronchography
CT scan of the chest has replaced bronchography for the investigation of bronchial abnormalities such as bronchiectasis, a trend that has been emphasized by the advent of 3-dimensional reconstruction. We have found on a number of occasions that the CT scan was not sensitive enough to provide details of the finer internal structure of bronchi, or their connections. In these cases we use segmental bronchography, in which the bronchoscope is advanced peripherally and wedged into the bronchus feeding the area of interest. The dye is hand injected through the working channel with a syringe under fluoroscopy, and images are taken in rapid sequence. Since lipid-based contrast materials (e.g. Lipiodol), the bronchography agents of old, are not readily available, we use arteriography contrast materials such as Ioversol (Optiray, Mallinckrodt Inc.). We have used 1:1 dilutions with normal saline, and varying amounts ranging from 20 to 40 ml depending on the size of the area to be studied. To date we have seen no side effects, such as significant bronchospasm. The resolution of the images with these contrast materials is substantially inferior to the older ones and they fade rapidly, but we typically obtain the information we seek. Figure 3 exemplifies segmental bronchography to diagnose a cardiac bronchus.

Bronchoscopy for Airway and Pulmonary Bleeding
The treatment of pulmonary bleeding is widely addressed in the adult literature, and the use of both flexible and rigid bronchoscopy to control such bleeding is common. Interventions include pulmonary lavage of cold epinephrine-saline solution, CO_2 laser therapy, Nd:YAG laser therapy, balloon occlusion of bronchi, insertion of an endoscopic Watanabe spigot and instillation of thrombin or fibrinogen-thrombin glue. Many of these are used for short-term stabilization until definitive measures can be applied [chapter 6, this vol., pp. 64–74].

The paediatric literature barely addresses the use of bronchoscopy for airway and lung bleeding. A review of pulmonary haemorrhagic syndromes in children lists iced saline, diluted solution of epinephrine and balloon tamponade as options to control bleeding [49]. However, more recent reviews such as on the use of bronchoscopy in the paediatric intensive-care

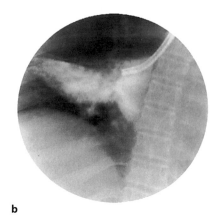

Fig. 3. Segmental bronchography. **a** Injection of a contrast agent through the wedged bronchoscope into an orifice that connects to a blind pouch identified as a cardiac bronchus. **b** The true middle lobe bronchus.

a

b

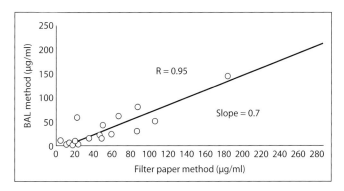

Fig. 4. Amiloride – measurement of airway deposition. Comparison of two methods to determine drug deposition to the airway. The BAL method utilizes a dilution measurement and is compared to direct absorption onto filter paper pledgets. Parallel measurements were undertaken in 17 individuals and found to be highly correlated (R = 0.95). Courtesy of Robert E. Wood, unpublished data.

unit [50] and on diffuse alveolar haemorrhage in children [51] do not list bronchoscopy-related interventions to control bleeding. The scant paediatric literature addressing direct airway treatment of airway bleeding largely relies on single-centre case reports, the largest being a series of 14 patients with ages ranging from 4 days to 11 years, with acute life-threatening pulmonary haemorrhage. The interventions included CO_2 laser bronchoscopy, Nd:YAG laser bronchoscopy, endoscopic balloon occlusion of a lobe or main bronchus, topical airway vasoconstrictors and endoscopic tumour excision [52].

An exciting phase in the interventions to control airway bleeding has recently emerged. The successful intrapulmonary instillation of activated recombinant factor VII to control diffuse alveolar haemorrhage has been reported in a series of adult patients [53]. Similarly tranexamic acid, a synthetic antifibrinolytic agent, has also been reported in a series of 6

patients [54]. The use of both agents is an extension of previous experience with their systemic administration to effectively treat patients with recalcitrant pulmonary bleeding.

We have recently used activated recombinant factor VII as an intervention of last resort to control an unremitting diffuse pulmonary haemorrhage of 4 weeks' duration, in a 16-year-old patient with acute myelogenous leukaemia [55]. We used the protocol of Heslet et al. [53]: activated recombinant factor VII was administered into both main stem bronchi at a dose of 50 μg/kg diluted in normal saline to 50 ml and divided into 2 aliquots of 25 ml per bronchus. The haemorrhage was visualized during the procedure, and its resolution following the treatment was immediate, unequivocal and definitive.

Direct Measurements of Drug Deposition to the Airway
Measurements of drug deposition to the lung have conventionally been obtained by using a urea-based correction factor for dilution applied to BAL fluid [56]. The concentration of drug deposited on the surface of airways at least 3 mm in diameter can also be measured by direct sampling. The fluid is collected by filter paper pledgets, carefully weighed and delivered through a flexible bronchoscope with a catheter plugged with wax to prevent contamination of the specimen [57]. The two methods were compared in paediatric patients and were found to be highly correlated (fig. 4).

Endoscopy-Assisted Tracheal Intubation and (Selective) Bronchial Intubation
Direct visualization of the airway via a flexible bronchoscope has been reported to be of assistance in the intubation of the patient with a difficult airway [58; chapter 5, this vol., pp. 54–63] and during placement of a bronchial blocker to enable single-lung ventilation during video-assisted thoracoscopic surgery [59].

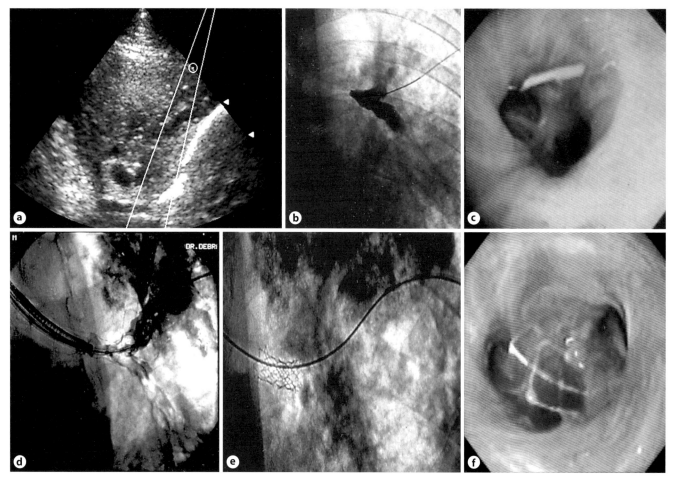

Fig. 5. Illustrative case of combined transthoracic and bronchoscopic treatment of an obliterative membrane of a bronchus in a young adult with CF [61]. **a** Ultrasonography demonstration of a fluid-filled left upper lobe bronchus distal to a (membranous) occlusion. **b** X-ray image of a percutaneous bronchogram outlining the intact left upper lobe bronchial tree distal to a membranous obstruction of the bronchus. **c** Bronchoscopic visualization of a percutaneous transthoracic needle puncturing a membranous occlusion of the left upper lobe bronchus. **d** X-ray image of bronchoscopic visualization of percutaneous transthoracic needle depicted in the photograph in **c**. **e** X-ray image of a Palmaz wire stent and transthoracic percutaneous catheter in the left upper lobe after successful repeat perforation of a membranous obstruction of the bronchus. **f** Bronchoscopic visualization of the patent left upper lobe bronchus (at 2 o'clock in the image) after placement of a Palmaz wire stent.

Treatment of Bronchitis Obliterans

Chang et al. [60] have described an obliterative-like lesion of the bronchus in children with chronic suppurative lung disease. We have observed similar lesions in young adults with CF which we have termed membranous obliterative bronchitis [61]. We breached the obstructive membranes via flexible bronchoscopy and restored airway patency [61]. Figure 5 depicts a combined transthoracic and bronchoscopic treatment of an obliterative membrane of a bronchus in a young adult with CF. For details of the case, refer to Colin et al. [61]. We think that this experience may be extrapolated to the paediatric population in the future.

Conclusions and Future Directions

EBB and TBB have both been shown to be safe procedures in paediatric pulmonology. The role of EBB appears to have been established for research. At this time there is no proven advantage to the acquisition of histological material via EBB towards the goal of improved patient management. As quality research into a variety of morbidities is performed, the clinical applications of the procedure will be better defined. The clinical role of TBB is well established and is particularly related to monitoring and management of patients after lung transplantation, although published reports suggest that diagnostic samples may also be obtained in the non-transplant setting, particularly in children with interstitial lung disease. Much of the technical limitation of EBB emanates from the small calibre of the working channel of the paediatric bronchoscopes. With improved miniaturization of the optical component of the bronchoscope, it is hoped that a larger proportion of the cross-section of the bronchoscope can be dedicated to the working channel. TBB will also benefit from technical optimization of the paediatric bronchoscope, as the yield of informative samples, while adequate, is lower with the use of smaller biopsy forceps.

The ambitious developments in adult invasive bronchoscopy include endobronchial ultrasonography and highly sophisticated methods to directly evaluate the cellular structure of the airways and parenchyma via confocal fluorescent laser microscopy (alveoloscopy). Because of the size limitation of the paediatric bronchoscope, these are at present outside the reach of the smaller instruments. As above, however, future miniaturization may bring these advanced investigative methodologies into the reach of the paediatric bronchoscopist.

References

1 Barbato A, Magarotto M, Crivellaro M, Novello A Jr, Cracco A, de Blic J, Warner JO, Zach M: Use of the paediatric bronchoscope, flexible and rigid, in 51 European centres. Eur Respir J 1997;10: 1761–1766.

2 Bolliger CT, Mathur PN: ERS/ATS statement on interventional pulmonology. Eur Respir J 2002; 19:356–373.

3 Midulla F, de Blic J, Barbato A, Bush A, Eber E, Kotecha S, Haxby E, Moretti C, Pohunek P, Ratjen F, ERS Task Force: Flexible endoscopy of paediatric airways. Eur Respir J 2003;22:698–708.

4 Bush A, Pohunek P: Brush biopsy and mucosal biopsy. Am J Respir Crit Care Med 2000;162: S18–S22.

5 Salva PS, Theroux C, Schwartz D: Safety of endobronchial biopsy in 170 children with chronic respiratory symptoms. Thorax 2003;58:1058–1060.

6 Colin AA, Ali-Dinar T: Endobronchial biopsy in childhood. Chest 2007;131:1626–1627.

7 Saglani S, Nicholson AG, Scallan M, Balfour-Lynn I, Rosenthal M, Payne DN, Bush A: Investigation of young children with severe recurrent wheeze: any clinical benefit? Eur Respir J 2006; 27:29–35.

8 Noone PG, Leigh MW, Sannuti A, Minnix SL, Carson JL, Hazucha M, Zariwala MA, Knowles MR: Primary ciliary dyskinesia: diagnostic and phenotypic features. Am J Respir Crit Care Med 2004;169:459–467.

9 Bush A, Chodhari R, Collins N, Copeland F, Hall P, Harcourt J, Hariri M, Hogg C, Lucas J, Mitchison HM, O'Callaghan C, Phillips G: Primary ciliary dyskinesia: current state of the art. Arch Dis Child 2007;92:1136–1140.

10 Jeffery P, Holgate S, Wenzel S, Endobronchial Biopsy Workshop: Methods for the assessment of endobronchial biopsies in clinical research: application to studies of pathogenesis and the effects of treatment. Am J Respir Crit Care Med 2003;168:S1–S17.

11 Baran R, Tor M, Tahaoglu K, Ozvaran K, Kir A, Kizkin O, Turker H: Intrathoracic tuberculous lymphadenopathy: clinical and bronchoscopic features in 17 adults without parenchymal lesions. Thorax 1996;51:87–89.

12 De Blic J, Azevedo I, Burren CP, Le Bourgeois M, Lallemand D, Scheinmann P: The value of flexible bronchoscopy in childhood pulmonary tuberculosis. Chest 1991;100:688–692.

13 Mullins D, Livne M, Mallory GB Jr, Kemp JS: A new technique for transbronchial biopsy in infants and small children. Pediatr Pulmonol 1995; 20:253–257.

14 Donato L, Helms P, Barats A, Lebris V: Bronchoscopy in childhood pulmonary tuberculosis (in French). Arch Pédiatr 2005;12(suppl 2):S127–S131.

15 Cakir E, Uyan ZS, Oktem S, Karakoc F, Ersu R, Karadag B, Dagli E: Flexible bronchoscopy for diagnosis and follow-up of childhood endobronchial tuberculosis. Pediatr Infect Dis J 2008;27: 783–787.

16 Regamey N, Hilliard TN, Saglani S, Zhu J, Balfour-Lynn IM, Rosenthal M, Jeffery PK, Alton EW, Bush A, Davies JC: Endobronchial biopsy in childhood. Chest 2008;133:312.

17 Cokugras H, Akcakaya N, Seckin, Camcioglu Y, Sarimurat N, Aksoy F: Ultrastructural examination of bronchial biopsy specimens from children with moderate asthma. Thorax 2001;56:25–29.

18 Barbato A, Turato G, Baraldo S, Bazzan E, Calabrese F, Tura M, Zuin R, Beghe B, Maestrelli P, Fabbri LM, Saetta M: Airway inflammation in childhood asthma. Am J Respir Crit Care Med 2003;168:798–803.

19 Payne DN, Rogers AV, Adelroth E, Bandi V, Guntupalli KK, Bush A, Jeffery PK: Early thickening of the reticular basement membrane in children with difficult asthma. Am J Respir Crit Care Med 2003;167:78–82.

20 Payne DN, Qiu Y, Zhu J, Peachey L, Scallan M, Bush A, Jeffery PK: Airway inflammation in children with difficult asthma: relationships with airflow limitation and persistent symptoms. Thorax 2004;59:862–869.

21 Regamey N, Ochs M, Hilliard TN, Muhlfeld C, Cornish N, Fleming L, Saglani S, Alton EW, Bush A, Jeffery PK, Davies JC: Increased airway smooth muscle mass in children with asthma, cystic fibrosis, and non-cystic fibrosis bronchiectasis. Am J Respir Crit Care Med 2008;177: 837–843.

22 Saglani S, Molyneux C, Gong H, Rogers A, Malmstrom K, Pelkonen A, Makela M, Adelroth E, Bush A, Payne DN, Jeffery PK: Ultrastructure of the reticular basement membrane in asthmatic adults, children and infants. Eur Respir J 2006; 28:505–512.

23 Pohunek P, Warner JO, Turzikova J, Kudrmann J, Roche WR: Markers of eosinophilic inflammation and tissue re-modelling in children before clinically diagnosed bronchial asthma. Pediatr Allergy Immunol 2005;16:43–51.

24 Saglani S, Malmstrom K, Pelkonen AS, Malmberg LP, Lindahl H, Kajosaari M, Turpeinen M, Rogers AV, Payne DN, Bush A, Haahtela T, Makela MJ, Jeffery PK: Airway remodeling and inflammation in symptomatic infants with reversible airflow obstruction. Am J Respir Crit Care Med 2005;171:722–727.

25 Saglani S, Payne DN, Zhu J, Wang Z, Nicholson AG, Bush A, Jeffery PK: Early detection of airway wall remodeling and eosinophilic inflammation in preschool wheezers. Am J Respir Crit Care Med 2007;176:858–864.

26 Turato G, Barbato A, Baraldo S, Zanin ME, Bazzan E, Lokar-Oliani K, Calabrese F, Panizzolo C, Snijders D, Maestrelli P, Zuin R, Fabbri LM, Saetta M: Nonatopic children with multitrigger wheezing have airway pathology comparable to atopic asthma. Am J Respir Crit Care Med 2008; 178:476–482.

27 Payne DN, Adcock IM, Wilson NM, Oates T, Scallan M, Bush A: Relationship between exhaled nitric oxide and mucosal eosinophilic inflammation in children with difficult asthma, after treatment with oral prednisolone. Am J Respir Crit Care Med 2001;164:1376–1381.

28 Lex C, Zacharasiewicz A, Payne DN, Wilson NM, Nicholson AG, Kharitonov SA, Barnes PJ, Bush A: Exhaled breath condensate cysteinyl leukotrienes and airway remodeling in childhood asthma: a pilot study. Respir Res 2006;7:63.

29 Saglani S, Papaioannou G, Khoo L, Ujita M, Jeffery PK, Owens C, Hansell DM, Payne DN, Bush A: Can HRCT be used as a marker of airway re-modelling in children with difficult asthma? Respir Res 2006;7:46.

30 Hilliard TN, Regamey N, Shute JK, Nicholson AG, Alton EW, Bush A, Davies JC: Airway remodelling in children with cystic fibrosis. Thorax 2007;62:1074–1080.

31 Payne D, McKenzie SA, Stacey S, Misra D, Haxby E, Bush A: Safety and ethics of bronchoscopy and endobronchial biopsy in difficult asthma. Arch Dis Child 2001;84:423–426.

32 Saglani S, Payne DN, Nicholson AG, Scallan M, Haxby E, Bush A: The safety and quality of endobronchial biopsy in children under five years old. Thorax 2003;58:1053–1057.

33 Regamey N, Balfour-Lynn I, Rosenthal M, Hogg C, Bush A, Davies JC: Time required to obtain endobronchial biopsies in children during fiberoptic bronchoscopy. Pediatr Pulmonol 2009;44:76–79.

34 Molina-Teran A, Hilliard TN, Saglani S, Haxby E, Scallan M, Bush A, Davies JC: Safety of endobronchial biopsy in children with cystic fibrosis. Pediatr Pulmonol 2006;41:1021–1024.

35 Scott JP, Higenbottam TW, Smyth RL, Whitehead B, Helms P, Fradet G, de Leval M, Wallwork J: Transbronchial biopsies in children after heart-lung transplantation. Pediatrics 1990;86:698–702.

36 Whitehead B, Scott JP, Helms P, Malone M, Macrae D, Higenbottam TW, Smyth RL, Wallwork J, Elliott M, de Leval M: Technique and use of transbronchial biopsy in children and adolescents. Pediatr Pulmonol 1992;12:240–246.

37 Kurland G, Noyes BE, Jaffe R, Atlas AB, Armitage J, Orenstein DM: Bronchoalveolar lavage and transbronchial biopsy in children following heart-lung and lung transplantation. Chest 1993;104:1043–1048.

38 Faro A, Visner G: The use of multiple transbronchial biopsies as the standard approach to evaluate lung allograft rejection. Pediatr Transplant 2004;8:322–328.

39 Benden C, Harpur-Sinclair O, Ranasinghe AS, Hartley JC, Elliott MJ, Aurora P: Surveillance bronchoscopy in children during the first year after lung transplantation: is it worth it? Thorax 2007;62:57–61.

40 Greene CL, Reemtsen B, Polimenakos A, Horn M, Wells W: Role of clinically indicated transbronchial lung biopsies in the management of pediatric post-lung transplant patients. Ann Thorac Surg 2008;86:198–203.

41 Fitzpatrick SB, Stokes DC, Marsh B, Wang KP: Transbronchial lung biopsy in pediatric and adolescent patients. Am J Dis Child 1985;139:46–49.

42 Fan LL, Kozinetz CA, Wojtczak HA, Chatfield BA, Cohen AH, Rothenberg SS: Diagnostic value of transbronchial, thoracoscopic, and open lung biopsy in immunocompetent children with chronic interstitial lung disease. J Pediatr 1997; 131:565–569.

43 Barbato A, Panizzolo C, Cracco A, De Blic J, Dinwiddie R, Zach M: Interstitial lung disease in children: a multicentre survey on diagnostic approach. Eur Respir J 2000;16:509–513.

44 Visner GA, Faro A, Zander DS: Role of transbronchial biopsies in pediatric lung diseases. Chest 2004;126:273–280.

45 Muntz HR, Wallace M, Lusk RP: Pediatric transbronchial lung biopsy. Ann Otol Rhinol Laryngol 1992;101:135–137.

46 Stacey S, Hurley E, Bush A: Sedation for pediatric bronchoscopy. Chest 2001;119:316–317.

47 Nussbaum E, Zagnoev M: Pediatric fiberoptic bronchoscopy with a laryngeal mask airway. Chest 2001;120:614–616.

48 Regamey N, Hilliard TN, Saglani S, Zhu J, Scallan M, Balfour-Lynn IM, Rosenthal M, Jeffery PK, Alton EW, Bush A, Davies JC: Quality, size, and composition of pediatric endobronchial biopsies in cystic fibrosis. Chest 2007;131:1710–1717.

49 Avital A, Springer C, Godfrey S: Pulmonary haemorrhagic syndromes in children. Paediatric Respiratory Reviews 2000;1:266–273.

50 Bush A: Bronchoscopy in paediatric intensive care. Paediatr Respir Rev 2003;4:67–73.

51 Susarla SC, Fan LL: Diffuse alveolar hemorrhage syndromes in children. Curr Opin Pediatr 2007; 19:314–320.

52 Sidman JD, Wheeler WB, Cabalka AK, Soumekh B, Brown CA, Wright GB: Management of acute pulmonary hemorrhage in children. Laryngoscope 2001;111:33–35.

53 Heslet L, Nielsen JD, Levi M, Sengelov H, Johansson PI: Successful pulmonary administration of activated recombinant factor VII in diffuse alveolar hemorrhage. Crit Care (Lond) 2006;10:R177.

54 Solomonov A, Fruchter O, Zuckerman T, Brenner B, Yigla M: Pulmonary hemorrhage: a novel mode of therapy. Respir Med 2009;103:1196–1200.

55 Colin AA, Shafieian M, Andreansky M: Bronchoscopic instillation of activated recombinant factor VII to treat diffuse alveolar hemorrhage in a child. Pediatr Pulmonol 2010;45:411.

56 Wagener JS, Rock MJ, McCubbin MM, Hamilton SD, Johnson CA, Ahrens RC: Aerosol delivery and safety of recombinant human deoxyribonuclease in young children with cystic fibrosis: a bronchoscopic study. Pulmozyme Pediatric Broncoscopy Study Group. J Pediatr 1998;133: 486–491.

57 Noone PG, Regnis JA, Liu X, Brouwer KL, Robinson M, Edwards L, Knowles MR: Airway deposition and clearance and systemic pharmacokinetics of amiloride following aerosolization with an ultrasonic nebulizer to normal airways. Chest 1997;112:1283–1290.

58 Finer NN, Muzyka D: Flexible endoscopic intubation of the neonate. Pediatr Pulmonol 1992;12: 48–51.

59 Hammer GB, Harrison TK, Vricella LA, Black MD, Krane EJ: Single lung ventilation in children using a new paediatric bronchial blocker. Paediatr Anaesth 2002;12:69–72.

60 Chang AB, Boyce NC, Masters IB, Torzillo PJ, Masel JP: Bronchoscopic findings in children with non-cystic fibrosis chronic suppurative lung disease. Thorax 2002;57:935–938.

61 Colin AA, Tsiligiannis T, Nose V, Waltz DA: Membranous obliterative bronchitis: a proposed unifying model. Pediatr Pulmonol 2006;41:126–132.

Andrew A. Colin, MD, Professor of Pediatrics
Chief, Division of Pediatric Pulmonology, Miller School of Medicine, University of Miami
1580 NW 10th Avenue
Miami, FL 33136 (USA)
Tel. +1 305 243 3176, Fax +1 305 243 1262, E-Mail acolin@med.miami.edu

Priftis KN, Anthracopoulos MB, Eber E, Koumbourlis AC, Wood RE (eds): Paediatric Bronchoscopy.
Prog Respir Res. Basel, Karger 2010, vol 38, pp 54–63

Flexible Fibre-Optic Bronchoscopy in the Intensive-Care Unit

Anastassios C. Koumbourlis

Division of Allergy, Pulmonary and Sleep Medicine, Children's National Medical Center, George Washington University, Washington, D.C., USA

Abstract

Flexible fibre-optic bronchoscopy and bronchoalveolar lavage have become important diagnostic tools for the evaluation and often for the treatment of infants and children with serious lung and airway problems causing respiratory insufficiency or failure. These patients are cared for in the paediatric or neonatal intensive-care units, and they usually require endotracheal intubation (or tracheostomy) and mechanical ventilation. Although the technique of the procedure and the equipment used do not differ from those used in the outpatient setting, the severity of illness and the lability of the patients pose unique challenges for the bronchoscopist. These challenges stem primarily from the fact that even the smallest bronchoscope causes significant obstruction of the artificial airway, which the patient may not be able to tolerate. The airway obstruction has various effects on the lung mechanics (especially on airway resistance), on the gas exchange (causing significant hypoxaemia and/or hypercapnia) and on the haemodynamic status of the patient. The following chapter discusses the range of possible problems as well as the precautions that should be taken in order to avoid severe adverse effects.   Copyright © 2010 S. Karger AG, Basel

In principle, flexible fibre-optic bronchoscopy (FFB) in the intensive-care unit (ICU) is not different from a bronchoscopy performed in an outpatient setting. The equipment as well as the basic technique are the same [1–5]. Yet, differences in the patient population and in the conditions under which the procedure is performed in the ICU demand very different considerations and precautions. The range of potential problems was very graphically summed up in the title of a recent editorial on the effects of FFB on mechanical ventilation: 'How to cause chaos with a bronchoscope in the ICU' [6]. The following chapter discusses the most common of these problems and provides tips on how to avoid 'causing chaos'.

Characteristics of the Critical-Care Setting

Patient Population

Patients undergoing an FFB in the ICU differ substantially from those who undergo the procedure in an outpatient setting (table 1). The latter tend to have a single condition or symptom involving the airways and/or the lung parenchyma (e.g. persistent wheezing or stridor, recurrent croup, persistent cough, recurrent pneumonia) but they are otherwise well or at least clinically stable. In contrast, patients in the ICU are either critically ill or at risk of becoming critically ill with conditions that often affect multiple organ systems. Their respiratory insufficiency or failure is often caused by the dysfunction or failure of organ systems other than the respiratory (e.g. cardiogenic or neurogenic pulmonary oedema, liver failure, major surgery or trauma). The vast majority of the ICU patients receive some form of mechanical ventilatory support either by non-invasive means such as continuous or biphasic positive airway pressure and more commonly via an endotracheal tube (ETT) or tracheostomy tube (T tube).

Airway Size

The insertion of a flexible fibre-optic bronchoscope into the trachea causes partial obstruction of its lumen, the degree of which depends on the diameter of the patient's trachea in relation to the diameter of the bronchoscope. This

Table 1. Differences between patient populations undergoing FFB in the ICU and undergoing FFB as outpatients

	Patients in the ICU	Outpatients
Clinical status	serious or critical	stable
Type of problem	often multisystem	primarily respiratory
Respiratory status	insufficiency or failure	stable or insufficiency
Haemodynamic status	labile	stable
Ventilation	usually mechanical	usually spontaneous breathing
Intubation/tracheostomy	usually yes	usually no

Table 2. Tracheal size, recommended ETT size and estimated increase in airway resistance (R_{aw}) during flexible bronchoscopy

Age group	Average tracheal size (AP/transverse diameter)[1] mm	ETT size (diameter) mm	Bronchoscope diameter mm	ETT obstruction %	Estimated R_{aw} increase from baseline[2] n-fold
Preterm newborn	~2.5–3.5	2.0–3.0	2.2	54	12.5
0–24 months (term)	5.3±1.0/6.4±1.2	3.5–4.5	2.2 2.8	54–19 64–31	8.52.5 63–3.5
2–4 years	7.4±0.8/8.1±0.7	4.5–5.5	2.8 3.8	39–26 71–52	7.5–3.5 ≥70–7.0
4–8 years	8.0±0.6 to 9.2±1.1/ 9.0±0.9 to 9.3±0.8	5.5–6.5	2.8 3.8 4.9	26–19 52–34 79–57	3.5–2.0 9.5–3.0 ≥70–≥15
8–18 years[3]	10.5±0.5 to 13.7±1.7/ 10.7±0.6 to 14.0±1.2	6.5–8.0	2.8 3.8 4.9 5.5	19–8 34–23 57–30 72–47	2.0–~1 5.0–3.0 ≥15–5.0 ≥70–~10

AP = Anteroposterior.
[1] Adapted from Griscom and Wohl [7].
[2] Adapted from Hsia et al. [8].
[3] Tracheal dimensions are slightly smaller in adolescent girls.

obstruction is rarely a problem for adult patients whose trachea is approximately 20–25 mm in diameter, whereas the diameter of flexible bronchoscopes does not exceed 6.3 mm. In contrast, the trachea of infants and children has a diameter that ranges from approximately 2.5 mm (among those born prematurely) to 5–10 mm in toddlers and young children [6]. When a patient has an artificial airway (ETT or T tube), the diameter of the airway is severely limited even in an adult-sized patient, and therefore even a small bronchoscope may obstruct a significant portion of the patient's airway (table 2). This not only compromises the ability to ventilate the patient, but it makes the procedure considerably more difficult for the bronchoscopist because the narrow artificial airway decreases the manoeuvrability of the bronchoscope. The manoeuvrability is further limited by the curve of the ETT (or the T tube; fig. 1a, b). Thus, although in theory a 2.8-mm bronchoscope should be able to pass through even a 3.0-mm ETT, in practice, one needs a substantially larger ETT in order to be able to advance the bronchoscope without difficulty while maintaining adequate ventilation [8]. When the size of the ETT is prohibitive for FFB and the patient is in a relatively stable condition, one might consider extubating the patient and temporarily placing a laryngeal mask that has a larger internal diameter than the ETT and allows adequate ventilation and better manoeuvrability for the bronchoscope. The patient can then

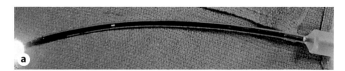

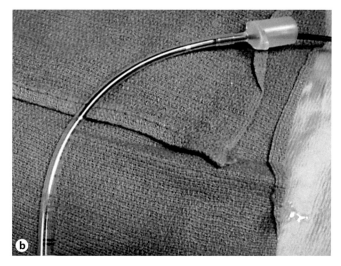

Fig. 1. **a** A 2.8-mm flexible fibre-optic bronchoscope can pass through a 3.0-mm ETT when it is in a straight position. **b** The same bronchoscope can move only halfway when the ETT is curved.

be re-intubated with the appropriate size ETT at the end of the procedure.

Neonatal versus Paediatric ICU
Patients in the neonatal ICU often develop respiratory conditions that would warrant an FFB and bronchoalveolar lavage (BAL), e.g. atelectasis or pneumonia, but most of them are not candidates due to the small size of their airways (especially when they are intubated) that prohibits the use of virtually all bronchoscopes with a suction channel. Thus, FFB in the neonatal ICU is performed primarily for inspection of the airways without BAL. Airway problems are congenital [chapters 10 and 11, this vol., pp. 114–119, 120–129] but also iatrogenic (e.g. airway abnormalities such as subglottic stenosis and/or tracheobronchomalacia due to prolonged intubation and mechanical ventilation). Because of the small size of the infant trachea, FFB in the neonatal ICU may often need to be performed with the 2.2-mm ultrathin bronchoscope that has no suction channel. It should be noted that even this size bronchoscope will almost completely obstruct the 2.5- to 3.0-mm ETTs that are commonly used in the extremely low-birth-weight neonates. In special circumstances (e.g. such as a difficult intubation or for a very quick inspection of the trachea and carina), the ultrathin bronchoscope can be used for a very brief period

of time (<1 min). In such cases, it is imperative to use an extra amount of lubrication to facilitate the advancement of the bronchoscope (and thus shorten the duration of the procedure), while minimizing the possibility of dislodging the ETT during the advancement or withdrawal. In contrast, FFB in the paediatric ICU almost always includes BAL for diagnostic purposes, and it is often performed for therapeutic purposes (e.g. removal of mucus plugs causing atelectasis) [1–5, 9, 10].

Pathophysiological Effects of Flexible Fibre-Optic Bronchoscopy

FFB is by definition an invasive procedure that may cause or trigger a series of undesirable responses from several organs that can be summarized as follows.

Effects on Lung Mechanics
The most profound effect on lung mechanics during FFB is undoubtedly the increase in airway resistance (R_{aw}) caused by the obstruction of the airway by the bronchoscope. Since the resistance to airflow is inversely proportional to the fourth power of the radius of the tube, the obstruction of the airway by the bronchoscope causes a marked increase in the R_{aw} (the actual increase in R_{aw} depends on other factors as well including the length of the tube). In an intubated and mechanically ventilated patient, the increase in R_{aw} will affect both the peak inspiratory (PIP) and the positive end-expiratory pressure (PEEP) as well as the tidal volume that is delivered to the patient. Which of these parameters and to what extent will be affected depends on the size of the bronchoscope in relation to the size of the airway as well as on the mode of mechanical ventilation [8, 11]. When the patient is ventilated in a volume control mode, the increase in R_{aw} will result in increases in the PIP and the PEEP. In a recent study evaluating the changes in R_{aw} with different combinations of bronchoscopes and ETTs, significant (and potentially clinically important) increases in the PIP (more than 20 cm H_2O) were found more frequently than significant increases in the PEEP (more than 5 cm H_2O) [8]. These pressure changes increase the risk for an air leak especially in patients with obstructive lung disease and significant air-trapping whereas they may cause significant haemodynamic instability in patients with impaired cardiovascular function. Pressure control ventilation has little effect on the pressures but it may severely limit the delivered tidal volume and thus may lead to significant respiratory decompensation (fig. 2a, b).

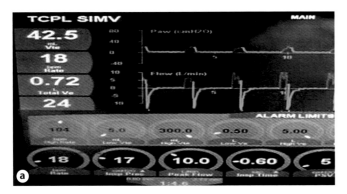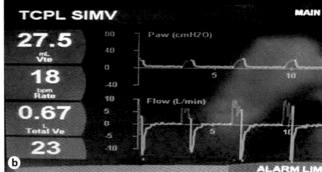

Fig. 2. **a** Ventilator display of the settings used in an infant in pressure control ventilation. The tidal volume is depicted in the upper left corner. **b** Upon insertion of the bronchoscope, the airway pressure remained the same but the tidal volume decreased by 35% (from 42.5 to 27.5 ml).

Changes in lung compliance are less common during FFB, but they do occur, primarily because of atelectasis that may develop as a result of suctioning (that may lead to alveolar collapse) and/or because of the instillation of normal saline during BAL that washes out surfactant. Suctioning is a necessary part of FFB (even when there is no BAL performed) in order to remove secretions that obscure the airways. A recent study has shown that even a single application of endotracheal suctioning may decrease temporarily but significantly the dynamic lung compliance [12]. On the other hand, the instillation of relatively large amounts of normal saline during BAL will at least temporarily decrease the static lung compliance. Considering that patients in the ICU tend to have conditions associated with very low lung compliance (e.g. acute respiratory distress syndrome, pneumonia, atelectasis), an additional decrease may have disproportionately severe effects.

Effects on Gas Exchange
Transient deterioration of gas exchange due to partial obstruction of the airway is one of the most common problems encountered during FFB. Hypoxaemia is probably the single most common gas exchange abnormality [2–5, 13]. The mechanisms that cause hypoxaemia are multiple, and they may differ from patient to patient. In critically ill patients with minimal or no pulmonary reserves, hypoxaemia can be caused simply by atelectasis due to the decrease in tidal volume. Patients who tolerate the decrease in tidal volume can become hypoxaemic from the depletion of intra-alveolar oxygen due to frequent suctioning during the procedure. Finally, hypoxaemia can be caused by the instillation of normal saline used for the BAL that washes out surfactant and causes localized 'flooding' of the alveoli [chapter 3, this vol., pp. 30–41].

Hypercapnia is primarily the result of the hypoventilation that is caused by the airway obstruction and cannot be compensated by increasing the frequency of respiration and/or the tidal volume on the ventilator. The hypercapnia is usually well tolerated by the majority of the patients, and it does not require any special interventions. Two notable exceptions are patients with pulmonary hypertension and patients with cerebral oedema. Hypercapnia may cause acute and severe pulmonary vasoconstriction in the former, thus raising the already increased pulmonary vascular resistance and worsening the pulmonary hypertension [14]. In contrast, hypercapnia causes cerebral vasodilatation worsening the cerebral oedema in the latter [15].

Cardiovascular Effects
Although FFB does not directly affect the cardiovascular system, it may cause significant cardiac or haemodynamic changes produced by a variety of indirect mechanisms. Such mechanisms include changes in the vascular tone caused by hypoxaemia and/or hypercapnia, as well as changes in the intrathoracic pressure (especially during coughing episodes) that may affect the venous return and/or the afterload of the left ventricle. Finally, increases in heart rate and in systemic blood pressure may be caused by anxiety and discomfort that are often associated with the procedure. All these effects are usually well tolerated by most patients but they can be very deleterious in patients with compromised cardiac function, increased systemic blood pressure or increased intracranial pressure. Among the various factors that can cause haemodynamic instability, the increase in PEEP is of special importance because of the profound effects it may have on cardiac output. The latter can be affected either due to an increase in the left ventricle afterload and/or due to an

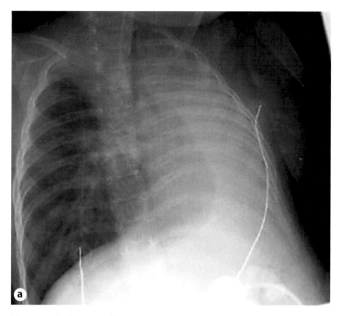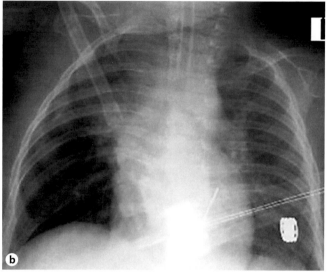

Fig. 3. a Left lung collapse in a patient intubated and mechanically ventilated. The lung failed to expand with manipulations of the ventilator settings and chest physical therapy. **b** Repeat chest radiograph 4 h after bronchoscopy and lavage shows re-expansion of the atelectatic lung.

increase in pulmonary vascular resistance [16, 17]. These effects are of particular importance for patients with non-pulsatile pulmonary circulation (i.e. patients who had the Glenn or Fontan procedures for correction of congenital heart defects) that is entirely dependent upon having an adequate systemic blood pressure and low pulmonary vascular resistance. Unfortunately, these patients are also likely to require a bronchoscopy due to the relatively high prevalence of congenital or acquired airway abnormalities associated with their condition. Last but not least is the increase in central venous pressure caused by high PEEP that in turn may cause a significant increase in the intracranial pressure.

Applications of Flexible Fibre-Optic Bronchoscopy in the Intensive-Care Unit

Persistent or Recurrent Atelectasis
Atelectasis is one of the most common causes of worsening of the respiratory status of patients in the ICU, and it often delays their recovery (especially those on mechanical ventilation). The causes of atelectasis differ from patient to patient [chapter 14, this vol., pp. 149–155]. In many patients, atelectasis is part of their disease process (e.g. extensive mucus plugging, surfactant deficiency, respiratory muscle weakness). In other patients, atelectasis is caused by

mechanical compression of the lung (e.g. development of pleural effusion, pressure from an enlarged liver) or of the airways (e.g. compression of the left main stem bronchus by an enlarged heart or vessel). Iatrogenic causes of atelectasis such as right (or less commonly left) main stem intubation or prolonged immobilization of the patient with subsequent collapse of the dependent regions of the lungs are among the most common causes. Often, non-invasive diagnostic methods such as chest radiography or CT scan can identify the cause of the atelectasis. However, FFB is the only method able to determine the severity of the problem (particularly valuable in cases of dynamic changes in the airways) and to provide real-time assessment of the effectiveness of an intervention (e.g. effect of an increase in the PEEP for the management of bronchomalacia). Moreover, FFB allows direct therapeutic interventions such as the removal of mucus plugs (fig. 3a, b; online suppl. video 1) [1–4, 18, 19]. **Vi**

Abnormal Breathing Sounds
This is probably the most common indication for FFB in the neonatal ICU. The abnormal breathing sounds include stridor, wheezing or a combination of both. Abnormalities in the newborn are mostly congenital (fig. 4) and virtually include the entire spectrum of airway abnormalities [20], primarily of the extrathoracic airways (e.g. laryngomalacia, laryngeal webs or cysts, congenital subglottic stenosis,

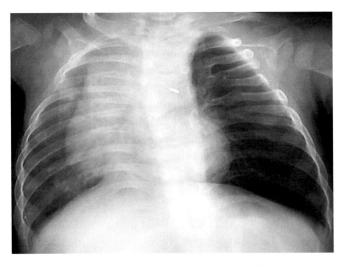

Fig. 4. Four-month-old infant with transposition of the great arteries repaired on day 5 of life. The patient presented with persistent wheezing and difficulty in breathing. A chest radiograph revealed severe air-trapping in the left lung.

airway haemangiomas, severe tracheomalacia or critical tracheal stenosis; online suppl. videos 2 and 3) [9, 10; chapter 11, this vol., pp. 120–129] Iatrogenic airway abnormalities can be seen in newborn infants and older children and may involve the extrathoracic and/or the intrathoracic airways. The former often involve the vocal cords that may be paretic or paralysed secondary to direct injury (e.g. traumatic intubation) or indirect injury (e.g. damage to the recurrent laryngeal nerve during cardiac surgery) [21, 22]. The subglottic area is probably the most commonly affected airway segment with acquired stenosis due to the narrow size of the airway (especially in prematurely born infants). Affected children almost invariably present with significant respiratory distress and stridor. When wheezing is present, it tends to be audible and biphasic suggesting presence of a fixed airway obstruction (e.g. tracheal compression by a vascular ring; online suppl. videos 4–8) [23; chapter 12, this vol., pp. 130–140].

ETT Placement
Proper position of the ETT is of the utmost importance for any critically ill patient in order to provide optimal ventilation and prevent complications such as atelectasis or even air leak in case that the ETT slips into one of the main stem bronchi or hits the carina. These risks are amplified in infants and young children because their trachea is by definition short and therefore small changes in the position of

the tube can have significant effects. In addition, most paediatric patients are intubated with uncuffed ETTs that can easily slide in and out.

Currently, the assessment of the proper position of the ETT in most ICUs is made by chest radiography performed at least daily. In theory, a quick inspection of the ETT under direct visualization via a flexible bronchoscope would be the ideal solution obviating the need for multiple chest radiographs. However, in practice this is not feasible because the bronchoscope has to be sterilized after its use. Therefore, in a big ICU, one would literally need dozens of bronchoscopes in order to provide this inspection in a timely fashion. Thus, bronchoscopy is reserved for cases in which high precision is required (e.g. placement of the ETT just above the carina in patients with very severe tracheomalacia or selective intubation of one lung) [24].

Difficult Intubation
Patients with congenital anatomical abnormalities or injuries that preclude the proper opening of the jaw for direct laryngoscopy can be intubated with the use of a flexible bronchoscope threaded through the ETT via a Seldinger-type technique [24; chapter 4, this vol., pp. 42–53].

Evaluation of Abnormalities
Patients in the ICU often present with radiographic findings and/or symptoms of unclear aetiology. FFB may help to identify the nature and severity of the problem, and guide its management. Figure 5 shows complete occlusion of the right upper lobe bronchus due to malacia causing persistent atelectasis and pneumonia in an infant with presumed asthma (online suppl. video 9). Application of higher PEEP allows the resolution of the atelectasis via improved clearance of secretions and eventually extubation. Online supplementary video 10 shows virtually complete occlusion of the lower trachea in a patient who suffered acute respiratory arrest. The patient had just been found to have extensive lymphoma. Removal of large amounts of thick secretions revealed severe compression of the trachea by the tumour.

Practical Considerations and Precautions

Several surveys have shown that the prevalence of complications from FFB in the ICU is very low [5]. This is because the ICU is a controlled environment, staffed with individuals with great expertise in the management of critically ill patients. The patients usually have a secure airway and are

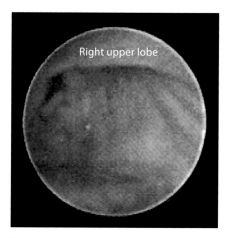

Fig. 5. Infant with history of recurrent episodes of wheezing and respiratory distress requiring intubation and mechanical ventilation. The patient could not be weaned off the ventilator due to persistent atelectasis of the right upper lobe. Bronchoscopy revealed virtually complete obstruction of the right upper lobe bronchus.

receiving ventilatory and haemodynamic support. Because intubated patients are being subjected to endotracheal suctioning on a routine basis, with catheters of similar or larger diameter than the bronchoscope, the bronchoscopist has also a much better idea as to how well the patient will tolerate the partial obstruction of the airway by the bronchoscope. On the other hand, critically ill patients may not be able to tolerate even the transient haemodynamic or gas exchange changes that may occur during the procedure, thus increasing its risks [1–5]. Fortunately, most of the potential complications are predictable and thus preventable if all the necessary precautions are taken. Some of the issues that require special attention and may be controversial include the following.

Sedation and Pain Control
FFB is not a painful procedure and therefore there is little need for pain control. However, it may often be associated with anxiety that can potentially cause significant increases in the heart rate and blood pressure which may be deleterious to a critically ill patient. Therefore, it is advisable to have the patient well sedated during the procedure [chapter 2, this vol., pp. 22–29]. Although the majority of intubated patients in the ICU tend to receive large doses of narcotics, they should not be assumed to be well sedated because they tend to develop tolerance. Thus, it is reasonable to give additional doses of narcotics and/or benzodiazepines when the procedure is about to begin. Alternatively, one could use intravenous propofol that in addition to an excellent

short-term anaesthetic effect provides an amnesic effect (an important feature for older children and adolescents) and usually causes no significant haemodynamic changes.

Muscle Relaxation
The use of muscle relaxants during performance of FFB makes the procedure 'easier' for the bronchoscopist and safer for the patient because it prevents: (a) sudden movements that may cause injury (especially when invasive interventions such as transbronchial biopsy are attempted), (b) abnormally laboured breathing due to partial obstruction of the ETT and (c) cough that could potentially raise the intrathoracic and intraluminal pressures to dangerous levels. On the other hand, muscle relaxation has certain disadvantages, especially the elimination of spontaneous breathing and cough which make the dynamic changes that take place in the airway lumen through the normal respiratory cycle difficult to assess. This is not a significant problem when FFB is performed primarily for BAL. However, when the procedure is performed to evaluate tracheobronchomalacia, its presence and severity may be grossly underestimated because of the positive airway pressure the patient receives (and which is further increased because of the presence of the bronchoscope). In such cases, the patient should be allowed to breathe (and cough) spontaneously in order to observe the dynamic changes in the airway lumen.

When muscle relaxants are administered specifically for the procedure, it is important to also give additional doses of narcotics/sedatives, because the patient will not be able to express his/her anxiety or discomfort (in such cases sudden increases in the heart rate and blood pressure are highly suggestive of inadequate sedation).

Size of the Bronchoscope
Although the larger bronchoscopes generally offer superior imaging and/or better suctioning capabilities, it is generally advisable to use the smallest possible bronchoscope in the intubated patient in order to facilitate its navigation and to minimize the degree of airway obstruction. According to a recent study, in order to maintain adequate tidal volumes and/or to prevent dangerous increases in the airway pressures, there needs to be a considerable difference between the diameter of the ETT and that of the bronchoscope. Based on their measurements in a lung model, Hsia et al. [8] concluded that the difference should be >1.3 mm for infants and toddlers, >2.0 mm for children and young adolescents and >2.5 mm for older adolescents and young adults.

Coagulation Status

FFB and BAL are generally non-traumatic procedures, and in this respect they could be safely performed even in patients who are coagulopathic (a fairly common problem in the ICU among patients with liver or multisystem organ failure). However, transfusion of platelets should be considered when the platelet count is <40,000/μL and should definitely be administered if the platelet count is <20,000/μL. It is advisable that platelets be transfused within 1 h or ideally just before and during the procedure.

Airway Protection

Dislodgement of the ETT and/or accidental extubation of the patient are some of the possible and potentially dangerous complications of FFB in intubated patients. Both of these conditions can cause acute and severe respiratory and haemodynamic changes. Therefore, it is strongly recommended that the ETT is kept at the level of the lip by an assistant (the tube should be held firmly but without being compressed) in order to avoid slipping in or out during insertion or withdrawal of the bronchoscope. This is especially important when there is a tight fit between the bronchoscope and the ETT. The assistant may also greatly help the movement of the bronchoscope by straightening the ETT and/or by carefully hyperextending the patient's head. We have found this to be very useful when the 2.8-mm bronchoscope is used in tubes of <4.0 mm diameter.

Use of Mucolytics

Mucolytics, such as N-acetylcysteine (Mucomyst), recombinant DNAse (dornase α) and hypertonic saline, have been used for the resolution and removal of mucus plugs in a variety of conditions associated with atelectasis and lobar collapse [25, 26]. In addition to the above substances we have often used the intravenous preparation of sodium bicarbonate diluted with normal saline in a ratio of 1:4 or 1:5 (e.g. 20 ml of $NaHCO_3$ diluted with 100 ml of normal saline). The mixture is then used for the lavage in aliquots of 5–15 ml depending on the size of the patient. It should be noted that despite their widespread use the efficacy of mucolytics has not been conclusively proven [26].

Ventilatory Management

Patients who are intubated and mechanically ventilated will probably require adjustments in their ventilator settings, and specific guidelines for the proper interventions are available [27]. In general, the FFB is expected to affect the following parameters:

Fraction of inspired oxygen: Patients should be given 100% oxygen during the procedure in order to prevent or minimize the possibility of clinically important desaturation.

Respiratory rate: In general when heavy sedation and/or muscle relaxation are used, the ventilator rate should be increased appropriate for the patient's age levels. However, when the FFB is performed through a very narrow airway, it may be necessary to decrease the frequency and/or the tidal volume, in order to allow for complete exhalation.

PEEP: The presence of the bronchoscope inside the airway increases the intraluminal pressure and therefore the PEEP by preventing complete passive exhalation. The actual increase in PEEP is difficult to calculate because it varies according to the size of the bronchoscope in relation to the size of the patient's airway. In our experience, the majority of the patients tend to tolerate the procedure well without the need to adjust PEEP. Nevertheless, we would consider decreasing PEEP by at least half in certain patients such as those who have already developed an air leak, those who may develop severe adverse effects due to increased PEEP (e.g. patients who underwent a Glenn or Fontan procedure) and those who are already receiving very high PEEP (>10 cm H_2O). When the objective of the FFB is the detection of possible tracheobronchomalacia, it is advisable to have the patient completely disconnected from the ventilator for a brief period (10–20 s) in order to better observe the dynamic changes under spontaneous breathing.

Tidal volume: Maintaining adequate tidal volume in a mechanically ventilated patient during FFB can be a challenge. If the patient is ventilated in the pressure control mode, the tidal volume will be decreased [8]. If the volume control mode is used, the tidal volume will theoretically remain unaffected but the PIP will increase. As a safety precaution, modern ventilators have an upper limit for pressure, and, when reached, the ventilator will automatically 'dump' the breath. This upper limit is usually set at approximately 10 cm H_2O above the required PIP. Because during FFB the PIP may increase by more than 20 cm H_2O, it is likely that the patient may not get ventilated at all. To avoid this problem, one can temporarily change the alarm settings. Alternatively, one can switch to pressure control ventilation with a prolonged inspiratory time (inspiration:expiration ratio of 2:1 or more) that requires relatively low airflows which can be accommodated through the narrow airway. In our experience, the safest and most efficient way to ventilate labile patients is by manual ventilation using the lowest possible respiratory rate and a very prolonged inspiratory time.

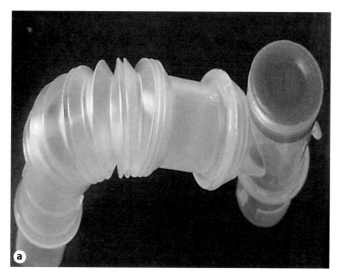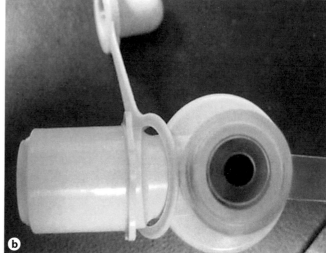

Fig. 6. **a** Adaptor for the insertion of the flexible bronchoscope into the ETT while maintaining the ventilatory support. The diaphragm provides a tight fit around the bronchoscope that does not allow any leak. **b** The opening of this type of adaptor is 4 mm in diameter, and as a result there is leaking of pressure and/or volume around bronchoscopes that are less than 4 mm in diameter.

Adaptor: The procedure should be performed through an adaptor connected to the ETT or the laryngeal mask airway that allows the continuation of the mechanical or manual ventilation. There are different commercial models. We have found that for paediatric patients the adaptors that have a 'slit diaphragm' (fig. 6a) provide a better seal around the bronchoscope than those with a fixed opening (fig. 6b) which allow a big leak around the paediatric bronchoscopes that may significantly reduce the ability to adequately ventilate the patient. The leak around the bronchoscope can be minimized or prevented by cutting off the 'finger' of a surgical glove and covering the opening.

Bronchoscopy in Non-Intubated ICU Patients
Often, patients are admitted to the ICU because of progressive hypoxaemia and increased work of breathing that are associated with a high probability for respiratory failure. In such cases, FFB with BAL could be very helpful in determining whether respiratory insufficiency is due to an infection (in which case isolating specific pathogens and determining their sensitivities could be very important) or due to other processes (e.g. pulmonary haemorrhage). However, it is also possible that the procedure itself may actually precipitate the respiratory failure leading to intubation and mechanical ventilation from which the patient may not be able to recover. This category includes patients with advanced cystic fibrosis, neuromuscular disorders and those after bone marrow transplantation. Although these are all high-risk

patients, respiratory failure should not be considered inevitable. In many cases, respiratory failure is the result of the combination of relative hypoventilation due to sedation, very poor pulmonary reserves due to the underlying illness and atelectasis caused by the washing-out of surfactant due to BAL. Many of these problems can be prevented or at least minimized. Specifically, non-invasive ventilation should be started as early as possible prior to FFB in order to recruit already atelectatic areas and to prevent further atelectasis. The procedure should be performed with a laryngeal mask that allows adequate ventilation during the FFB, and the patient should be placed on non-invasive ventilation immediately after the end of the procedure [28].

Is FFB Safe?
Despite the considerable risks of any invasive procedure performed in critically ill patients, several studies that have reviewed the rate of complications during and after FFB both in adults and children have shown a rather remarkably low rate of complications [4, 5, 29]. Overall, if all necessary precautions are taken, FFB can be safely performed even in critically ill infants and children.

Is FFB Always Necessary?
Although FFB can be safely performed even in very labile critically ill patients, possible alternatives should be carefully considered. If the main objective of the procedure is to obtain BAL fluid for cultures from patients who have

a diffuse disease process, one might consider performing a non-bronchoscopic BAL. The latter can be easily performed with the use of an 8-french feeding catheter that has a suction channel larger than that of the paediatric bronchoscopes, thus yielding better results [30]. Recent technological advancements have already made 'virtual bronchoscopy' and other 3-dimensional techniques a non-invasive alternative that can be considered when structural airway anomalies are suspected [chapter 9, this vol., pp. 95–112]. However, these techniques require that the patient be transported to a different part of the hospital, a condition which for many critically ill patients may be more hazardous than the bedside invasive procedure. Of course, there is currently no alternative to FFB for obtaining specimens or for removing mucus plugs from specific areas of the lung.

References

1 Nicolai T: Pediatric bronchoscopy. Pediatr Pulmonol 2001;31:150–164.
2 Bush A: Bronchoscopy in paediatric intensive care. Paediatr Respir Rev 2003;4:67–73.
3 Midulla F, de Blic J, Barbato A, Bush A, Eber E, Kotecha S, Haxby E, Moretti C, Pohunek P, Ratjen F: Flexible endoscopy of paediatric airways. Eur Respir J 2003;22:698–708.
4 Davidson MG, Coutts J, Bell G: Flexible bronchoscopy in pediatric intensive care. Pediatr Pulmonol 2008;43:1188–1192.
5 Geraci G, Pisello F, Sciume C, Li Volsi F, Romeo M, Modica G: Complication of flexible fiberoptic bronchoscopy: literature review. Ann Ital Chir 2007;78:183–192.
6 Bush A: Primum non nocere: how to cause chaos with a bronchoscope in the ICU. Chest 2009;135:2–4.
7 Griscom NT, Wohl ME: Dimensions of the growing trachea related to age and gender. AJR Am J Rheumatol 1986;146:233–237.
8 Hsia D, Di Blasi RM, Richardson P, Crotwell D, Debley J, Carter E: The effects of flexible bronchoscopy on mechanical ventilation in a pediatric lung model. Chest 2009;135:33–40.
9 Wood RE: Flexible bronchoscopy in infants. Int Anesthesiol Clin 1992;30:125–132.
10 Bush A: Neonatal bronchoscopy. Eur J Pediatr 1994;153(suppl 2):S27–S29.
11 Tung A, Morgan SE: Modeling the effect of progressive endotracheal tube occlusion on tidal volume in pressure-control mode. Anesth Analg 2002;95:192–197.
12 Morrow B, Futter M, Argent A: Effect of endotracheal suction on lung dynamics in mechanically ventilated paediatric patients. Aust J Physiother 2006;52:121–126.
13 Schellhase DE, Fawcett DD, Schultz GE, Lensing SY, Tryka AF: Clinical utility of flexible bronchoscopy and bronchoalveolar lavage in young children with recurrent wheezing. J Pediatr 1998;132:312–318.
14 Bush A, Busst CM, Knight WB, Shinebourne EA: Interactions between alveolar hypercapnia and epoprostenol on the pulmonary circulation: clinical and pharmacologic implications. Pulm Pharmacol 1990;3:167–170.
15 Kerwin AJ, Croce MA, Timmons SD, Maxwell RA, Malhotra AK, Fabian TC: Effects of fiberoptic bronchoscopy on intracranial pressure in patients with brain injury: a prospective clinical study. J Trauma 2000;48:878–882.
16 Lindholm CE, Ollman B, Snyder JV, Millen EG, Grenvik A: Cardiorespiratory effects of flexible fiberoptic bronchoscopy in critically ill patients. Chest 1978;74:362–368.
17 Feihl F, Broccard AF: Interactions between respiration and systemic hemodynamics. I. Basic concepts. Intensive Care Med 2009;35:45–54.
18 Bar-Zohar D, Sivan Y: The yield of flexible fiberoptic bronchoscopy in pediatric intensive care patients. Chest 2004;126:1353–1359.
19 Kreider ME, Lipson DA: Bronchoscopy for atelectasis in the ICU: a case report and review of the literature. Chest 2003;124:344–350.
20 Fan LL, Sparks LM, Fix FJ: Flexible fiberoptic endoscopy for airway problems in a pediatric intensive care unit. Chest 188;93:556–560.
21 Smith MM, Kuhl G, Carvalho PR, Marostica PJ: Flexible fiber-optic laryngoscopy in the first hours after extubation for the evaluation of laryngeal lesions due to intubation in the pediatric intensive care unit. Int J Pediatr Otorhinolaryngol 2007;71:1423–1428.
22 Valletta EA, Pregarz M, Bergamo-Andreis IA, Boner AL: Tracheoesophageal compression due to congenital vascular anomalies (vascular rings). Pediatr Pulmonol 1997;24:93–105.
23 Wood RE: Pitfalls in the use of the flexible bronchoscope in pediatric patients. Chest 1990;97:199–203
24 Frei FJ, Ummendhofer W: Difficult intubation in pediatrics. Paediatr Anaesth 1996;6:251–263.
25 Eifinger F, Welzing L, Lange L, Rietschel E, Himbert U: Successful mucolysis in pertussis using bronchoscopically applied dornase alfa. Pediatr Pulmonol 2008;43:305–306.
26 Jelic S, Cunningham JA, Factor P: Clinical review: airway hygiene in the intensive care unit. Crit Care 2008;12:209.
27 Trachsel D, Erb TO, Frei FJ, Hammer J, Swiss Paediatric Respiratory Research Group: Use of continuous positive airway pressure during flexible bronchoscopy in young children. Eur Respir J 2005;26:773–777.
28 Nussbaum E, Zagnoev M: Pediatric fiberoptic bronchoscopy with a laryngeal mask airway. Chest 2001;120:614–616.
29 Efrati O, Sadeh-Gornik U, Modan-Moses D, Barak A, Szeinberg A, Vardi A, Paret G, Toren A, Vilozni D, Yahav Y: Flexible bronchoscopy and bronchoalveolar lavage in pediatric patients with lung disease. Pediatr Crit Care Med 2009;10:80–84.
30 Koumbourlis AC, Kurland G: Nonbronchoscopic bronchoalveolar lavage in mechanically ventilated infants: technique, efficacy and applications. Pediatr Pulmonol 1993;15:257–262.

Anastassios C. Koumbourlis, MD, MPH
Chief, Division of Allergy, Pulmonary and Sleep Medicine, Children's National Medical Center
Professor of Clinical Pediatrics
George Washington University
Suite 1030, 111 Michigan Avenue, N.W.
Washington, DC 20010–2970 (USA)
Tel. +1 202 476 2642, Fax +1 202 476 5864, E-Mail AKoumbou@cnmc.org

Priftis KN, Anthracopoulos MB, Eber E, Koumbourlis AC, Wood RE (eds): Paediatric Bronchoscopy.
Prog Respir Res. Basel, Karger 2010, vol 38, pp 64–74

Interventional Bronchoscopy

Leonardo Donato[a] · Thi Mai Hong Tran[b] · Eleni Mihailidou[c]

[a]Medicosurgical Paediatric Department, University Hospital Strasbourg, Strasbourg, France; [b]Pulmonary Department, Hanoi National Hospital of Paediatrics, Hanoi, Vietnam; [c]Department of Paediatrics, University Hospital of Crete, Heraklion, Greece

Abstract

The miniaturization of rigid and flexible endoscopes and their accessories has paved the way for the wider use of bronchoscopy as therapeutic intervention in paediatric patients in a broader spectrum of airway diseases. The purpose of this chapter is to describe and evaluate specific interventional techniques applicable to children such as: dilatation of central airway stenoses, laser photoresection and tracheobronchial stenting. The indications for, and the methodologies used in paediatric interventional bronchoscopy (IB) differ from those in adults. In the latter group, lung cancer is the most common indication for intervention, which is performed in a setting of reduced life expectancy. Conversely, in children, the main indication is a congenital or acquired structural abnormality of the airway. Another important difference is that IB in children is often limited by the lack of experience among bronchoscopists as well as the lack of size-appropriate equipment. The decision to proceed with an IB procedure requires a multidisciplinary approach and the weighing of benefits versus risks of more conventional therapies such as surgery, tracheostomy, long-term ventilatory support or even abstention from any intervention if growth-related spontaneous improvement is reasonably expected.   Copyright © 2010 S. Karger AG, Basel

Bronchoscopy has been used therapeutically from its very beginning, in 1897, when George Killian removed a pork bone from the right main bronchus of a 63-year-old farmer. In 1905, Killian placed the first tracheal stent. During the first decades of the 20th century, Chevalier Jackson designed a series of small tubes, thus extending the technique of bronchoscopy to children. The primary application was relief of airway obstruction due to foreign-body aspiration, removal of thick purulent secretions in bronchopulmonary infections, and endobronchial tuberculosis. The subsequent evolution of paediatric pulmonary medicine and of cardiothoracic surgery expanded the field of therapeutic bronchoscopy to include various tracheobronchial malformations and acquired injuries.

Interventional bronchoscopy (IB) is usually a therapeutic rather than a diagnostic procedure, the primary purpose of which is to restore airway patency. IB can be useful in a variety of clinical conditions such as foreign-body removal [chapter 8, this vol., pp. 83–94], guided aspiration of mucus plugs and clots from the bronchi, assistance to tracheal intubation when larynx exposure is critical [chapters 4 and 5, this vol., pp. 42–53 and 54–63], dilatation of tracheobronchial stenoses, placement of airway stents, laser photoresection of mucosal injuries, and transtracheal fine-needle aspiration of cysts or nodes. Other indications include whole-lung lavage [chapter 7, this vol., pp. 75–82], endoscopic closure of bronchopleural fistula and peri-operative bronchoscopy (e.g. airway inspection during thoracic surgery, selective intubation for single-lung ventilation, detection and repair of tracheo-oesophageal fistula) [chapter 4, this vol., pp. 42–53].

Endoscopic Management of Airway Stenosis

Assessment of Airway Stenosis

The endoscopic findings and classification of congenital and acquired central airway stenoses are described in chapters 12 and 16 [this vol., pp. 130–140 and 173–181]. The extent and consistency of a stenosis are usually assessed by rigid tube examination under general anaesthesia. Chest CT scanning is often necessary to determine the relationship of abnormal airways to adjacent mediastinal structures (e.g. vessels and lymph nodes) as well as the degree of the stenosis. However, an axial CT scan may underestimate the degree of obstruction in cases of mucosal involvement or of dynamic collapse if a forced expiratory technique is not utilized [1; chapter 9, this vol., pp. 95–112].

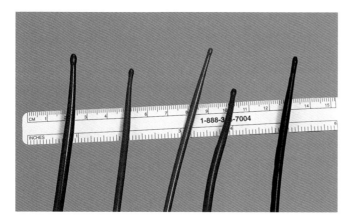

Fig. 1. Set of thin gum elastic bougies (Nelaton®). They can be used to determine the diameter of a rigid stenosis. It is not recommended to use them for dilatation (risk of airway wall perforation or laceration).

A more accurate measurement of the cross-sectional area is made with the use of a lubricated instrument of known outer diameter. Determination of the size of stenosis is based on the largest rigid tube that can be passed through the stricture, as well as by a gum elastic bougie set (fig. 1) or a long-shape balloon catheter. The length of the stenosis is measured by moving an optical telescope from the distal to the proximal end of the narrowing and drawing a felt-tip line on the barrel at both points. For most authors rigid bronchoscopy remains the gold standard for the assessment of central airway stenosis.

Repair of Airway Stenosis
IB procedures are usually best suited for segmental stenoses caused by the presence of tumours, granulomas etc. obstructing the airway lumen. Choosing the most appropriate method for treating a narrowed airway depends on the nature of the lesion, and one could consider the following options:

(a) mucosal lesions with soft consistency are best treated by laser photoresection (e.g. web-like lesions, bulky granulomas, mural cysts and tumours);

(b) segmental tracheobronchomalacia, extrinsic compression or postoperative twisting of the airway may be managed by tracheobronchial stenting, which can be used as an alternative to surgery or tracheostomy;

(c) fibrocartilaginous rigid lesions can be dilated by using various rigid bronchoscopic procedures (e.g. congenital cartilage rings, ischaemic stricture and anastomotic stenosis);

(d) a combination of the methods described above can be used in case of complex lesions (e.g. laser photoresection of mucosal injury and then stenting, or stenting of

segmental collapse induced by endoscopic dilatation of a fixed stenosis).

Interventional Bronchoscopic Techniques

Airway Dilatation
Long-segment and funnel-shaped stenoses usually require surgical correction by tracheoplasty, and they are not amenable to bronchoscopic interventions, although successful dilatations have been reported using elongated balloon catheters [2]. On the other hand, in cases of either congenital or acquired short-segment stenoses, bronchoscopic airway dilatation is often the preferable alternative to surgery as the latter is often associated with severe complications due to the poor quality of the ischaemic airway wall.

Endoluminal pneumatic dilatation is the most often used method for the treatment of acquired tracheobronchial stenosis and should be considered prior to attempting more invasive surgical procedures [3–5]. The method is as follows: a balloon catheter is inserted through the stenosis and is inflated with saline or air. High pressure levels are delivered to the maximum balloon capacity, either manually or by means of a pressure inflator. The balloon remains inflated for 15–60 s and then is deflated and withdrawn to allow the child to recover and the mucosa to reperfuse. The stricture is dilated in increments with different balloon diameters (from 4 to 8 mm in infants) in order to avoid tracheobronchial rupture or laceration. The procedure is usually carried out under visual control with an optical telescope passed through a rigid tube (fig. 2). The balloon catheter can be advanced over a radiopaque guidewire which is positioned in the airway under fluoroscopic control. Bronchographic contrast is used to locate the area to be dilated, and the balloon is inflated with diluted contrast [6]. Long-shaped balloon catheters are more suitable than round-shaped ones that tend to bulge centrally or distally to the rigid stenotic segment when inflated, risking adjacent airway laceration. If unsuccessful, the procedure can be repeated after a few minutes. Relapses are frequently reported following balloon dilatation, and most patients require multiple interventions.

The *balloon dilatation method* is suitable for cicatricial stenoses with fibrocartilaginous involvement. Endoscopic balloon dilatation is also used in the management of children with postoperative anastomotic stricture and in those with metal airway stents which need to be redilated.

Balloon dilatation has been used experimentally in children with segmental congenital tracheal stenosis, in which the stricture is composed of 2 or 3 complete 'O-shaped'

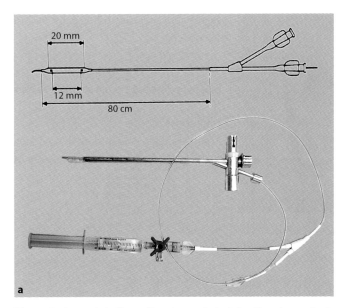
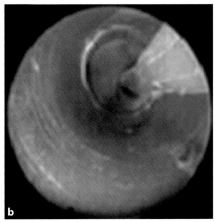

Fig. 2. Endoscopic balloon dilatation technical details. **a** An angioplasty-type balloon catheter is inserted through the side port of the rigid tube. **b** The balloon is placed through the stenosis under visual control and then inflated.

cartilage rings (Cantrell type III). However, several authors report immediate recollapse after balloon dilatation, and the need for additional invasive procedures to restore the airway patency [7–10]. In our experience, complete cartilaginous rings are resistant to the radial expansion force of the balloon, and therefore we do not recommend the use of the balloon dilatation. Instead, one could use a rigid bronchoscope as a 'bougie'. The rigid tubes are passed repeatedly through the stenosis in increasing diameters. The procedure aims to break the cartilaginous rings at their lowest resistance point, i.e. adjacent to the pars membranacea. This is achieved by starting with the smallest-diameter tube (Storz 2.5®); the bevel is sprayed with silicone and placed vertically in order to exert the maximum stress point at the level where the posterior wall should be. The tube is then carefully but firmly pushed forward into the axis of the trachea, usually giving the endoscopist the feeling of an elastic stop followed by a sudden sliding forward motion. The tube's motion should be immediately restrained in order to avoid injuring the main carina. Fluoroscopy may be used during the procedure if the distance between the tube and the carina cannot be determined by telescope. At this time, the optical telescope control shows circumferential stretching of the cartilage rings without any perceived split. Larger-diameter tubes are successively inserted until a brief crack is felt, indicating cartilage ring fracture (fig. 3 and online suppl. video 1). It is essential to keep the tube's motion along the axis of the airway, and to stop it as soon as the stenosis has been crossed;

otherwise severe complications may occur. Once the cartilaginous ring is broken, it will never heal again because of its avascular nature; thus, the stenosis will not recur. In our institution, rigid tube dilatation has been applied in 5 infants with segmental congenital tracheal stenosis. The procedure was successful in 4 cases, and no complications were observed. In the remaining case, the smallest-diameter tube could not be passed through the rings, and a surgical resection with end-to-end anastomosis was eventually carried out. Surprisingly, scarcely any evidence of such a procedure can be found in the literature. Only a recent review on the current state of congenital tracheal stenosis mentions conservative management as an alternative to surgery in segmental stenosis [11]. It is clear that some patients with mild stenosis can be managed conservatively [12]. Children who are candidates for early surgery are at high risk of peri-operative morbidity [1, 13]. Therefore, selected cases could benefit if therapeutic bronchoscopy is attempted prior to the invasive surgical correction.

Endobronchial Laser Therapy

Lasers produce a beam of monochromatic, phased, collimated light that can induce tissue vaporization, coagulation, haemostasis and necrosis. Biological effects depend on the wavelength emitted by the laser source. Adults' interventional pulmonologists mainly use YAG laser for endoluminal recanalization in patients with malignant tumours that obstruct the major airway. Complications of YAG laser

Video

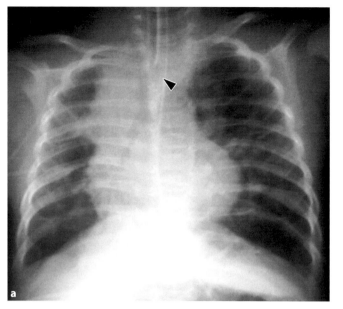

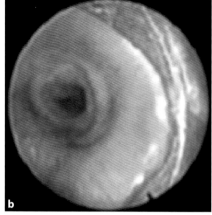

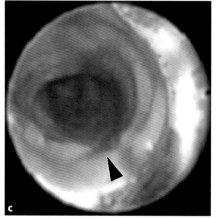

Fig. 3. Six-week-old female with severe respiratory distress. **a** Jamming of the endotracheal tube into the upper part of the trachea (arrowhead) and chest overdistension: tracheal stenosis. **b** The course of the rigid tube is hindered by a rigid circumferential stenosis: complete cartilage rings (Storz 3 tube – outer diameter 5 mm; the cross-sectional area of the stenosis is measured and found to be 3 mm). **c** Successive intubation of the stenosis with Storz 2.5, 3 and 3.5 tubes; 3 cartilage rings have been broken (arrowhead) at the level of the posterior wall. (Watch the whole procedure in video 1.)

therapy include perforation of the airway with severe bleeding or gas leak. In infants and toddlers, the damaged airway is fragile and closely surrounded by large vascular structures. It makes sense to deliver energy with low diffusion and haemostatic properties.

Several types of laser are currently used in paediatric interventional pulmonology:

- The *CO$_2$ laser* allows shallow penetration of tissues and precise cutting, but the system is cumbersome for use [14–17]. The CO$_2$ laser beam is air-transmitted via a set of articulated mirrors connected to dedicated rigid tubes; the beam is targeted onto a red light spot and energy is delivered by pressing a foot pedal. Specific wavelength filter glasses are required for the endoscopist and staff.
- The *KTP laser* (kalium-titanium-phosphate) seems more suitable for paediatric use since the beam is transmitted fibre-optically and is compatible with standard rigid tubes or even with a fibre-optic bronchoscope with shielded working channel [18, 19].

The KTP specific wavelength is obtained by doubling the frequency emitted by a YAG laser chamber through a crystal of potassium-titanyl-phosphate so that the system can be operated either in a YAG or KTP mode. Having a KTP source which allows usage by other specialists is an advantage in a multipurpose suite as laser equipment is expensive.

- The *argon laser* exhibits interesting properties but its cost may be prohibitive.

The KTP laser energy is delivered at the tip of a thin coated optical fibre. Since metal guide devices do not fit the small paediatric tubes, the easiest way to proceed is to tape the laser fibre onto the outside of the optical telescope (fig. 4a). Compared to other bronchoscopic interventions, laser procedures require extra precautions that can be summarized as follows:

1. Deep sedation levels are required to avoid inaccurate targeting due to the child's movement.
2. The fractional inspired oxygen has to be lowered to below 0.5 before activating the laser beam because of

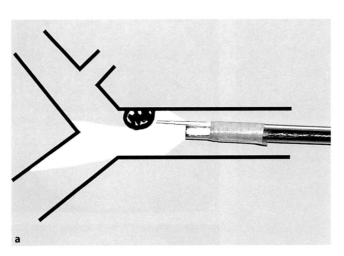
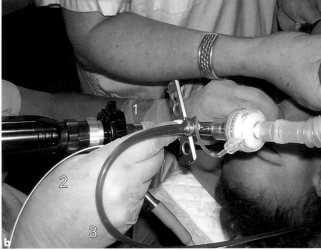

Fig. 4. KTP laser mounting. **a** The KTP optical fibre is taped onto the outside of the telescope, protruding 1 cm ahead of the telescope tip in order to ensure an appropriate field of view. **b** The telescope (1) and the fibre (2) are passed together through the front port of the broncho-scope. Note the green colour of the fibre that indicates laser beam activation. A pipe for continuous suction (3) is plugged to the side port.

the potential of ignition of the gas and/or the char.

3 It is necessary to plug a gas exhaustion pipe on the side port of the rigid tube in order to avoid smoke inhalation (fig. 4b). Moreover, gas suction greatly improves visualization during the procedure as the KTP produces green flashlights due to smoke reflection that can be dazzling to the operator (online suppl. video 2).

4 Any flammable material has to be removed from the target area, including suction probes, endotracheal or tracheostomy tubes, and airway stents. If needed, ventilating tubes can be protected from laser ignition by wrapping in aluminium foil tape [20].

Laser procedures have a high potential for untoward effects that can be avoided if the operator strictly follows the required procedures:

- The laser fibre should always be aimed parallel to the airway wall to avoid transmural injury. Areas that require extra attention include: the anterior part of the middle trachea (close to aortic arch and innominate artery), the posterior wall (close to the oesophagus) and the anterior parts of the main bronchi (close to the pulmonary artery branches). A CT scan prior to the laser procedure is advisable in order to avoid target errors. This is especially important in patients with cardiomegaly, abnormalities of the great vessels or masses that cause displacement of the mediastinal structures.
- Circumferential lasing or exposure of cartilages should be avoided. The aim of endobronchial debulking is to

restore airway patency, irrespective of the anatomical result (fig. 5).

- Web-like diaphragms are treated using radial incisions, leaving bridges of intact mucosa between the burns (fig. 6a). In our experience one laser photoresection course is enough for web removal, thus making it more effective than balloon dilatation.
- Resection of bulky granuloma is achieved by running the fibre tip on the protruding area (fig. 6b). The laser vaporizes or carbonizes the lesions precisely and bloodlessly. We prefer this method to forceps granuloma excision which is more imprecise and haemorrhagic. The KTP laser energy can be modulated, thus varying the depth of absorption. The procedure should begin with the laser source set at a low power range (e.g. 5 W) that can be subsequently adjusted by 2-watt steps according to its effect on the tissue. While the photoresection is in progress, it is important to keep in mind that the burn causes mucosal necrosis at the basis of the lesion and that a healing process will subsequently take place. Re-epithelization is initiated underneath a substantial fibrin layer, and its role is crucial for the prevention of recurrent stenosis. Indeed, it acts as an endogenous stent that allows flat mucosal healing. Spontaneous clearing occurs within 15 days, and mucosal repair is complete after several weeks (fig. 7).

The broncholaser can be used in several airway problems, mostly iatrogenic ones, such as subglottic stenosis in

Video

Fig. 5. Eighteen-month-old male with endobronchial tuberculosis. **a** The intermediate bronchus is completely obstructed by subcarinal lymphadenopathy; the chest X-ray (not shown) revealed middle and right lower lobe atelectasis. **b** Endoscopic view after KTP laser photoresection. Reventilation of the intermediate bronchus (relief of atelectasis) has been established. The laser fibre is seen at the bottom of the picture. (Watch the whole procedure in video 2.)

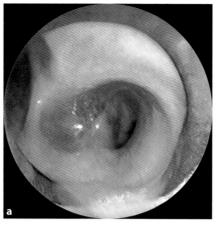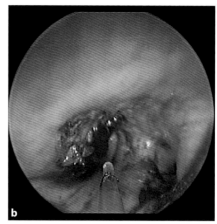

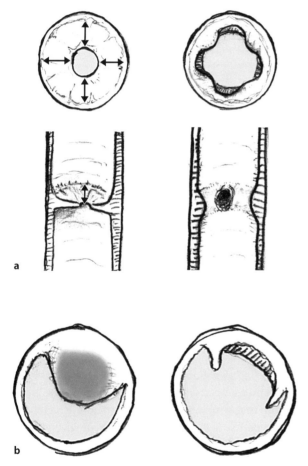

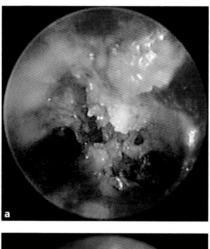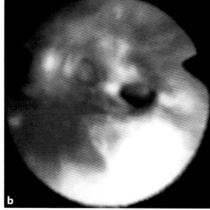

Fig. 6. General principles of laser photoresection. **a** Radial incisions on a web-like lesion (arrows), leaving tissue bridges of intact mucosa between the burns to avoid recurrence of stenosis. **b** Resection of bulky granuloma. The laser energy is delivered to the protruding area of the lesion (greyed), leaving the margin intact.

Fig. 7. Thirteen-month-old female with obstructive granuloma arising from the RB9 segmental bronchus due to peripheral foreign-body retention. **a** Endoscopic view after KTP laser photoresection and foreign-body release. RB8 and RB10 segmental bronchi can be visualized, but RB9 appears to be completely obstructed (Hopkins 2.8 telescope rod lens). **b** Endoscopic view 3 months later. The mucosal healing process is completed, and RB9 is now ventilating (Olympus BFXP40 fibre-optic bronchoscope).

intubated patients or suprastomal granulomas in patients with tracheostomy. Excision of the granulomas prior to decannulation is probably the most frequent indication of endobronchial laser therapy in paediatric patients [18, 21, 22]. Endobronchial laser therapy has also been suggested for the splitting of complete cartilage rings, the marsupialization of tracheobronchial cysts, even for sealing small tracheo-oesophageal fistulas [19, 23]. Laser photoresection is not recommended for tumours that obstruct the airways (e.g. aggressive mediastinal lymphoma) because bronchoscopic manoeuvres can at least temporarily worsen the airway obstruction. Aggressive mediastinal lymphoma quickly responds to corticosteroids and chemotherapy. Endobronchial carcinoid, which is virtually unheard of among young children but can occur in young teenagers, is amenable to laser photoresection with successful control of bleeding. However, the procedure does not allow for the evaluation of lymph nodes in order to investigate the possibility of metastases; therefore, the choice between laser photoresection and conventional surgery remains controversial.

Laser photoresection can be used for certain benign tumours of the airways [24, 25] and for congenital cysts with a transmural component; there is no evidence of superiority of fine-needle aspiration in the latter. Mediastinal dysembryoplastic tumours require removal by open surgery.

Primary tuberculosis sometimes produces huge mediastinal lymph nodes in infants and toddlers, and significant endobronchial involvement [chapter 16, this vol., pp. 173–181]. Endoscopic debulking may be required if chemotherapy and corticosteroids fail to relieve the obstruction. Particular attention should be paid to the risk of induced bleeding in this situation. Laser photoresection provides recanalization and haemostasis at the same time [17]. However, the anatomical relationship between enlarged lymph nodes and pulmonary arteries has to be carefully studied by CT scans before proceeding (online suppl. video 2). The laser fibre should always be kept away from great vessels as lasing through a previously weakened airway wall may cause unexpected vascular injury very quickly.

To date, there are no well-defined indications for laser intervention in the paediatric airway. Novel applications are expected with the evolution of newer laser sources (e.g. photodynamic therapy with photosensitizing agents, pulsed-dye laser, excimer). Endoscopists in training in the broncholaser technique should be exposed to various methods on butcher's meat or liver in order to understand the power of photoresection and its limitations before applying the technique to the paediatric population.

Tracheobronchial Stenting

Stents are prosthetic devices designed to maintain the integrity of hollow tubular structures. In children, airway stents were first used during surgical procedures, but there are currently two types of tracheobronchial stents (silicone tubes and metal meshes or coils) that can be inserted via a bronchoscope. Airway stents have been used in various clinical situations including tracheobronchomalacia, twisting or compression of the airway following cardiothoracic surgery, stenosis in the area of the anastomosis after lung transplantation, and congenital or acquired intrinsic stenosis. In young children severe tracheobronchomalacia is probably the most 'common' indication for airway stenting. Although no comparative study is available, anterior aortopexy is widely considered to be the gold standard in this condition [26, 27]. However, surgery is not always possible and airway stenting can be proposed as an alternative. There are few paediatric series in the literature, and the number of reported cases is limited. Moreover, the various authors' criteria to judge success or failure are heterogeneous, leading to striking discordances in the conclusions [28]. Nevertheless, a comparison of the basic advantages and disadvantages of each type of stent can be made when studying these series (table 1) [8, 29–34].

The use of the *Palmaz®* prosthesis, initially designed for endovascular stenting, was the first to be reported in paediatric patients with airway obstruction. It is a tubular mesh made of stainless steel and comes in a collapsed form. The stent is mounted on a balloon catheter which is inserted into the airway via a rigid bronchoscope or endotracheal tube under fluoroscopic guidance. It is then expanded to the desired diameter by inflation of the balloon. Several stents can be combined to form a Y-shaped structure in order to reconstruct the carinal region, thus ensuring collateral ventilation (e.g. of the right upper or middle lobe) through the mesh [29].

Self-expanding metal airway stents are also available in paediatric dimensions. As severe complications have been reported with first-generation steel self-expanding metal airway stents, their use is not recommended in children today. More recently, nitinol self-expanding metal airway stents have been developed (Ultraflex®) and described in paediatric series. Nitinol is a titanium-based alloy with thermal-shape-memory-specific properties. A small coil is enclosed in a thin introducer sheath; once released into the airway, the stent warms up to body temperature and subsequently expands to the memorized diameter [35].

Silicone stents have better biocompatibility than their metal counterparts and are widely used in adults. The

Table 1. Paediatric case series on endoscopic airway stenting.

Reference	Stent type	N age	Location	Stenting duration	Tissue tolerance	Migration	Outcome
Filler et al. [29]	Palmaz®	16 cases 9 mo [0–26]	Tr = 18 Br = 12	14 mo [2–56]	gran = 6 erosion = 2 embed = 1	2	death = 3 remov = 6
Furman et al. [30]	Palmaz®	6 cases 10 mo [2–38]	Tr = 6 Br = 6	21 mo [5–38]	gran = 2 embed = 4	0	death = 2 remov = 0
Nicolai et al. [31]	Strecker® nitinol Ultraflex®	7 cases 15 mo [3–108]	Tr = 6 Br = 13	50 mo [36–72]	gran = 2 erosion = 1	2	death = 4 remov = 0
Maeda et al. [8]	Palmaz®	5 cases 5 mo [2–12]	Tr = 8	36 mo [24–40]	gran = 2 embed = 5	0	death = 1 remov = 0
Fayon et al. [32]	Tracheo-bronxane®	14 cases 7 mo [2–69]	Tr = 16 Br = 10	7 mo [3–15]	gran = 0 embed = 0	5	death = 3 remov = 13
Vinograd et al. [33]	Palmaz® nitinol	32 cases 5 mo [1–64]	Tr = 20 Br = 22	9 mo [2–72]	gran = 26 erosion = 1 embed = 6	2	death = 15 remov = 11
Shin et al. [34]	nitinol covered	7 cases 12 yrs [0–14]	Tr = 5 Br = 3	24 mo [17–28]	gran = 3 erosion = 2 embed = 0	0	death = 3 remov = 5

Age: median and range in months.
Location: Tr = trachea; Br = main bronchus; total number of stents inserted.
mo: months
N: number of cases.
Outcome: remov = number of alive unstented children at the end of the study.
References: in chronological order of publication.
Stenting duration: median and range in months (death excluded).
Tissue tolerance: gran = significant granulation tissue development; embed = embedding

'Dumon stent' is a smooth silicone molded tube, the outer surface of which is studded. The stent is first threaded through a dedicated applicator and is inserted into the airway by rigid bronchoscopy; it is then released by withdrawing the applicator. The silicone radial expansive force ensures that the stent remains in place whilst the studs enhance stability by becoming anchored to the tracheobronchial cartilage. Dumon stents are suitable for infants and children (fig. 8), and a paediatric introducer has recently been manufactured. It should be noted that, unlike metal stents, silicone tubes have a continuous surface that does not allow for collateral ventilation if bronchial openings are covered. Moreover, small-sized Y-shaped silicone stents are not yet available due to current manufacturing limitations. Thus, in infants and toddlers silicone stents can only be placed into the trachea or the left main bronchus [32].

Metal stents afford good stability, do not significantly impair mucociliary clearance or collateral ventilation, but have a strong tendency to become embedded into the airway wall. Development of granulation tissue is commonly observed and can be responsible for major obstruction and residual stenosis after the removal of the stent. Parietal erosion, vascular perforation and migration to surrounding organs have been described. Mucosal embedding can make stent removal hazardous with the possibility of lethal outcome; case reports mention the need for surgical removal under cardiopulmonary bypass. Many authors consider

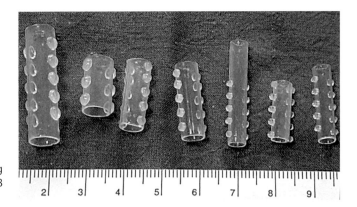

Fig. 8. Small straight silicone stents. Scaling is in centimetres (Tracheobronxane® BB series, Novatech SA, France).

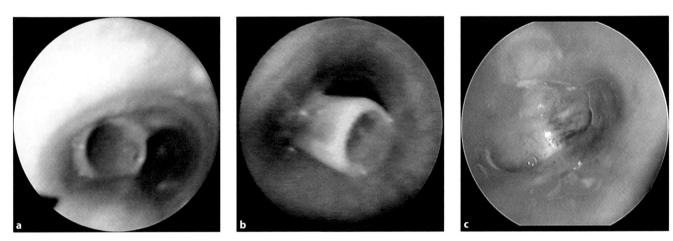

Fig. 9. Behaviour of silicone stents in the paediatric airway. **a** Four-month-old male with vascular compression of left main bronchus after surgical repair of tetralogy of Fallot. The stent has been left in place for 15 months with no complications. **b** Four-year-old male with vascular compression of left main bronchus after surgical repair of aortic hypoplasia. Upward stent migration (tracheal view) after 1 month was manifested by cough but no symptoms of obstruction (courtesy of A. Labbe, Hôtel-Dieu, Clermont-Ferrand, France). **c** Two-year-old-male with severe segmental tracheomalacia. Immediate placement of tracheal stent relieved the symptoms of obstruction. However, severe dyspnoea and bilateral lung overdistension are observed 24 h later. The stent has migrated distally, and both main bronchi are partially obstructed by the distal end of the silicone tube.

metal stents as permanent implants that have to be dilated on a regular basis in growing children.

Silicone stents are relatively easy to insert and remove, and have satisfactory tissue compatibility. In a recent report, the duration of silicone stenting was notably shorter compared with that of metal stents [32], which often remain in situ indefinitely. Nevertheless, silicone stents also cause substantial complications such as mucociliary clearance impairment that requires daily aerosol administration and chest physiotherapy. Mucus plugging can occur, and repeated bronchoscopic interventions are needed in some patients.

In our series, one child died from mucus inspissation and plugging. Moreover, silicone stents are more prone to migration and technical failure than their metal counterpart (fig. 9). It is therefore mandatory that such patients live close to a centre where bronchoscopic interventions can be carried out quickly.

Clearly the ideal, entirely complication-free stent does not exist. Attempts have been made to combine the advantages of metal and silicone stents by covering metal meshes with polymer sheaths. Recent reports on polyurethane-covered nitinol stents showed that, when compared to the

Donato · Tran · Mihailidou

standard metal stents, they were better tolerated by the epithelial tissue and could be removed successfully, without complications. Nevertheless, they also resulted in formation of granulation tissue and impairment of mucociliary clearance [34]. There is very little information about the long-term outcome of airway stenting, especially in children [36]. Similarly, there are only few guidelines regarding their selection in paediatric populations. For example, the Food and Drug Administration has issued a warning against the use of metal stents in adult patients with airway obstruction due to benign disease; silicone stents are widely used instead. In children, the only unequivocal 'guideline' is that airway stenting is a second-line therapy and should be restricted to selected cases where conventional management has failed. Further developments are expected with polymer-covered stents and bioresorbable materials. Improvements in both biocompatibility and stability may expand the field of paediatric airway stenting beyond the range of rescue indications.

Contraindications to Interventional Bronchoscopy

IB is an invasive procedure that caries the potential of serious complications; therefore its use should be carefully weighed against the overall health status of the patient. In general, IB is not recommended in the following conditions:

(a) in cases of severe multisystem anatomical or functional abnormalities that will not improve even after an IB procedure has been performed (e.g. multiple severe airway or other malformations, severe brain injury and refractory heart failure);

(b) in cases where there is a reasonable chance that the airway lesion may improve spontaneously over time (e.g. tracheomalacia after repair of a tracheo-oesophageal fistula, postintubation subglottic stenosis) provided of course that in the interim the patient can maintain an adequate, although not necessarily optimal, level of ventilation; spontaneous improvement usually occurs not as a result of improvement of the cartilages (these actually remain defective), but due to the increase in the endoluminal diameter with advancing age and the fact that the great vessels move progressively away from the central airways;

(c) in cases when the patient may not be able to tolerate the conditions under which the procedure has to be performed (e.g. occlusion of the airway during balloon dilatation or the low oxygen concentration required during laser procedures);

(d) in cases of severe coagulopathy and/or haemodynamic instability that would dramatically increase the probability of serious complications;

(e) last but not least, even when a skilled bronchoscopist is available, IB procedures should not be undertaken if a multidisciplinary team is not available; such a team should include skilful paediatric anaesthesiologists, critical-care physicians, surgeons and appropriately trained supporting staff.

Conclusion

IB holds great promise for the future but its current applications in paediatric practice are limited by a variety of factors such as lack of size-appropriate equipment and the relatively small number of cases that have been performed. These limitations prevent the training of more bronchoscopists in the acquisition of the necessary skills and the collection of sufficient data, which will permit the development of evidence-based standards and guidelines for performing the various procedures. Technological advancements and co-operation between centres in the context of multicentre trials is urgently needed to overcome these limitations.

Acknowledgements

Special thanks go to Andreas Margioris (School of Health Science, University Hospital of Crete) and to Iain Edwards (ICTR Arusha, Tanzania) for the English-language review.

References

1 Chiu PP, Kim PC, Forte V, Holtby H, Caldarone CA, Coles J, Cox P, Bohn D, Edgell D, Foreman F, Gruenwald C: The Airway Reconstruction Team – recent challenges in the management of congenital tracheal stenosis: an individualized approach. J Pediatr Surg 2005;40:774–780.

2 Bagwell CE, Talbert JL, Tepas JJ: Balloon dilatation of long-segment tracheal stenoses. J Pediatr Surg 1991;26:153–159.

3 Messineo A, Narne S, Mognato G, Giusti F, Guglielmi M: Endoscopic dilation of acquired tracheobronchial stenosis in infants. Pediatr Pulmonol 1997;23:101–104.

4 Elkerbout SC, van Lingen RA, Gerritsen J, Roorda RJ: Endoscopic balloon dilation of acquired airway stenosis in newborn infants: a promising treatment. Arch Dis Child 1993;68:37–40.

5 Rimell FL, Stool SE: Diagnosis and management of pediatric tracheal stenosis. Otolaryngol Clin North Am 1995;28:809–827.

6 McLaren CA, Elliot MJ, Roebuck DJ: Tracheobronchial intervention in children. Eur J Radiol 2005;53:22–34.

7 Elliot M, Roebuck D, Noctor C, McLaren C, Hartley B, Mok Q, Dunne C, Pigott N, Patel C, Patel A, Wallis C: The management of congenital tracheal stenosis. Int J Pediatr Otorhinolaryngol 2003;67(suppl 1):S183–S192.

8 Maeda K, Yasufuku M, Yamamoto T: A new approach to the treatment of congenital tracheal stenosis: balloon tracheoplasty and expandable metallic stenting. J Pediatr Surg 2001;36:1646–1649.

9 Tôrer B, Gülcan H, Oguzkurt L, Oguzkurt P, Tarcan A: Use of balloon-expandable metallic stent in a premature infant with congenital tracheal stenosis. Pediatr Pulmonol 2008;43:414–417.

10 Anton-Pacheco JL, Cano I, Comas J, Galletti L, Polo L, Garcia A, Lopez M, Cabezali D: Management of congenital tracheal stenosis in infancy. Eur J Cardiothorac Surg 2006;29:991–996.

11 Herrera P, Caldarone C, Forte V, Campisi P, Holtby H, Chait P, Chiu P, Cox P, Yoo SJ, Manson D, Kim PC: The current state of congenital tracheal stenosis. Pediatr Surg Int 2007;23:1033–1044.

12 Cheng W, Manson DE, Forte V, Ein SH, McLusky I, Papsin BC, Hechter S, Kim PC: The role of conservative management in congenital tracheal stenosis: an evidence-based long-term follow-up study. J Pediatr Surg 2006;41:1203–1207.

13 Chiu PP, Kim PC: Prognostic factors in the surgical treatment of congenital tracheal stenosis: a multicenter analysis of the literature. J Pediatr Surg 2006;41:221–225.

14 Bagwell CE: CO_2 laser excision of pediatric airway lesions. J Pediatr Surg 1990;25:1152–1156.

15 Halstead LA: The use of lasers in the pediatric airway; in Othersen BH (ed): The Pediatric Airway. Philadelphia, Saunders, 1991, pp 186–196.

16 Monnier P, George M, Monod ML, Lang F: The role of the CO_2 laser in the management of laryngotracheal stenosis: a survey of 100 cases. Eur Arch Otorhinolaryngol 2005;262:602–608.

17 Ayache D, Wagner I, Denoyelle F, Garabedian EN: Use of the carbon dioxide laser for tracheobronchial pathology in children. Eur Arch Otorhinolaryngol 2000;257:287–289.

18 Rimell FL, Shapiro AM, Mitskavich MT, Modreck P, Post JC, Maisel RH: Pediatric fiberoptic laser rigid bronchoscopy. Otolaryngol Head Neck Surg 1996;114:413–417.

19 Ishman SL, Kerschner JE, Rudolph CD: The KTP laser: an emerging tool in pediatric otolaryngology. Int J Pediatr Otorhinolaryngol 2006;70:677–682.

20 Walker P, Temperley A, Thelfo S, Hazelgrove A: Avoidance of laser ignition of endotracheal tubes by wrapping in aluminium foil tapes. Anaesth Intensive Care 2004;32:108–112.

21 Sharp HR, Hartley BE: KTP laser treatment of suprastomal obstruction prior to decannulation in paediatric tracheostomy. Int J Pediatr Otorhinolaryngol 2002;66:125–130.

22 Mandell DL, Yellon RF: Endoscopic KTP laser excision of severe tracheotomy-associated suprastomal collapse. Int J Pediatr Otorhinolaryngol 2004;68:1423–1428.

23 Othersen HB, Hebra A, Tagge EP: A new method of treatment for complete tracheal rings in an infant: endoscopic laser division and balloon dilation. J Pediatr Surg 2000;35:262–264.

24 Conforti S, Bonacina E, Ravini M, Torre M: A case of fibrous histiocytoma of the trachea in an infant treated by endobronchial Nd:YAG laser. Lung Cancer 2007;57:112–114.

25 Breen DP, Dubus JC, Chetaille B, Payan MJ, Dutau H: A rare cause of an endobronchial tumour in children: the role of interventional bronchoscopy in the diagnosis and treatment of tumours while preserving anatomy and lung function. Respiration 2008;76:444–448.

26 Dave S, Currie BG: The role of aortopexy in severe tracheomalacia. J Pediatr Surg 2006;41:533–537.

27 Masters IB, Chang AB: Interventions for primary (intrinsic) tracheomalacia in children. Cochrane Database Syst Rev 2005;4:CD005304.

28 Nicolai T: Airway stents in children. Pediatr Pulmonol 2008;43:330–344.

29 Filler RM, Forte V, Chait P: Tracheobronchial stenting for the treatment of airway obstruction. J Pediatr Surg 1998;33:304–311.

30 Furman RH, Backer CL, Dunham ME, Donaldson J, Mavroudis C, Holinger LD: The use of balloon-expandable metallic stents in the treatment of pediatric tracheomalacia and bronchomalacia. Arch Otolaryngol Head Neck Surg 1999;125:203–207.

31 Nicolai T, Huber RM, Reiter K, Merkenschlager A, Hautmann H, Mantel K: Metal airway stent implantation in children: follow-up of seven children. Pediatr Pulmonol 2001;31:289–296.

32 Fayon M, Donato L, de Blic J, Labbe A, Becmeur F, Mely L, Dutau H: French experience of silicone tracheobronchial stenting in children. Pediatr Pulmonol 2005;39:21–27.

33 Vinograd I, Keidar S, Weinberg M, Silbiger A: Treatment of airway obstruction by metallic stents in infants and children. J Thorac Cardiovasc Surg 2005;130:146–150.

34 Shin JH, Hong SJ, Park SJ, Ko GY, Lee SY, Kim HB, Jang JY: Placement of covered retrievable expandable metallic stents for pediatric tracheobronchial obstruction. J Vasc Interv Radiol 2006;17:309–317.

35 Tsugawa C, Nishijima E, Muraji T, Yoshimura M, Tsubota N, Asano H: A shape memory airway stent for tracheobronchomalacia in children: an experimental and clinical study. J Pediatr Surg 1997;32:50–53.

36 Kumar P, Bush AP, Ladas GP, Goldstraw P: Tracheobronchial obstruction in children: experience with endoscopic airway stenting. Ann Thorac Surg 2003;75:1579–1586.

L. Donato
Service de Pédiatrie 2, Hôpital Hautepierre
Avenue Molière
FR–67098 Strasbourg (France)
Tel. +33 388 127 786, Fax +33 388 127 132, E-Mail leonard.donato@chru-strasbourg.fr

Chapter 7

Priftis KN, Anthracopoulos MB, Eber E, Koumbourlis AC, Wood RE (eds): Paediatric Bronchoscopy.
Prog Respir Res. Basel, Karger 2010, vol 38, pp 75–82

Whole-Lung Lavage

Robert E. Wood

Division of Pulmonary Medicine, Cincinnati Children's Hospital Medical Center, University of Cincinnati College of Medicine,
Cincinnati, Ohio, USA

Abstract

Whole-lung lavage (WLL) is a therapeutic technique for the clearance from alveolar spaces of abnormal material in conditions such as pulmonary alveolar proteinosis. The technique requires the repetitive filling and emptying of the lung with fluid (saline), thus clearing the particulate matter from the alveolar space. The technique involves isolation of the lung that is being lavaged while preserving ventilation for the other lung. While this can be achieved relatively easily in adult patients with the use of a double-lumen endotracheal tube, it poses many challenges when the procedure has to be performed in infants and young children. The following chapter describes the pathophysiological changes that take place during WLL, the technical aspects of the technique with emphasis on its modification for use in infants and young children, as well as the possible alternatives.   Copyright © 2010 S. Karger AG, Basel

Whole-lung lavage (WLL, also called 'bronchopulmonary lavage') is a therapeutic technique applicable to certain conditions in which the alveolar spaces must be cleared of abnormal material. Although it is most commonly used in the treatment of pulmonary alveolar proteinosis [1, 2], there have been reports of its successful use in entities such as lipoid pneumonia [3] or pneumoconiosis [4]. Because during the procedure one of the lungs is completely filled with fluid, WLL is limited to patients who are able to tolerate one-lung ventilation. Simultaneous double-lung lavage can be performed only if a patient is placed on extracorporeal membrane oxygenation (ECMO).

History

Therapeutic lung lavage was first reported during the 1960s, in adults. Initial reports involved segmental or lobar lavage with a cuffed endobronchial catheter positioned with the aid of fluoroscopy [5]. By 1965, Ramirez and Campbell [6] reported WLL in adult patients with alveolar proteinosis, using a double-lumen endotracheal tube. This technique remains the standard approach today [7, 8]. Serial/sequential segmental or lobar lavage, using a flexible bronchoscope, has been reported by a number of authors [9, 10] and may be useful in patients with severe lung disease who cannot tolerate unilateral WLL.

Paediatric applications of WLL developed slowly, because of the rarity of conditions mandating such lavage and the small size of the paediatric airway. Sporadic cases of paediatric alveolar proteinosis began to be reported in the 1970s, but therapeutic options were few. WLL has been performed with ECMO [11, 12], but this technique involves major risks and cannot be repeated many times, as is necessary for the treatment of a chronic condition such as alveolar proteinosis. Unilateral WLL in an infant, utilizing a Swan-Ganz catheter, was reported by Moazam et al. [13]. This technique, while innovative, is very inefficient, due to the small size of the catheter. Sequential segmental/lobar lavage has been performed with a paediatric flexible bronchoscope [12, 14] in children.

My first attempt to lavage the lungs of a child with alveolar proteinosis was in 1974, in which serial segmental lavages were performed in a 6-year-old girl with a 6-mm bronchoscope (at the time, the smallest with suction channel). Although a reasonable amount of alveolar sediment was removed, the procedure was very slow and inefficient. The possibility of placing 2 endotracheal tubes into the child's trachea (one for ventilation, the other for lavage) was not adopted, because the tubes would have to be very small, with much wasted space between them and the airway wall. In 1975, using a 3.5-mm flexible bronchoscope (with no suction channel) a long, cuffed, 4.5-mm

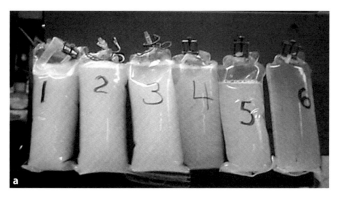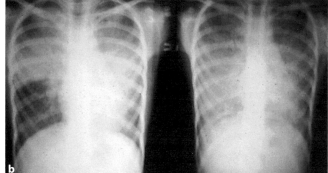

Fig. 1. a, b Results of 6-litre lavage via single-lumen tube in a child with pulmonary alveolar proteinosis. This procedure was performed via a single-lumen 4.5-mm cuffed endobronchial tube positioned in the right main bronchus. With this technique, it is not feasible to include the right upper lobe. Note the marked clearing of the turbidity of the effluent (**a**).

endotracheal tube was guided into the patient's main stem bronchi. The lavage was performed through the endotracheal tube while the patient was breathing spontaneously through the residual airway surrounding the tube. The technique allowed a 6-litre lavage of one lung in approximately 30 min (fig. 1). Subsequently, the technique was adopted for much smaller patients who were under general anaesthesia [15].

The Physiology of Whole-Lung Lavage

Surfactant Issues

Pulmonary surfactant readily and rapidly redistributes into any available air-liquid interface. Therefore, WLL has the potential to significantly deplete the available surfactant, leaving the postlavage lung with very poor compliance until new surfactant can be produced. However, if no air-liquid interface is available, the normal surfactant will mostly remain in situ, thus making postlavage recovery much easier. It is therefore important to perform WLL in such a way as to minimize surfactant loss.

At the beginning of WLL, the lungs should be ventilated with 100% oxygen for a sufficient time to remove the majority of the nitrogen from the alveolar spaces. As the lung is initially filled with fluid, time should be allowed for the alveolar gas (now consisting mostly of oxygen and carbon dioxide) to be absorbed, leaving no air-liquid interface. While it is not feasible to monitor this process in real time, in general, the lung should initially be filled with fluid slowly, over a period of approximately 10 min. Subsequent volume exchanges are done as rapidly as the equipment will allow.

Pulmonary Perfusion

Unless and until sufficient hypoxic pulmonary vasoconstriction has occurred, perfusion of the non-ventilated lung will result in at least some degree of systemic oxygen desaturation. Once the lung has been filled to the point that the fluid pressure within the airways and alveoli exceeds capillary perfusion pressure, however, this physiological shunting stops, and the oxygen saturation rises. The nadir of saturation depends on the relative degree of shunting as well as the residual function of the ventilated lung. Some desaturation must be expected and accepted; in otherwise healthy patients, no adverse effects should be expected from brief desaturations. Some institutions have routinely performed WLL in a hyperbaric chamber so that oxygenation can be better maintained in the face of severe dysfunction of the ventilated lung [16].

Technical Issues of Whole-Lung Lavage

Anaesthesia and Intra-Operative Monitoring

Although lung lavage on spontaneously breathing patients is feasible [17], the procedure is usually done under general anaesthesia and muscle relaxation. Continuous monitoring of the oxyhaemoglobin saturation, end-tidal CO_2 and EKG are required, whereas placement of an arterial line for continuous monitoring of blood pressure and evaluation of blood gases may be considered.

Airway Management

Older Children and Adolescents

WLL requires a secure airway for ventilation and effective separation of the ventilated and the lavaged lung. In patients who are large enough, this is best achieved with a double-lumen endotracheal tube. In general, the largest double-lumen tube that can be readily passed into the patient's trachea should be utilized, to facilitate both ventilation and lavage. Because the smallest such tube currently available is 26 Fr (outer diameter of approx. 8.3 mm), it cannot be used in children younger than 10–12 years of age. The double-lumen endotracheal tube is placed by a conventional technique, and its positioning should be verified by flexible bronchoscopy through both sides of the tube. Separation of the lungs is then achieved by inflation of the tracheal and bronchial cuffs. The patient is ventilated with 100% oxygen for at least 10 min before the beginning of the lavage.

Infants and Small Children

Smaller patients whose airway cannot accommodate a double-lumen endotracheal tube present a special challenge. It is essential to have an effective and functional airway during the procedure; it is also essential to have a stable and secure route for the ingress and egress of fluid from the lung being lavaged. This can be achieved by a single-lumen, cuffed, endotracheal tube, while ventilation is maintained through the residual airway outside the endotracheal tube [15]. Because there is no commercial source of cuffed paediatric endotracheal tubes of sufficient length, one must also fashion a longer tube for the procedure. The critical factors here are to have a tube large enough to achieve effective fluid exchange, yet small enough to allow effective ventilation around the outside of the tube. This may require some trial and error on the part of the operator.

Preparation of the Tube

A cuffed endotracheal tube is lengthened with a segment of uncuffed tube of the same diameter (fig. 2). The tubes are joined with the tip of a 15-mm endotracheal tube anaesthesia adapter, cut off and tapered at the cut end. In very small patients, it may be important to trim the taper from the distal end of the cuffed tube; this requires smoothing of the cut edges and may require melting the cut edges to seal the pilot tube of the balloon cuff. It must be confirmed that the balloon cuff will hold pressure.

The patient is placed under anaesthesia, and a nasopharyngeal (NP) tube is passed through one nostril (fig. 3).

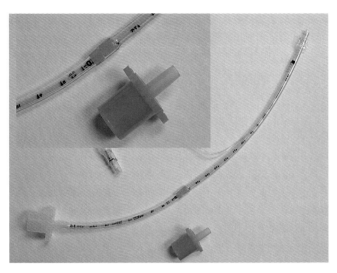

Fig. 2. The extended endotracheal tube as described in the text. The connection between the two segments of tube is made from the 15-mm adapter, and the two segments are force-fitted together.

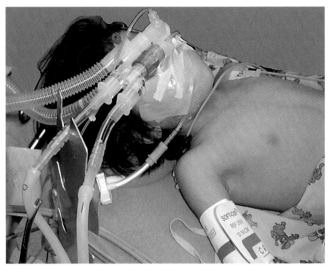

Fig. 3. Child undergoing WLL with the single-tube technique. Ventilation is achieved via an NP tube; the nose and mouth are tightly sealed with non-porous tape, and an orogastric tube is placed to relieve any gas passing into the stomach. A Y-adapter is attached to the cuffed endobronchial tube positioned in the left main bronchus for instillation and drainage of saline.

Ventilation is thereafter maintained via the NP tube. The modified endotracheal tube is passed into the trachea, *via the opposite nostril*, over a suitable flexible bronchoscope. The endotracheal tube is then positioned in the distal trachea, and the flexible bronchoscope is removed. The tube is clamped, and it is confirmed that there is sufficient room around the outside of the tube to achieve ventilation via the NP tube (by observation of chest rise, auscultation etc.). If there is too much resistance, the tube is removed and replaced by a smaller-diameter tube. Because it is essential to position the tube precisely with the use of a flexible bronchoscope, the smallest tube that can be used with this technique is a 2.5-mm endotracheal tube that can allow the passing of a 2.2-mm flexible bronchoscope. When it is confirmed that the patient can ventilate adequately around the tube, the flexible bronchoscope is re-inserted into the tube, and the tip of the tube is advanced beyond the carina and positioned in the appropriate location. The tube is very securely taped at the nostril (and care must now be taken to ensure that the position of the head and neck are not changed throughout the procedure, as this may dislodge the tube). An orogastric tube is placed for the decompression of the stomach, and the mouth is sealed with non-porous tape. The nostrils are also taped securely, to eliminate a leak through the nose. The adequacy of ventilation is again confirmed with the cuff of the (endobronchial) tube inflated. Note that in small patients, there is a potential problem of the cuff obstructing the distal trachea, if the proximal end of the cuff extends too far proximally. An endotracheal tube with the shortest cuff available should be used (and any extension of the tube beyond the distal margin of the cuff may need to be removed). It may be useful to pass a 2.2-mm flexible bronchoscope through the NP tube and through the glottis (alongside the endotracheal tube) to directly inspect the distal trachea.

Technique of the Lavage

The lumen of the endotracheal tube that enters the lung to be lavaged is connected to a Y-adapter that is connected to 2 cystoscopy irrigating sets (fig. 4). A bag of warmed (40°C), non-pyrogenic irrigating saline is connected to the first irrigating set at a height such that the filling pressure is in the order of 30–40 cm. Higher pressures can result in transudation of fluid across the pleura, with formation of a hydrothorax. The other limb of the Y-adapter is connected to an empty bag on the floor.

The initial instillation of saline should be done slowly (approx. over 10 min) allowing time for re-absorption of alveolar gas. The amount and rate of the influx are based on the estimated capacity of the lavaged lung. It is not necessary to try to instill a premeasured volume of saline, because the volume the lung will accept cannot be accurately predicted. Fluid is allowed to flow into the lung until the flow stops.

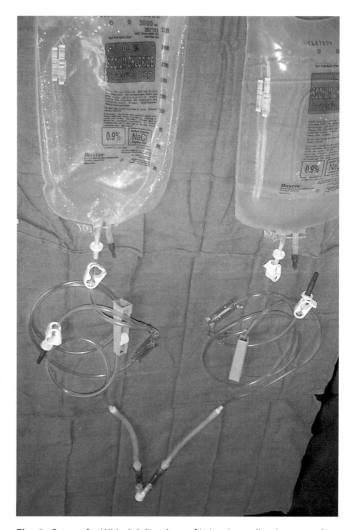

Fig. 4. Set-up for WLL. A 3-litre bag of irrigating saline is warmed to 40°C and connected to a cystoscopy irrigating set, which is in turn connected to the endobronchial tube. An empty bag is connected to the other side to receive the effluent. Gravity is used to fill and empty the lung (40 cm for inflow, table height for outflow) as the sides of the Y-adapter are alternately clamped.

Once the lung is filled, the intake line is clamped and the effluent line (consisting of a second irrigation set connected to the other limb of the Y-adapter) is unclamped, allowing the fluid to drain by gravity into the reservoir on the floor. As one bag is emptied of saline, it is moved to the effluent side. The drainage should be allowed to continue until the flow essentially stops. Then the effluent line is clamped, and the intake line is unclamped, allowing the lung to fill again. This process is repeated until it has been determined that maximal benefit has been reached. Typical volumes used for WLL in adolescents and adults range between 15 and 25 litres.

Lung lavage is continued until the effluent clears satisfactorily, or until it is otherwise determined that the procedure has achieved its 'maximal' benefit. The saline is then drained as completely as possible, and the endotracheal tube is suctioned deeply with a catheter. The lung is then inflated with oxygen, holding pressure of 30–40 cm for 30–60 s to achieve alveolar recruitment. Suctioning can be repeated if there seems to be fluid in the tube, and then both sides of the double-lumen tube are connected to the anaesthesia circuit so that both lungs can be simultaneously ventilated. The balloon cuff on the bronchial side is deflated. Muscle relaxation, if used, is reversed, and the patient is extubated when appropriate. Electively, the double-lumen tube can be removed and replaced temporarily with a single-lumen tube if it appears that the patient will require support for a longer time.

At some centres, upon completion of the lavage of the left lung, the patient will be ventilated for 1 h or 2, and then the right lung will be lavaged, during the same anaesthesia session. Despite the appeal of finishing everything in one session, this approach has significant downsides. Specifically, the procedure extends from an average of 2–2.5 h to as long as 6–8 h. The long procedure is exhausting for the operator as well, there are logistical problems associated with scheduling long operating room times, and the prolonged anaesthesia usually precludes the extubation of the patient at the end of the procedure and makes at least a brief hospitalization rather inevitable. Our practice is to perform 2 separate procedures, with an interval of 3–4 days between; each procedure takes 2–2.5 h, the patients are extubated before leaving the operating room, and the procedures are done on an ambulatory basis. The patients can usually be discharged within 3–4 h after completion of the procedure.

One significant limitation of the lavage technique in infants and young children is that it makes the lavage of the right upper lobe virtually impossible because the orifice of the right upper lobe is too close to the carina to allow fluid to enter the upper lobe without obstructing the distal trachea with the balloon cuff. If the patient is positioned in a full decubitus position, with the lavaged lung up, there is a significant risk that the weight of the lung when filled with saline will push the proximal portion of the endobronchial tube over the orifice of the other lung, reducing or preventing ventilation.

Alveolar Clearance
In order to achieve clearance of particulate material from the alveoli, there must be effective exchange of fluid and mixing and not merely flooding of the alveoli with fluid.

In practice, at least several exchanges of fluid are needed before physiologically meaningful clearance is achieved. The degree of clearance from the alveoli of the offending substance depends on the volume of fluid entering and leaving the alveoli as well as the mixing that can be achieved during the fill/empty cycles. Much more effective alveolar mixing/clearance can be achieved by mechanically agitating the alveoli/fluid during the lavage [18]. In practice, this is done by manual or mechanical chest percussion. While the optimal frequency and/or intensity of the percussive blows are unclear, theoretical considerations would suggest that higher frequencies might be more effective at the alveolar level. Mechanical percussion devices can achieve relatively high frequencies (and are also much easier on the operators than manual percussion), but there is little data upon which to base comparisons. Nevertheless, it can be dramatic to see the increased turbidity of the effluent upon initiating chest percussion after initial clearing when percussion is not done from the beginning.

The most effective alveolar clearance will be obtained if the lung is allowed to empty as completely as feasible on each cycle. This will allow pulmonary perfusion, and thus some degree of desaturation, during part of the lavage cycle. However, in most cases, the desaturation will be brief.

The effect of body position during WLL is unclear. If the patient is placed in a lateral decubitus position with the lavaged lung *up*, the entire hemithorax is exposed for mechanical percussion. However, the weight of the saline-filled lung may compress the dependent lung and compromise ventilation. It is unknown whether gravitational forces play any role in the egress of particulate material from the fluid-filled alveoli. If the patient remains in a recumbent position, not all the surface of the hemithorax can be reached by mechanical percussion, and one could postulate that this would decrease the efficiency of the alveolar clearance in the regions not directly percussed. In our experience, when patients were rotated during the course of WLL in order to deliver percussion to formerly dependent regions, there had been no visible increase in the turbidity of the effluent. However, CT scans of patients with pulmonary alveolar proteinosis following WLL may show much more clearing of non-dependent areas (fig. 5).

Site of the Lavage
In general, it is reasonable to lavage the left lung first, as it is usually smaller than the right and therefore there will be less ventilation/perfusion mismatch and more ventilatory

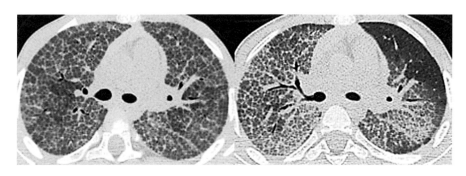

Fig. 5. CT scan showing preferential clearing of the non-dependent portion of the lung in a child with pulmonary alveolar proteinosis. **a** Before lavage. **b** After lavage of the left lung; the procedure was done with the child in a supine position, making it difficult to perform mechanical percussion of the dependent portions of the lung.

capacity available even though both lungs are dysfunctional. The right lung is lavaged after the left lung has recovered from the lavage process and (presumably) has improved from the disease process for which the WLL is being performed.

Results of Whole-Lung Lavage

Patients with pulmonary alveolar proteinosis usually respond well to WLL. There are, however, some exceptions, and the reasons for failure are not obvious but may include patients with abnormal surfactant and forms of secondary alveolar proteinosis. Children as small as 3.5 kg have been successfully lavaged in our institution with volumes of approximately 1 litre and produced effluent that has a large amount of sediment. However, there have been also a few children, in whom there was no sediment in the effluent, and not surprisingly such children do not appear to benefit from the procedure.

The duration of beneficial effect depends on a number of variables, including the underlying disease state and its natural history, and the efficacy of the lavage procedure. Certain patients may require lavage as often as every 4–6 weeks, while others may not require another lavage for 2–3 years. In our experience, the lavage can be postponed until the patient begins to become symptomatic but should not wait until there is severe hypoxaemia and impeding respiratory failure.

When all necessary precautions are taken, the procedure can be performed safely without any serious complications. However, it should be avoided shortly after a surgical procedure in the lung (e.g. a lung biopsy). I have seen at least 1 case, in which the combination of a partially healed surgical wound together with high hydrostatc pressure resulted in a hydrothorax (although interestingly not a pneumothorax). Intra-operative changes in the tube position may cause complications such as leakage of saline or obstruction of the contralateral lung. Such problems tend to get corrected

relatively easily without harm to the patient, but understandably causing transient tachycardia in the operator and anaesthesiologist…

Optimization of Oxygenation

Because hypoxaemia is one of the most common and potentially severe complications during WLL, several techniques have been proposed for the improvement of oxygenation during the procedure. Such techniques have included the use of hyperoxygenated solution for improved oxygen supply [19] and the use of inhaled nitric oxide combined with pulmonary artery balloon inflation [20]. Although the outcome of these modifications has been reportedly successful, they have not fundamentally changed the way the WLL is performed. One method that could theoretically greatly improve the oxygenation during WLL would be to use perfluorochemical liquid for the lavage because of its high solubility of oxygen and carbon dioxide, and a relative low surface tension [21, 22].

WLL with the patient on ECMO has been tried on several occasions. Its major advantage is that both lungs can be lavaged simultaneously with a single-lumen tube while the patient remains fully oxygenated [23]. Repeat lavages under cardiopulmonary bypass have also been reported [24]. However, this technique is quite radical and with high potential for complications (bleeding, stroke, infection, trauma to major vessels), and therefore it is not recommended as the first choice. It should probably be reserved for situations in which a single lavage session can reasonably be expected to result in a definitive resolution of the patient's problem or when the patient's condition is so severe that survival during single-lung lavage is in serious doubt. An alternative to full cardiopulmonary bypass via veno-arterial ECMO would be to use venovenous ECMO but to our knowledge there is no experience with it in this particular situation.

Alternatives to Whole-Lung Lavage

In some patients, WLL may not be safe or technically feasible. In such cases, one has to consider alternative techniques, which may be utilized at least as a stopgap measure in hopes of improving the baseline lung function until WLL or some other definitive treatment can be applied. The most conventional and practical approach is to treat small(er) areas of the lung, using a flexible bronchoscope to perform segmental or subsegmental bronchoalveolar lavage [14, 25]. The goal is to try to clear a few small areas while leaving the largest possible lung volume available for gas exchange during the process, instead of only one lung. The flexible bronchoscope is passed through an endotracheal tube and wedged into a peripheral position. Saline is then instilled and removed sequentially until the effluent seems reasonably clear. It is most effective to place the patient in a decubitus position with the lavaged lung down, as this minimizes spillover into the other lung. This technique can surely be beneficial but has numerous limitations. It is slow, and it is difficult to perform mechanical chest percussion during the procedure. There is loss of active surfactant both from the area lavaged and also from other areas into which saline may spill over. Some such spillover is inevitable and can result in substantial drops in oxygen saturation. It can be difficult to access and lavage every subsegmental bronchus (or, for that matter, to keep track of what bronchi have already been lavaged). Regardless of the limitations, however, in selected patients, this technique is clearly beneficial, and it may be the only feasible technique available for a given patient.

Conclusion

WLL can be applied in almost any patient, given proper indications and careful attention to technique and the patient's physiology. Recent advances in the understanding of the pathophysiology of pulmonary alveolar proteinosis and other surfactant-related conditions have opened the door to the introduction of medical therapies such as granulocyte-macrophage colony-stimulating factor [2] that may be able to control or even treat the disease, thus obviating the need for WLL. Until this day comes, pulmonologists should be familiar with the technique and complications of WLL.

References

1 Rosen S, Castleman B, Liebow A: Pulmonary alveolar proteinosis. N Engl J Med 1958;258:1123–1142.
2 Trapnell BC, Carey BC, Uchida K, Suzuki T: Pulmonary alveolar proteinosis, a primary immunodeficiency of impaired GM-CSF stimulation of macrophages. Curr Opin Immunol 2009;21:514–521.
3 Chang H, Chen C, Chen C, Hsuie T, Chen C, Lei W, Wu M, Jin Y: Successful treatment of diffuse lipoid pneumonitis with whole lung lavage. Thorax 1993;48:947–948.
4 Wilt J, Banks D, Weissman D, Parker J, Vallyathan V, Castranova V, Dedhia H, Stulken E, Ma J, Ma J, Cruzzavala J, Shumaker J, Childress C, Lapp N: Reduction of lung dust burden in pneumoconiosis by whole-lung lavage. J Occup Environ Med 1996;38:619–624.
5 Ramirez J, Schultz R, Dutton R: Pulmonary alveolar proteinosis: a new technique and rationale for treatment. Arch Intern Med 1963;112:419–431.
6 Ramirez J, Campbell G: Pulmonary alveolar proteinosis: endobronchial treatment. Ann Intern Med 1965;63:429–441.
7 Selecky P, Wasserman K, Benfield J, Lippmann M: The clinical and physiological effect of whole-lung lavage in pulmonary alveolar proteinosis: a ten-year experience. Ann Thorac Surg 1977;24:451–461.

8 Paschen C, Reiter K, Stanzel F, Teschler H, Griese M: Therapeutic lung lavages in children and adults. Respir Res 2005;6:138.
9 Brach B, Harrell J, Moser K: Alveolar proteinosis: lobar lavage by fiberoptic bronchoscopic technique. Chest 1976;69:224–227.
10 Garvey J, Guarneri J, Khan F, Goldstein J: Clinical evaluation of bronchopulmonary lavage using the flexible fiberoptic bronchoscope. Ann Thorac Surg 1980;30:427–432.
11 Hiratzka L, Swan D, Rose E, Ahrens R: Bilateral simultaneous lung lavage utilizing membrane oxygenator for pulmonary alveolar proteinosis in an 8-month-old infant. Ann Thorac Surg 1983;35:313–317.
12 Mahut B, de Blic J, Le Bourgeois M, Beringer A, Chevalier J, Scheinmann P: Partial and massive lung lavages in an infant with severe pulmonary alveolar proteinosis. Pediatr Pulmonol 1992;13:50–53.
13 Moazam F, Schmidt J, Chesrown S, Graves S, Sauder R, Drummond J, Heard S, Talbert J: Total lung lavage for pulmonary alveolar proteinosis in an infant without the use of cardiopulmonary bypass. J Pediatr Surg 1985;J Pediatr Surg:398–401.
14 Mahut B, Delacourt C, Scheinmann P, de Blic J, Mani T, Fournet J, Bellon G: Pulmonary alveolar proteinosis: experience with eight pediatric cases and a review. Pediatrics 1996;97:117–122.

15 McKenzie B, Wood R, Bailey A: Airway management for unilateral lung lavage in children. Anesthesiology 1989;70:550–553.
16 Jansen H, Zuurmond W, Roos C, Schreuder J, Bakker D: Whole-lung lavage under hyperbaric oxygen conditions for alveolar proteinosis with respiratory failure. Chest 1987;91:829–832.
17 Froudarakis ME, Koutsopoulos A, Mihailidou HP: Total lung lavage by awake flexible fiberoptic bronchoscope in a 13-year-old girl with pulmonary alveolar proteinosis. Respir Med 2007;101:366–369.
18 Perez A, Rogers R: Enhanced alveolar clearance with chest percussion therapy and positional changes during whole-lung lavage for alveolar proteinosis. Chest 2004;125:2351–2356.
19 Zhou B, Zhou HY, Xu PH, Wang HM, Lin XM, Wang XD: Hyperoxygenated solution for improved oxygen supply in patients undergoing lung lavage for pulmonary alveolar proteinosis. Chin Med J (Engl) 2009;122:1780–1783.
20 Nadeau MJ, Côté D, Bussières JS: The combination of inhaled nitric oxide and pulmonary artery balloon inflation improves oxygenation during whole-lung lavage. Anesth Analg 2004;99:676–679.

21   Lindemann R, Rajka T, Henrichsen T, Vinorum OG, de Lange C, Erichsen A, Fugelseth D: Bronchioalveolar lavage with perfluorochemical liquid during conventional ventilation. Pediatr Crit Care Med 2007;8:486–488.

22   Jeng MJ, Soong WJ, Lee YS, Chang HL, Shen CM, Wang CH, Yang SS, Hwang B: Effects of therapeutic bronchoalveolar lavage and partial liquid ventilation on meconium-aspirated newborn piglets. Crit Care Med 2006;34:1099–1105.

23   Sihoe AD, Ng VM, Liu RW, Cheng LC: Pulmonary alveolar proteinosis in extremis: the case for aggressive whole lung lavage with extracorporeal membrane oxygenation support. Heart Lung Circ 2008;17:69–72.

24   Centella T, Oliva E, Andrade IG, Epeldegui A: The use of a membrane oxygenator with extracorporeal circulation in bronchoalveolar lavage for alveolar proteinosis. Interact Cardiovasc Thorac Surg 2005;4:447–449.

25   Doğru D, Yalçin E, Aslan AT, Ocal T, Ozçelik U, Güçer S, Kale G, Haliloglu M, Kiper N: Successful unilateral partial lung lavage in a child with pulmonary alveolar proteinosis. J Clin Anesth 2009;21:127–130.

Robert E. Wood, PhD, MD
Professor of Pediatrics and Otolaryngology
Cincinnati Children's Hospital Medical Center
University of Cincinnati College of Medicine
3333 Burnet Avenue MLC 2021
Cincinnati, OH 45229-3039 (USA)
Tel. +1 513 636 2776, Fax +1 513 636 3845, E-Mail rewood@cchmc.org

Priftis KN, Anthracopoulos MB, Eber E, Koumbourlis AC, Wood RE (eds): Paediatric Bronchoscopy.
Prog Respir Res. Basel, Karger 2010, vol 38, pp 83–94

Rigid Bronchoscopy

Alice Hitter · Alexandre Karkas · Sébastien Schmerber · Christian Adrien Righini

Department of Otorhinolaryngology, Head and Neck Surgery, Albert Michallon University Hospital, Grenoble, France

Abstract

Paediatric bronchoscopy entails two endoscopic techniques: flexible and rigid bronchoscopy. Flexible bronchoscopy is mainly performed by pulmonologists, whereas rigid bronchoscopy is a more invasive procedure usually carried out by otorhinolaryngologists. Each method has advantages and drawbacks. The selection of flexible or rigid bronchoscopy depends on the indication, the clinical context and the expertise of each medical centre. Flexible bronchoscopy has an essential role in the diagnosis of airway disease. On the other hand, rigid bronchoscopy is more efficient in the interventional management of airway lesions. Foreign-body removal is the most frequent indication for paediatric rigid bronchoscopy. Rigid tubes (laryngoscope and bronchoscope) are also used for the treatment of laryngeal and tracheal lesions thanks to the continuous evolution of various endoscopic techniques such as stenting, dilatation, debulking with laser or microdebrider, and intralesional injections. The rigid tube can secure the airway in case of obstruction, thus allowing for concomitant assisted ventilation. Rigid and flexible instruments complement each other in the evaluation of paediatric airways, and the close collaboration between otorhinolaryngologists and paediatric pulmonologists helps to ensure the selection of the most efficient and safe procedure.   Copyright © 2010 S. Karger AG, Basel

The respiratory tract can be explored using two endoscopic methods: flexible (fig. 1) and rigid (fig. 2) laryngoscopy and bronchoscopy. This chapter discusses the methods of and the indications for rigid (tube) airway exploration in the paediatric population as well as the differences between flexible and rigid laryngotracheobronchoscopy.

Flexible bronchoscopy is carried out under light sedation or general anaesthesia usually by a pulmonologist whereas rigid bronchoscopy is invariably performed in the operating theatre under general anaesthesia, usually by an otorhinolaryngologist. Complications of either procedure are rare but paediatric rigid bronchoscopy in particular necessitates anaesthesia and careful monitoring, and good cooperation

between the anaesthetist and otorhinolaryngologist. During rigid endoscopy, two surgical instruments are used for visualizing the respiratory tract: the rigid laryngoscope (assisted by rod lens telescope; fig. 3) and the rigid bronchoscope (also assisted by the rod lens telescope; fig. 4). The external diameter of the rigid bronchoscope is selected according to the weight of the child (table 1). There are several types of rigid telescopes, e.g. direct (0°) or angled vision (30° and 70°), and two main diameters, i.e. 2.7 and 4 mm. The main advantage of the rigid bronchoscope is that it secures the airway and allows for assisted ventilation during the procedure (fig. 4), whereas the rigid laryngoscope does not allow for simultaneous assisted ventilation.

Thanks to recent technological advancements, the therapeutic use of rigid endoscopy has expanded in the last 10 years. Current treatment of upper respiratory tract diseases by means of rigid bronchoscopy may render the performance of tracheostomy unnecessary, a procedure which is associated with high mortality (0.5–4%) and morbidity (44–70%) rates in neonates and children [1, 2].

Complete exploration of the airway with the rigid endoscope includes visualization of the larynx, the trachea and the proximal bronchi, i.e. the main and lobar bronchi, and the orifices of the segmental bronchi. The indications for laryngotracheoscopy will be detailed in the first part, and those of tracheobronchoscopy in the second part of this chapter.

Rigid Laryngoscopy

Flexible laryngoscopy is an excellent method for exploring lesions that cause stridor and respiratory distress in neonates and infants, with some notable exceptions such as laryngeal clefts and anomalies of the posterior aspect of the larynx (e.g. postcricoid haemangiomas) [3]. Yet, rigid laryngoscopy

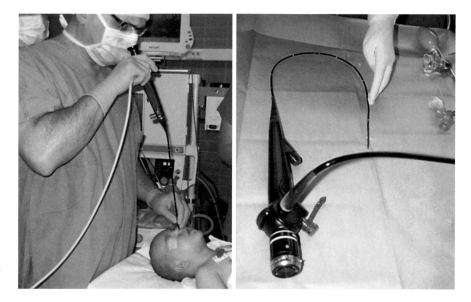

Fig. 1. Flexible laryngoscopy under general anaesthesia and spontaneous ventilation.

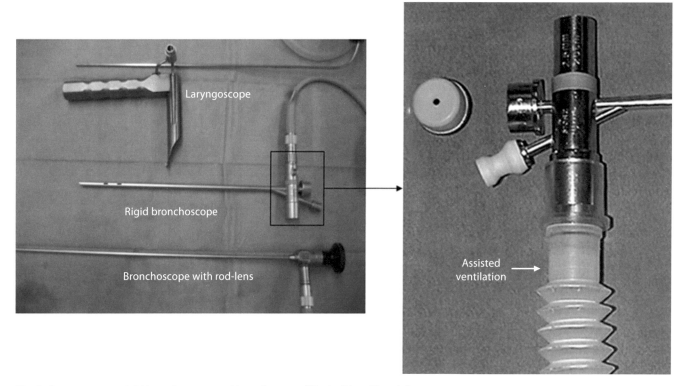

Laryngoscope

Rigid bronchoscope

Bronchoscope with rod-lens

Assisted ventilation

Fig. 2. Laryngoscope, rigid bronchoscope and bronchoscope fitted with rod lens telescope.

is useful when flexible laryngoscopy is normal despite a high suspicion of disease, or when an endoscopic treatment is considered.

Rigid laryngotracheoscopy is performed under general anaesthesia with spontaneous respiration without endotracheal intubation [chapter 2, this vol., pp. 22–29]. Induction is made with gas, and local anaesthesia (lidocaine) is applied topically onto the larynx. Direct laryngoscopy is performed with rigid 0- and 30-degree telescopes. This method allows exploration of the supraglottis, the

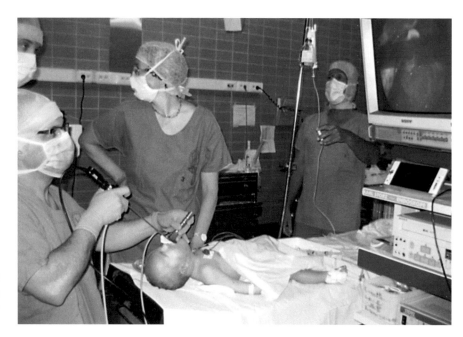

Fig. 3. Laryngotracheoscopy with rigid endoscope assisted by rod lens telescope under general anaesthesia and spontaneous ventilation.

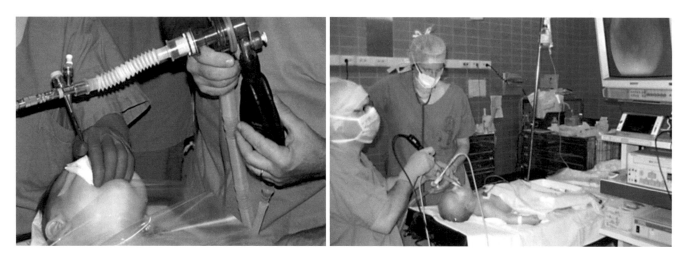

Fig. 4. Rigid bronchoscopy under general anaesthesia and assisted ventilation.

Table 1. Diameters of rigid bronchoscopes

Weight of patient	External diameter mm	Internal diameter mm	Size number (Storz)
<3 kg	4.2	3.5	2.5
3–6 kg	5	4.3	3
6–15 kg	5.7	5	3.5
15–20 kg	6.7	6	4
20–25 kg	7.8	7.1	5
25–35 kg	8.2	7.5	6

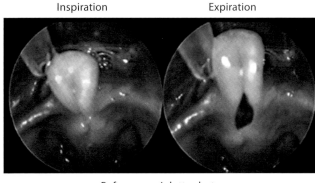

Before aryepiglottoplasty

After aryepiglottoplasty

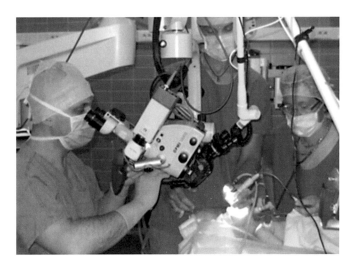

Fig. 5. Laryngoscopy and laser CO_2 microsurgery. Laryngomalacia before and after aryepiglottoplasty.

glottis, the subglottis and the trachea, as well as the superior oesophagus. If necessary, endoscopic surgical treatment can be performed during rigid laryngotracheoscopy. The main paediatric laryngeal pathologies [chapter 11, this vol., pp. 120–129] are discussed below with an emphasis on the use of rigid laryngoscopy in their diagnosis and treatment.

Laryngomalacia

Laryngomalacia constitutes the major cause of congenital stridor, accounting for approximately 75% of all cases [4]. Laryngomalacia is usually diagnosed by flexible laryngoscopy. Rigid laryngoscopy is useful in the evaluation of laryngomalacia: firstly when an associated airway anomaly such as a laryngeal cleft is suspected, and secondly when laryngomalacia requires endoscopic surgical treatment.

In most cases, laryngomalacia resolves spontaneously by 2 years of age. Yet, in 11.6% of cases, surgery is still required when symptoms indicating severe disease such as chronic respiratory insufficiency, growth delay or apnoeic spells are present [5].

Aryepiglottoplasty is currently the standard procedure for severe laryngomalacia; it entails resection of

aryepiglottic folds and the mucosa over the arytenoids and excision of accessory arytenoid cartilages or of the lateral border of the epiglottis (fig. 5). The extent of the procedure depends on the location of tissue prolapsing into the airway. Several methods have been described to perform aryepiglottoplasty: cold steel dissection, CO_2 laser, KTP (potassium-titanyl-phosphate) laser and microdebrider. Other surgical techniques used to treat laryngomalacia include laser epiglottopexy and epiglottic suturing [6, 7]. The aim of the latter methods is to reduce epiglottic obstruction. Thanks to the development of endoscopic surgical procedures, severe laryngomalacia rarely requires tracheostomy.

Vocal Cord Paralysis

This is the second most frequent cause of stridor in neonates after laryngomalacia [8]. Laryngeal paralysis can be unilateral or bilateral. Diagnosis can be made either by flexible or by rigid laryngoscopy under general anaesthesia with spontaneous breathing.

Bilateral abductor muscle paralysis results in adduction of both vocal cords and closure of the glottis with severe dyspnoea that requires urgent treatment. In half of the cases, paediatric bilateral laryngeal paralysis resolves spontaneously but tracheostomy may still be required sometimes [8]. Several surgical treatments have been suggested to avoid tracheostomy: enlarged laryngoplasty, arytenoidopexy, arytenoidectomy and lateral posterior partial cordotomy. Rigid laryngoscopy is used to perform arytenoidectomy or cordotomy. This endoscopic technique uses CO_2 laser (online suppl. video 1) or KTP laser [9, 10]. Because of the relatively small size of the larynx in children, cordotomy usually suffices for airway enlargement. A second cordotomy, ipsilateral or bilateral, is indicated if one surgical session is not sufficient.

Endoscopic cordotomy is currently the procedure of choice for the treatment of bilateral abductor paralysis. This is a minimally invasive technique that provides no functional sequelae. It can be proposed even if the patient is expected to recover later [10]. Cordotomy is preferred to tracheostomy because of the deleterious effects of tracheostomy in the child such as tracheal stenosis and tracheomalacia.

Haemangioma
Usually symptoms of airway obstruction due to haemangiomas are not present at birth but arise in the first 3 months of life because of the haemangioma's natural history (a phase of rapid growth between 3 and 12 months of age, then a gradual involution leading to complete resolution before the age of 7 years in 70% of cases) [11].

Laryngoscopy (rigid or flexible) establishes the diagnosis and assesses the size and the location of the haemangioma. In many cases, the lesion is located in the left posterolateral wall of the subglottis (fig. 6). Laryngoscopy should not be preceded by systemic corticosteroid administration because corticosteroids can lead to virtually complete transient regression of the haemangioma, thus making the diagnosis difficult.

Because of the natural evolution and benign character of the lesion, some cases do not require treatment. Tracheostomy was initially the treatment of choice in cases of severe airway obstruction. A variety of medical and surgical treatment options exist but no consensus has yet been established. Many patients undergo different types of treatments during the course of their disease. Currently, endoscopic treatment is the best surgical option for symptomatic non-circumferential haemangiomas. Open surgical excision or medical treatment (corticosteroids, interferon, vincristine and, recently, propanolol) are preferred in case of symptomatic bilateral or circumferential haemangiomas [12]. Rigid laryngoscopy is used to perform several types of endoscopic treatment: laser, microdebrider and intralesional injection. Commonly

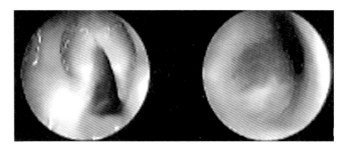

Fig. 6. Left subglottic haemangioma.

used methods include CO_2, YAG (yttrium-aluminium-garnet), KTP, thulium and diode (formed from a positive-negative junction and powered by injected electric current) laser [chapter 6, this vol., pp. 64–74]. The YAG laser and KTP laser are preferentially absorbed by haemoglobin. Therefore, they are preferred for the treatment of haemangiomas as they theoretically decrease the risk of stenosis [13]. Laser treatment requires several endoscopic sessions to obtain complete resection or to excise granulomas or adhesions. The use of the endoscopic microdebrider to excise haemangiomas appears to reduce the risk of subglottic stenosis [14]. Intralesional steroid injection through the rigid laryngoscope has also been reported to be successful but administration of systemic steroids and intubation for variable lengths of time may be required when using this treatment modality [15].

Papillomatosis
Recurrent respiratory papillomatosis is the most common benign tumour of the larynx among children, whereas haemangioma is the most common paediatric tumour when all other possible localizations (e.g. skin, oral mucosa) are considered [11]. Laryngeal papillomas are very challenging to manage because of their tendency to recur [16].

Following voice change, stridor is the second most common symptom. Other symptoms include cough, recurrent pneumonia, dyspnoea, acute respiratory distress, dysphagia and failure to thrive.

Rigid laryngoscopy allows biopsy and then removal of the lesion (fig. 7). Repeated endoscopic debulking is currently the treatment of choice. The goal is to maintain a safe airway with preservation of normal vocal cord anatomy and avoid complications such as stenosis or web formation. Several methods of debulking can be used that entail use of cold instruments, microdebrider, CO_2 laser, KTP laser, argon laser and thulium laser. However, no treatment is entirely effective in eradicating respiratory papillomatosis. Indeed, the latent virus remains in the tissue even when

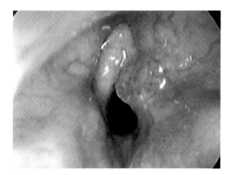

Fig. 7. Laryngeal papillomatosis at the supraglottic and glottic level.

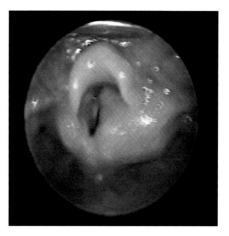

Fig. 8. Supraglottic cyst involving the right aryepiglottic cord and arytenoid.

Table 2. Benjamin and Inglis [20] classification of laryngotracheal clefts

Type	Laryngotracheal defect
I	Supraglottic interarytenoid defect; the level of the cleft remains above the level of the (true) vocal cords
II	The cleft extends below the level of the (true) vocal cords and partially into the cricoid cartilage
III	The cleft extends completely through the posterior cricoid cartilage, with or without further extension into the cervical tracheo-oesophageal wall
IV	Common tracheo-oesophagus that extends into the thorax and may extend all the way down the carina

all the clinically apparent papilloma has been removed. Adjuvant therapy should be considered when the patient needs more than 4 surgical debulking procedures per year [17]. Intralesional injection of cidofovir (an antiviral agent) through a rigid laryngoscope may help control regrowth of papillomas [18].

Laryngotracheal Cleft

Laryngotracheal cleft is an uncommon congenital malformation defined by an anomalous connexion between the larynx or trachea and the oesophagus. This malformation is associated with other congenital abnormalities in 50% of cases [19].

Four types of posterior laryngeal clefts of increasing gravity are distinguished (table 2) [20]. Diagnosis of type I laryngeal clefts is difficult because symptoms are usually non-specific and include delayed aspiration with fluid ingestion (due to excessive passage of fluids into the glottis through the defect of the interarytenoid region, even with intact vocal cords), chronic cough and stridor. For the other types, symptoms are severer, including recurrent pneumonia and cyanotic attacks during feeds. Type I laryngeal clefts may be difficult to visualize during endoscopy and necessitate suspension laryngoscopy with bimanual interarytenoid palpation.

Management of type I laryngeal clefts is controversial and may require either medical treatment (antireflux therapy, thickened fluids, nasogastric tube feeding and gastrostomy) or endoscopic repair via rigid laryngoscopy [21]. Laryngeal cleft types II–IV require either rigid-tube endoscopy or open surgical repair. Endoscopic repair has low morbidity and complication rates, whereas open surgery is reserved for extensive clefts and revision surgery. Various endoscopic techniques have been described for treating laryngeal clefts: endoscopic mucosal resection with suturing of the interarytenoid region, and CO_2 laser excision of the posterior side of the arytenoids with Gelfoam injection [21, 22]. Rigid airway endoscopy is essential in order to establish the diagnosis, perform endoscopic treatment, and check the larynx and trachea after surgery in case of open surgical repair of the cleft.

Laryngeal Cyst

Prematurity and a history of prolonged intubation in the neonatal period are the two risk factors for the development of laryngeal cysts; consequently the incidence of this disorder is increasing [23].

Rigid laryngoscopy is the gold standard for the management of laryngeal cysts (fig. 8). Treatment consists of

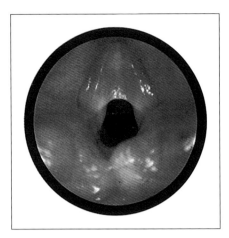

Fig. 9. Type II laryngeal web.

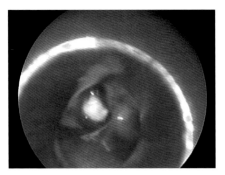

Fig. 10. Foreign body (fragment of a nut) in the right lower lobe bronchus (online suppl. video 2).   ▮ideo

Table 3. Classification of Cohen [26] of laryngeal webs

Type	Glottic web
I	Anterior glottic web involving less than 1/3 of the vocal cords, without subglottic extension
II	Anterior glottic web involving up to 50% of the vocal cords, with anterior subglottic extension
III	Glottic web involving up to 75% of the vocal cords, with subglottic extension
IV	Glottic web involving up to 90% of the vocal cords which appear fused; it can be associated with cricoid cartilage or laryngotracheal anomalies (laryngeal atresia)

marsupialization, which entails wide opening of the walls of the cyst by using cold steel micro-instruments, CO_2 laser or microdebrider. Nevertheless, despite adequate marsupialization, cysts are recurrent in nature with a recurrence rate of up to 43% [24, 25].

Laryngeal Web
Laryngeal webs are congenital malformations in which there is abnormal tissue between two structures within the larynx. The most common site of involvement is the anterior glottis (fig. 9).

Cohen [26] proposed a classification (table 3) based on web location and grade of airway obstruction. Endoscopic treatment through a rigid laryngoscope is the method of choice for type I and for some type II laryngeal webs.

Rigid Bronchoscopy

Rigid bronchoscopy is performed under general anaesthesia with spontaneous or assisted ventilation (fig. 4) [chapter 2, this vol., pp. 22–29]. The size of the bronchoscope is selected according to the weight of the child in order to avoid trauma of the airway (table 1).

Flexible bronchoscopy is able to diagnose most tracheobronchial abnormalities [chapter 12, this vol., pp. 130–140]; therefore, the main benefit of rigid bronchoscopy in children is currently its therapeutic use. There are two advantages of rigid bronchoscopy over its flexible counterpart: the large diameter of the working channel and the ability to maintain proper ventilation during surgery.

Extraction of aspirated foreign bodies is the most frequent indication for paediatric rigid bronchoscopy.

Foreign-Body Aspiration
Foreign-body aspiration is a frequent cause of acute respiratory distress in children. Therefore, early diagnosis and prompt extraction of the foreign body can be life-saving.

Foreign bodies are most frequently of vegetable origin, lodged in the right main or lower lobe bronchus (fig. 10) [27]. More than two thirds of the cases occur in children younger than 3 years of age, and there is male predominance. The clinical presentation is characterized by the foreign-body aspiration syndrome (choking and cyanotic spell, followed by cough and subsequent symptom relief). If the foreign body is lodged in one of the main stem bronchi, clinical examination reveals unilaterally decreased breath sounds and/or localized wheezing and crackles. Chest radiographs in inspiration and expiration can demonstrate air-trapping, atelectasis, pulmonary infiltrates or a radio-opaque foreign body [28]. Yet, confirmation or ruling-out of the diagnosis requires airway inspection, especially in cases of suspected aspiration with lack of clinical and/or radiographic changes. Flexible bronchoscopy has a diagnostic accuracy of 100% but a very limited therapeutic role, with a case resolution of only 10.7% [29]. On the other hand, rigid bronchoscopy has a high rate of negative findings when performed for suspected foreign-body aspiration in the absence of relevant clinical and radiological signs [29]. Consequently, when the diagnosis is equivocal, flexible bronchoscopy should be performed first. The role of multidetector computed tomography (CT) and virtual bronchoscopy in the diagnosis of foreign bodies is discussed in chapter 9 of this volume. Briefly, although virtual bronchoscopy has a sensitivity of 100% in diagnosing foreign body aspiration, there are false-positive findings (e.g. obstruction by mucus plug); however, normal multidetector CT findings essentially rule out foreign-body aspiration [30].

Rigid bronchoscopy under general anaesthesia is currently the standard treatment for aspirated foreign bodies. Extraction is carried out with the rigid bronchoscope using a large range of grasping forceps according to the nature and the dimensions of the foreign body, under telescopic guidance, while the airway is secured. After extraction of the foreign body, the bronchoscope is reinserted to look for retained fragments or mucus (online suppl. video 2). For extraction of more peripheral foreign bodies, inaccessible by the rigid-tube bronchoscope, the flexible bronchoscope can be introduced into the lumen of the rigid tube, thus allowing simultaneous ventilation through the rigid bronchoscope.

Complications of rigid bronchoscopy for aspirated foreign bodies are rare; they include pneumothorax, pneumomediastinum, tracheal laceration, subglottic oedema and hypoxic arrest [28].

Tracheo-Oesophageal Fistula
Congenital tracheo-oesophageal fistula (TOF) is most commonly associated with oesophageal atresia (fig. 11). The Gross anatomical classification of congenital tracheo-oesophageal anomalies includes 5 types of disorders (table 4) [31]. Additional congenital abnormalities occur in one third to one half of cases [chapter 12, this vol., pp. 130–140].

The classical triad of symptoms of the H-type TOF includes: cough and cyanosis during feeding, abdominal distension and recurrent pneumonia or bronchitis. Diagnosis is most commonly made with an oesophagogram performed using a contrast agent administered orally or by a feeding tube. Repeat studies are sometimes required to visualize the TOF so at least 2 examinations are

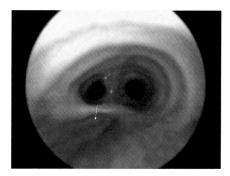

Fig. 11. Tracheomalacia and TOF (arrow) associated with oesophageal atresia (online suppl. video 4).

Table 4. Gross classification of oesophageal atresia (OA) and TOF

Type	Lesion
A	Isolated OA
B	OA with proximal TOF
C	OA with distal TOF
D	OA with proximal and distal TOF
E	Isolated H-type TOF (without OA)

recommended to increase the sensitivity of the oesophagogram. Rigid or flexible endoscopy (tracheobronchoscopy and oesophagoscopy) may also be diagnostic of H-type TOF (online suppl. video 3). Pre-operative rigid bronchoscopy is useful for catheterizing the TOF in order to help intra-operative localization. Oesophagography and endoscopy complement each other in the diagnosis and management of TOF [32].

Open surgical repair is the standard treatment of H-type TOF; however, repeat repair via an open thoracotomy is associated with 50% morbidity and a 10–22% refistulization rate [33]. Endoscopic repair of H-type TOF has been reported recently. Rigid bronchoscopy allows laser closing (KTP) or fibrin glue injection [33, 34]. The endoscopic approach as compared to the open procedure appears to decrease morbidity and allows rapid recovery.

Tracheobronchial Obstruction
Obstruction of the tracheobronchial tree can appear in a variety of situations such as tracheomalacia, bronchomalacia, external compression, stenosis and internal lesion [chapter 12, this vol., pp. 130–140]. Airway malacia and stenosis are the most frequent diagnoses in the paediatric population.

Video

Tracheomalacia, Bronchomalacia, External Compression
Paediatric tracheo- and/or bronchomalacia can be acquired or congenital. Acquired malacia is usually caused by long-term tracheostomy. Congenital malacia is sometimes isolated but most commonly associated with oesophageal atresia (fig. 11) or external compression of the airway. Vascular rings are the most common cause of external compression. The diagnosis of a vascular ring can be suspected with bronchoscopy, either flexible or rigid, but its anatomy is described by CT scan or magnetic resonance imaging [chapter 9, this vol., pp. 95–112]. Airway endoscopy can diagnose coexisting airway lesions such as laryngomalacia and evaluate pre-operative vocal cord motion. Surgical treatment of vascular rings can be accomplished by open thoracotomy or thoracoscopic repair.

Symptoms of tracheo- and/or bronchomalacia are variable and non-specific, and include recurrent wheeze, cough, recurrent lower airway infections, exercise intolerance, severe dyspnoea and respiratory insufficiency. Therefore, airway malacia may be confused with asthma; therefore, bronchoscopy is recommended in patients with therapy-resistant or atypical asthma. Flexible bronchoscopy is the method of choice for diagnosing malacia. Malacia is defined as a collapse of at least 50% of the airway lumen during expiration, cough or spontaneous breathing, or a ratio of cartilage to membranous wall area of less than 3:1 [chapter 9, this vol., pp. 95–112].

In most cases, symptoms are moderate, and conservative management is sufficient. However, management of severe malacia remains challenging. Correction of associated oesophageal atresia, relief of external compression, tracheostomy and aortopexy (a surgical procedure in which the aortic arch is fixated to the sternum and results in the tracheal lumen being pulled open) are current surgical options in the treatment of severe tracheo- and/or bronchomalacia. Airway stent placement during rigid bronchoscopy has been recently introduced in paediatrics [35]. Several types of stents are available such as metallic, balloon-expandable and silicone stents. However, complications including granulation tissue formation and stent migration are not uncommon. This method is still experimental and cannot be considered as a substitute for open surgical treatment as yet. Airway stenting can be considered when aortopexy has failed [36].

Tracheal Stenosis
Tracheal stenosis is the narrowing of the tracheal lumen and can be long- or short-segment, congenital or acquired. Congenital tracheal stenosis is often associated with

Table 5. Cantrell and Guild [37] classification of congenital tracheal stenosis

Type	Stenosis
I	Generalized hypoplasia; total tracheal involvement with normal bronchi and distal airway
II	Funnel-like stenosis; gradual tapering of the airway with normal subglottis and stenotic carinal end of the trachea
III	Segmental stenosis; involvement of 2–3 cartilage rings

cardiovascular and/or other respiratory anomalies. The anatomical classification by Cantrell and Guild [37] has identified three types of tracheal stenosis (table 5). The clinical presentation of congenital tracheal stenosis is variable, and the severity of symptoms correlates with the degree of airway obstruction, ranging from asymptomatic to respiratory distress. Bronchoscopy, either flexible or rigid, is the gold standard for establishing a definitive diagnosis; it can visualize the presence of complete cartilage rings and provide information on the length and the diameter of the stenosis. Multidetector CT with external rendering and virtual bronchoscopy can accurately describe the stenosis [36; chapter 9, this vol., pp. 95–112].

The management of tracheal stenosis depends on clinical expression, the anatomical pattern of the stenosis and associated anomalies [38]. Conservative treatment is often an option, while surgical treatment includes segmental resection with end-to-end anastomosis for short-segment stenosis and tracheoplasty for long-segment stenosis. Endoscopic techniques through the rigid bronchoscope are mainly used for the management of postoperative complications such as recurrence of stenosis and formation of granulation tissue. These methods include endoscopic dilatation, laser resection and tracheal stenting. Endoscopic dilatation and laser resection (online suppl. video 4) can be attempted first in ■Video selected cases of short-segment tracheal stenosis [38]. Airway stenting after laryngotracheoplasty has recently been developed using silicone prostheses. These stents seem to be well tolerated, avoiding granulation tissue and recurrence of stenosis [39].

Tracheal granuloma is a frequent cause of failure to decannulate the child with tracheostomy. Several endoscopic methods have been described for the management of such granulomas by rigid bronchoscopy, which include cold steel micro-instruments, KTP laser, YAG laser and, more recently, CO_2 laser with a fibre-optic carrier [40].

Table 6. Advantages and disadvantages of flexible (FB) and rigid bronchoscopy (RB)

	Advantages	Drawbacks
FB	Better exploration of distal airway May avoid general anaesthesia Useful for less invasive therapeutic procedure	Lower lighting and quality of images Not efficient for complex therapeutic procedures (extraction of foreign bodies, debulking)
RB	Better exploration of proximal airway Secures the airway in case of obstruction Useful for complex therapeutic procedures	General anaesthesia required Increased risk of complications Impossible to perform in case of cervical spine lesions

Tracheal tumours are rare in childhood. Rigid bronchoscopy may be useful for the diagnosis and treatment of these tumours. The treatment of choice is removal of the tumor via open thoracotomy. Endoscopic excision can be used when open surgery is not feasible [41, 42].

Tracheal Trauma

Tracheal injury is rare in children because of their anatomical characteristics (short neck and soft cartilages) but the small size of the paediatric airway increases the risk of obstruction. Causes are multiple: blunt trauma (bicycle handle bar), penetrating trauma or an aspirated foreign body. However, in most cases the trauma is iatrogenic, i.e. due to intubation or endoscopy [43].

The most frequent symptoms are respiratory distress, subcutaneous emphysema, stridor and haemoptysis. Chest radiography and CT scan may reveal pneumomediastinum and tracheal rupture. As a rule, any suspicion of airway rupture associated with respiratory distress is an indication of immediate tracheobronchoscopy, even before performing any imaging examination. Rigid bronchoscopy is preferred to flexible bronchoscopy because the former can secure the airway, while ventilating the patient and removing blood clots. Moreover, oesophagoscopy can be performed at the same time. It is worth noting that blunt cervical trauma can result in cervical spinal lesions, which have to be excluded prior to any manipulation of the neck. The severity of tracheal lesions can vary from mucosal laceration to laryngotracheal separation. Treatment depends on the severity of the lesions and clinical stability of the patient. Simple observation is possible in cases of minor injury without respiratory or infectious complications [44, 45]. Alternative approaches include endotracheal intubation beyond the lesion under laryngoscopic control, tracheostomy and open surgical repair with or without airway stenting [45].

Thus, rigid bronchoscopy is useful in the management of tracheal trauma in several ways: primary evaluation of the lesion, securing of the airway and treatment of long-term complications such as granulation tissue and stenosis.

Flexible versus Rigid Bronchoscopy

Flexible bronchoscopy is a more appropriate procedure to explore the distal airway, whereas rigid bronchoscopy allows more complete visualization of the proximal airway (posterior aspects of the larynx and trachea).

Flexible bronchoscopy is more efficient than rigid bronchoscopy for diagnostic exploration and for less invasive therapeutic procedures such as biopsy [chapter 4, this vol., pp. 42–53], bronchoalveolar lavage [chapter 3, this vol., pp. 30–41], aspiration of blood clots or mucus plugs [chapter 4] and endoscopic intubation [chapter 4]. This technique may avoid general anaesthesia and the potential complications of rigid bronchoscopy [chapter 2, this vol., pp. 22–29].

Rigid bronchoscopy in children is an ideal method for securing the airway in case of obstruction because the hollow rigid bronchoscope allows ventilation through its lumen. Moreover, complex therapeutic procedures such as extraction of foreign bodies, laser treatment, dilatation, tumour debulking and stenting can only be performed with the rigid bronchoscope. However, rigid bronchoscopy may expose the child to important complications, i.e. pneumothorax, pneumomediastinum, subglottic oedema or bronchospasm, and complications of general anaesthesia; these are, fortunately, quite rare.

Hence, the indications for flexible bronchoscopy are mainly diagnostic whereas the role of rigid bronchoscopy is principally therapeutic. The selection of flexible versus rigid bronchoscopy depends on the indication (diagnosis vs. therapy) and disease location (proximal vs. distal airway; table 6). The two endoscopic methods often complement each other. Paediatric rigid bronchoscopy presents certain risks and requires an experienced team. Therefore, the best approach for pre-operative airway exploration and endoscopic treatment has to be discussed on a case-by-case basis by a multidisciplinary team that includes the paediatric pulmonologist, the otorhinolaryngologist and the anaesthetist.

Future Trends

In the last decade, the development of various technologies has improved the therapeutic role of rigid bronchoscopy. However, the management of paediatric pathologies such as tracheobronchomalacia and tracheal stenosis remains a challenge. Airway stents, especially silicone-type stents, seem to be an effective and safe option in the treatment of such pathologies. In our opinion, endoscopic airway stenting through rigid bronchoscopy is a promising technique for the management of complex cases of tracheobronchial obstruction in children. In addition, virtual bronchoscopy is increasingly utilized in the diagnosis of airway disease,

especially in suspected foreign-body aspiration; its use may help to rule out foreign body, thus avoiding an invasive procedure such as bronchoscopy in selected cases.

Of course, new diagnostic and therapeutic technologies or their paediatric applications are not readily available in many medical institutions due to their high cost and the expertise required. Their broader dissemination in the future will help to optimize the management of children with airway disease.

Acknowledgements

We gratefully acknowledge Dr. Yves Pra and Dr. Victoria North for their contribution to this work.

Conflict of Interest

The authors declare no conflict of interest whatsoever with any company.

References

1 Carron JD, Derkay CS, Strope GL, Nosonchuk JE, Darrow DH: Pediatric tracheotomies: changing indications and outcomes. Laryngoscope 2000;110:1099–1104.

2 Carr MM, Poje CP, Kingston L, Kielma D, Heard C: Complications in pediatric tracheostomies. Laryngoscope 2001;111:1925–1928.

3 Zur KB, Wood RE, Elluru RG: Pediatric postcricoid vascular malformation: a diagnostic and treatment challenge. Int J Pediatr Otorhinolaryngol 2005;69:1697–1701.

4 Zoumalan R, Maddalozzo J, Holinger LD: Etiology of stridor in infants. Ann Otol Rhinol Laryngol 2007;116:329–334.

5 Roger G, Denoyelle F, Triglia JM, Garabedian EN: Severe laryngomalacia: surgical indications and results in 115 patients. Laryngoscope 1995;105:1111–1117.

6 Whymark AD, Clement WA, Kubba H, Geddes NK: Laser epiglottopexy for laryngomalacia: 10 years' experience in the west of Scotland. Arch Otolaryngol Head Neck Surg 2006;132:978–982.

7 Fajdiga I, Beden AB, Krivec U, Iglic C: Epiglottic suture for treatment of laryngomalacia. Int J Pediatr Otorhinolaryngol 2008;72:1345–1351.

8 De Gaudemar I, Roudaire M, François M, Narcy P: Outcome of laryngeal paralysis in neonates: a long term retrospective study of 113 cases. Int J Pediatr Otorhinolaryngol 1996;34:101–110.

9 Friedman EM, de Jong AL, Sulek M: Pediatric bilateral vocal fold immobility: the role of carbon dioxide laser posterior transverse partial cordectomy. Ann Otol Rhinol Laryngol 2001;110:723–728.

10 Lagier A, Nicollas R, Sanjuan M, Benoit L, Triglia JM: Laser cordotomy for the treatment of bilateral vocal cord paralysis in infants. Int J Pediatr Otorhinolaryngol 2009;73:9–13.

11 Denoyelle F (ed): Angiome sous-glottique et tracheal du nourrisson. ORL de l'enfant, éd 2. Paris, Médecine-Science Flammarion, 2006.

12 Denoyelle F, Leboulanger N, Enjolras O, Harris R, Roger G, Garabedian EN: Role of propanolol in the therapeutic strategy of infantile laryngotracheal haemangioma. Int J Pediatr Otorhinolaryngol 2009;73:1168–1172.

13 Rahbar R, Nicolas R, Roger G, Triglia JM, Garabedian EN, McGill TJ, Healy GB: The biology and management of subglottic haemangioma: past, present, future. Laryngoscope 2004;114:1880–1891.

14 Pransky SM, Canto C: Management of subglottic hemangioma. Curr Opin Otolaryngol Head Neck Surg 2004;12:509–512.

15 Bitar MA, Moukarbel RV, Zalzal GH: Management of congenital subglottic hemangioma: trends and success over the past 17 years. Otolaryngol Head Neck Surg 2005;132:226–231.

16 Pransky SM, Kang DR: Tumors of the Larynx and Bronchi; in Bluestone CD, Stool SE, Kenna MA (eds): Pediatric Otolaryngology, ed 3. Philadelphia, WB Saunders Co., 2003, vol 2.

17 Derkay CS, Wiatrak B: Recurrent respiratory papillomatosis: a review. Laryngoscope 2008;118:1236–1247.

18 Bielecki I, Mniszek J, Cofala M: Intralesional injection of cidofovir for recurrent respiratory papillomatosis in children. Int J Pediatr Otorhinolaryngol 2009;73:681–684.

19 Rahbar R, Rouillon I, Roger G, Lin A, Nuss RC, Denoyelle F, McGill TJ, Healy GB, Garabedian EN: The presentation and management of laryngeal cleft: a 10-year experience. Arch Otolaryngol Head Neck Surg 2006;132:1335–1341.

20 Benjamin B, Inglis A: Minor congenital laryngeal clefts: diagnosis and classification. Ann Otol Rhinol Laryngol 1989;98:417–420.

21 Chien W, Ashland J, Haver K, Hardy SC, Curren P, Hartnick CJ: Type 1 laryngeal cleft: establishing a functional diagnostic and management algorithm. Int J Pediatr Otorhinolaryngol 2006;70:2073–2079.

22 Rahbar R, Chen JL, Rosen RL, Lowry KC, Simon DM, Perez JA, Buonomo C, Ferrari LR, Katz ES: Endoscopic repair of laryngeal cleft type I and type II: when and why? Laryngoscope 2009;119:1797–1802.

23 Watson GJ, Malik TH, Khan NA, Sheehan PZ, Rothera MP: Acquired pediatric subglottic cyst: a series from Manchester. Int J Pediatr Otorhinolaryngol 2007;71:533–538.

24 Jaryszak EM, Collins WO: Microdebrider resection of bilateral subglottic cysts in a pre-term infant: a novel approach. Int J Pediatr Otorhinolaryngol 2009;73:139–142.

25 Lim J, Hellier W, Harcourt J, Leighton S, Albert D: Subglottic cysts: the Great Ormond Street experience. Int J Pediatr Otorhinolaryngol 2003;67:461–465.

26 Cohen SR: Congenital glottic webs in children: a retrospective review of 51 patients. Ann Otol Rhinol Laryngol 1985;121:2–16.

27 Heyer CM, Bollmeier ME, Rossler L, Nuesslein TG, Stephan V, Bauer TT, Rieger CH: Evaluation of clinical, radiologic and laboratory prebronchoscopy findings in children with suspected foreign body aspiration. J Pediatr Surg 2006;41:1882–1888.

28 Divisi D, Di Tommaso S, Garramone M, Di Francescantonio W, Crisci RM, Costa AM, Gravina GL, Crisci R: Foreign bodies aspirated in children: role of bronchoscopy. Thorac Cardiovasc Surg 2007;55:249–252.

29 Righini CA, Morel N, Karkas A, Reyt E, Ferretti K, Pin I, Schmerber S: What is the diagnostic value of flexible bronchoscopy in the initial investigation of children with suspected foreign body aspiration? Int J Pediatr Otorhinolaryngol 2007;71:1383–1390.

30 Cevizci N, Dokucu AI, Baskin D, Karadağ CA, Sever N, Yalçin M, Bahadir E, Başak M: Virtual bronchoscopy as a dynamic modality in the diagnosis and treatment of suspected foreign body aspiration. Eur J Pediatr Surg 2008;18:398–401.

31 Gross R: Tracheoesophageal fistula in newborn infants and infants. Pol Przegl Chir 1976;48:45–49.

32 Willetts IE, Dudley NE, Tam PK: Endoscopic treatment of recurrent tracheo-oesophageal fistulae: long-term results. Pediatr Surg Int 1998;13:256–258.

33 Meier JD, Sulman CG, Almond PS, Holinger LD: Endoscopic management of recurrent congenital tracheoesophageal fistula: a review of techniques and results. Int J Pediatr Otorhinolaryngol 2007;71:691–697.

34 Ishman SL, Kerschner JE, Rudolph CD: The KTP laser: an emerging tool in pediatric otolaryngology. Int J Pediatr Otorhinolaryngol 2006;70:677–682.

35 Anton-Pacheco JL, Cabezali D, Tejedor R, Lopez M, Luna C, Comas JV, de Miguel E: The role of airway stenting in pediatric tracheobronchial obstruction. Eur J Cardiothorac Surg 2008;33:1069–1075.

36 Hoppe H, Dinkel HP, Walder B, von Allmen G, Gugger M, Vock P: Grading airway stenosis down to the segmental level using virtual bronchoscopy. Chest 2004;125:704–711.

37 Cantrell JR, Guild HG: Congenital stenosis of the trachea. Am J Surg 1964;108:297–305.

38 Anton-Pacheco JL, Garcia-Hernandez G, Villafruela MA: The management of tracheobronchial obstruction in children. Minerva Pediatr 2009;61:39–52.

39 Monnier P: Airway stenting with the LT-Mold: experience in 30 pediatric cases. Int J Pediatr Otorhinolaryngol 2007;71:1351–1359.

40 Shires CB, Shete MM, Thompson JW: Management of suprastomal tracheal fibroma: introduction of a new technique and comparison with other techniques. Int J Pediatr Otorhinolaryngol 2009;73:67–72.

41 Pernas FG, Younis RT, Lehman DA, Robinson PG: Management of pediatric airway granular cell tumor: role of laryngotracheal reconstruction. Int J Pediatr Otorhinolaryngol 2006;70:957–963.

42 Conforti S, Bonacina E, Ravini M, Torre M: A case of fibrous histiocytoma of the trachea in an infant treated by endobronchial Nd:YAG laser. Lung Cancer 2007;57:112–114.

43 Borasio P, Ardissone F, Chiampo G: Post-intubation tracheal rupture: a report on ten cases. Eur J Cardiothorac Surg 1997;12:98–100.

44 d'Odemont JP, Pringot J, Goncette L, Goenen M, Rodenstein DO: Spontaneous favorable outcome of tracheal laceration. Chest 1991;99:1290–1292.

45 Kelley R, Reynders A, Seidberg N: Nonsurgical management of pediatric tracheal perforation. Ann Otol Rhinol Laryngol 2006;115:408–411.

Christian Adrien Righini
Department of Otorhinolaryngology, Head and Neck Surgery
Albert Michallon University Hospital
FR–38043 Grenoble Cedex 09 (France)
Tel. +33 4 76 76 56 93, Fax +33 4 76 76 51 20, E-Mail CRighini@chu-grenoble.fr

Chapter 9

Priftis KN, Anthracopoulos MB, Eber E, Koumbourlis AC, Wood RE (eds): Paediatric Bronchoscopy.
Prog Respir Res. Basel, Karger 2010, vol 38, pp 95–112

Virtual Bronchoscopy and Other Three-Dimensional Imaging Methods

Michael B. Anthracopoulos[a] · Efthymia Alexopoulou[c] · George C. Kagadis[b]

[a]Respiratory Unit, Department of Paediatrics, University Hospital of Patras, and [b]Department of Medical Physics, School of Medicine, University of Patras, Patras, and [c]2nd Department of Radiology, Attikon University Hospital, Medical School of Athens, Athens, Greece

Abstract

Flexible bronchoscopy (FB) is the only method that permits real-time direct visualization and dynamic evaluation of the tracheobronchial system. Multidetector computed tomography (MDCT) scanners can generate accurate 2-dimensional (multiplanar reformation) and 3-dimensional (multiplanar volume reconstruction, external volume rendering, VR, and virtual bronchoscopy, VB) images of the airways. Patient breath-holding in suspended inspiration is important but with the new faster scanners volume coverage during quiet breathing can achieve high-quality images. The new imaging techniques offer distinct advantages over FB that include: accurate mapping of airway compression or stenosis, visualization of the airway beyond the area of obstruction, evaluation of smaller airways, and imaging of parenchymal and mediastinal abnormalities. External VR and VB can delineate congenital defects such as pulmonary underdevelopment spectrum, tracheobronchial branching anomalies, tracheo-oesophageal fistula, sequestration spectrum and vascular rings. High-resolution CT is used to evaluate bronchiectasis and air-trapping due to small-airway disease. Newer-generation MDCT scanners can be used to assess dynamic collapse of the airways. Radiation exposure remains a concern in CT; patient- and disease-specific dose reduction should be implemented according to the ALARA ('as low as reasonably achievable') principle. Alternative techniques such as magnetic resonance imaging should be considered.

Flexible bronchoscopy (FB) is considered the gold standard for the detection and diagnosis of tracheobronchial disorders in children permitting direct visualization and dynamic evaluation of the airway lumen. Although safe, it is still an invasive procedure that requires patient sedation and cannot be used to evaluate airway morphology beyond high-grade stenosis of the bronchial lumen [1; chapter 2, this vol., pp. 22–29]. In clinical practice, FB is often combined with computed tomography (CT) scanning of the chest for more comprehensive evaluation of the airways and lung parenchyma.

In the last 20 years, a true revolution in CT technology has made possible non-invasive imaging of the airways. Conventional 'stop-and-shoot' CT that required long scan times with a single data set per breath-hold evolved into helical (spiral) CT that reduced acquisition time and minimized misregistration due to variation in the depth of respiration as well as respiratory and cardiac motion artefacts. More recently, multidetector (multislice) CT (MDCT) that employs multiple rows of detectors – currently 16- and 64-slice MDCT scanners are widely used, while 128-, 256- and, recently, 320-slice scanners are being actively marketed – along with other technical advancements have made true isotropic imaging of large volumes possible within a few seconds [2, 3]. MDCT provides continuous and complete sets of raw data that are transferred to a picture-archiving and communication system or 3-dimensional workstation for post-processing and analysis. Once the final volumetric data set is obtained, a variety of computer algorithms can be applied to generate accurate 2- or 3-dimensional images by utilizing the information obtained by the scan [2, 4]. The radiological technical terms used in this chapter are explained, in alphabetical order, in the Appendix.

Magnetic resonance imaging (MRI) is an attractive alternative to MDCT because of lack of patient exposure to radiation, fewer adverse reactions to intravenous contrast material (due to the use of non-iodine-based contrast materials), inherently higher soft tissue contrast and ability to perform functional studies. Its main drawbacks are a considerably

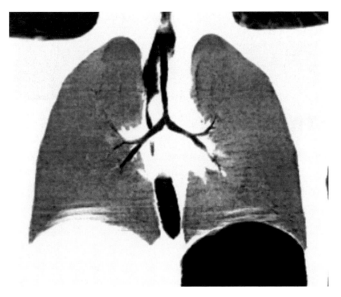

Fig. 1. Curved plane minimum intensity projection image showing the trachea and major bronchi of a 4-year-old girl with ring-sling syndrome. There is progressive worsening of tracheal stenosis from the central part of the trachea down to the level of the main carina. The calibres of the main bronchi appear normal.

longer acquisition time that requires sedation (and in prolonged examinations general anaesthesia) of young children, inferior spatial resolution of lung parenchyma (even with the most current state-of-the-art MRI technology), higher compromise in the presence of metallic devices and a relatively high cost. With technical evolution, MRI may one day replace CT in the evaluation of various congenital and acquired lung disorders but currently it is not commonly used in the evaluation of childhood airway disease [2].

Multidetector Computed Tomography Imaging of the Airways

The axial images obtained with MDCT contain the entire volume data set but have several limitations, including: (a) limited ability to detect subtle airway stenosis; (b) underestimation of the craniocaudad extent of disease; (c) difficulty displaying complex 3-dimensional structures and their relationship to the airway; (d) insufficient representation of airways oriented obliquely (or, even worse, parallel) to the axial plane, and (e) generation of a very large number (MDCT scanners produce hundreds) of images that are very difficult to review. In essence, 3-dimensionally rendered images are creative software solutions to the challenge of depicting 3-dimensional data – organized in a 3-dimensional matrix of volume elements (voxels)

– on the 2-dimensional surface of a computer monitor composed of picture elements (pixels). The reformatting process uses the CT voxels in 'off-axis views' (without changing them in any way), thus displaying the images produced from the original reconstruction process in an orientation other than the one they were originally generated.

Four basic postprocessing techniques of the volumetrically acquired data are used to enhance imaging of airway anatomy: 2-dimensional multiplanar reformation (MPR), 3-dimensional multiplanar volume reconstruction (MPVR), 3-dimensional shaded-surface display (SSD) and 3-dimensional volume rendering (VR) [2, 4, 5].

Multiplanar Reformation
MPRs are 1-voxel-thick 2-dimensional tomographic sections that are as accurate as axial images. By using dedicated algorithms, they can be interpolated along any arbitrary plane (usually coronal, sagittal or parasagittal) or a 'curved' tomographic surface (e.g. axis of the trachea, a bronchus or a feeding vessel). Precise cross-sectional and longitudinal images can be constructed along central and segmental bronchi, thus allowing 'lesion-oriented' reformations. MPRs have the advantage of high computational speed, thus incorporating information from a large number of axial frames while offering real-time images almost simultaneously with the axial sections. Most importantly, they can detect focal narrowing that may be missed when reading only the axial frames, and they can accurately depict the degree and longitudinal extent of bronchial stenosis. However, the potential decrease in spatial resolution due to partial volume averaging may result in overestimation of the degree of stenosis. This problem can be overcome by the overlapping of thin axial cuts and careful centring of the trace of the airway lumen of interest with concomitant inspection of the axial images is essential for their interpretation.

Multiplanar Volume Reconstruction
MPVR is a 3-dimensional rendering (volume-editing) technique that closely resembles 2-dimensional MPR. It was initially introduced as 'sliding thin-slab projections' to improve visualization of blood vessels and airways by 'stacking' several contiguous planar images. The method adds 'depth' to the anatomical display of airways and blood vessels and allows smoother and quicker visualization of the entire sequence of thin images (fig. 1). The technique allows reformatting under different protocols that enhance specific aspects of the airways or lung parenchyma. For example, the minimum intensity projection takes advantage of the lowest intensity voxels to evaluate airway lumen and areas of uneven attenuation of lung parenchyma (e.g. mild air-trapping), while

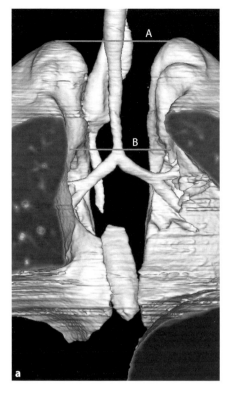
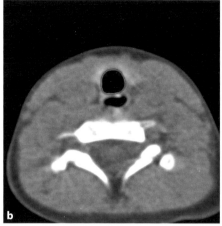
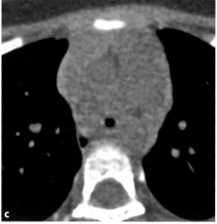

Fig. 2. a Three-dimensional SSD image of the patient presented in figure 1 that demonstrates the long segment concentric carrot-like tracheal stenosis (from line A to B) down to the level of the carina. The abnormally wide-angle (108°) bifurcation of the trachea and the normally sized main bronchi are clearly shown. An oesophageal indentation is visualized immediately above the level of the carina, most likely the result of the anomalous left pulmonary artery. There is no tracheal indentation due to the aberrant vessel, and no focal pulsation was visualized in FB. CT angiography was not performed in this patient (modified from Kagadis et al. [6], with permission). **b** CT axial image that corresponds to line A at the level of the T_1 vertebral body at the beginning of the tracheal stenosis; the cross-sectional tracheal area is normally sized (shortest diameter = 9.5 mm, area = 77.5 mm²). **c** CT axial image that corresponds to line B at the T_5 vertebral body, i.e. the level of maximum luminal stenosis; the cross-sectional tracheal area is markedly decreased (shortest diameter = 3.4 mm, area = 15.9 mm²), with the patent cross-sectional lumen constricted by 80% as compared to that of the non-stenotic portion.

the maximum intensity projection (highest intensity voxels) allows better visualization of the bronchial wall, improves nodule detection and differentiates between small nodules and vessels. MPVR may be used in selected cases to aid the interpretation of high-resolution CT (HRCT) as it offers an excellent ('bronchographic') display of segmental bronchiectasis, or to evaluate small-airway disease.

Shaded-Surface Display

This is an external rendering technique which is based on a predetermined threshold that is chosen to display the organ of interest. Each voxel is classified as either 0 or 100% (0 or 1) of a tissue type. The technique offers striking external 3-dimensional images of the central airways but is susceptible to noise and artefacts due to partial volume averaging (fig. 2).

Volume Rendering

Contrary to surface-rendering techniques that reflect voxel boundaries and not true interfaces, VR is a true volume-rendering technique that offers continuous scaling. Thus, while maximum intensity projection, minimum intensity projection and SSD make use of about only 10% of the

acquired CT data, VR incorporates the entire data set into a 3-dimensional image. This technique maintains the original spatial relationships of the volume data, adds depth and enhances detail allowing the reproduction of life-like images. However, despite its sophistication some information is still lost. Therefore, axial images remain indispensable in the evaluation of extraluminal disease. VR can be applied to the airways from both external ('fly-around' – virtual bronchography) and internal ('fly-through' – virtual endoscopy) perspectives.

External VR

This technique is extremely useful in depicting structures that do not course vertically to the transverse (axial) plane and offers accurate displays of overlapping structures and complex anomalies that extend into multiple planes. It constitutes a 'clinician-friendly' imaging modality that is able to detect short-segment airway narrowing, estimate the craniocaudad extent of tracheobronchial stenoses, describe complex tracheobronchial and cardiovascular congenital anomalies, and guide conventional and video-assisted thoracic surgery (fig. 3).

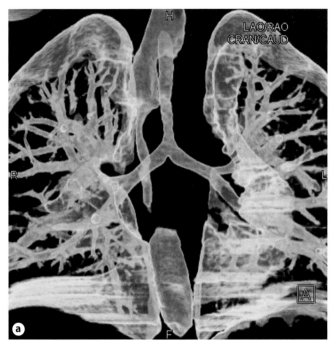

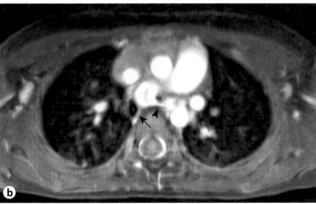

Fig. 3. a External VR image of the patient presented in figure 1. H = Head; F = feet; LAO/RAO = left/right anterior oblique; cran/caud = cranial/caudal; R = right; L = left; A = anterior view. **b** Cardiac MRI of the same patient shows a transverse view immediately above the level of the bifurcation of the trachea. The anomalous left pulmonary artery can be visualized encircling the trachea posteriorly (arrowhead). The oesophagus is displaced to the right (arrow).

Virtual Bronchoscopy

With the use of dedicated software, intraluminal navigation through the airways by an operator can provide additional information to other established techniques. Due to the non-collapsible air-filled tracheobronchial tree, virtual endoluminal visualization of the airways is much more easily achieved as compared to that of other hollow organs, thus making the demonstration of a variety of tracheobronchial anomalies possible. The main goal of virtual bronchoscopy

(VB) is to offer to the clinician a non-invasive diagnostic and follow-up tool, which provides images that closely resemble those of FB (fig. 4–6; online suppl. videos 1 and 2) and is well tolerated by the majority of patients [6, 7]. Although VB images can be obtained from MRI or the digital image of FB itself, MDCT is the most common data source. Current MDCT scanners produce virtual endoscopic images that closely resemble those obtained from conventional bronchoscopy [2, 6–8].

Submillimetre collimation of new MDCT technology can achieve deeper penetration making it possible for VB to accurately depict 6th- to 7th-order airways in adults and 3rd- to 4th-order (segmental/subsegmental) airways in children [8]. VB is of the greatest value in cases where FB is contraindicated or simply not possible [chapter 2, this vol., pp. 22–29]. It is also accurate in the evaluation of significant airway stenosis and, unlike FB, it is able to 'cross' such stenosis and assess the integrity of the peripheral airway. In addition, it can be useful in the evaluation of suspected foreign-body aspiration, tracheo-oesophageal fistula and other congenital airway abnormalities (see section on clinical applications of MDCT in paediatric patients) [4, 5]. Similarly to other 3-dimensional reconstruction techniques, VB findings should always be interpreted in conjunction with the axial sections as accurate measurement of lesions as well as of the diameter and length of stenoses is possible only on 2-dimensional images. Selection of the threshold level is of great importance for simulation as VB tends to overestimate airway stenosis and may display severe stenosis as complete occlusion due to partial volume averaging. In an early study using 4-row MDCT, Sorantin et al. [9] showed that, when using FB as gold standard, simultaneous display of axial cuts, MPR and VB on the workstation monitor raised sensitivity, precision and accuracy of the radiological findings in a group of 15 children with various causes of airway stenosis, while 4 additional patients were evaluated for diseases not involving the airways and were used as controls. The advantages and disadvantages of VB vs. FB are summarized in table 1. Adult research has shown that VB can be combined with ultrathin bronchoscopes to enable bronchoscopic biopsy of peripheral lesions by successful previewing and planning of the bronchoscopic routes to the areas of interest [10]; similar use of 3-dimensional technology may prove useful in paediatric cases. The indications of airway stenting for paediatric tracheobronchial obstruction are currently under investigation [chapter 6, this vol., pp. 64–74]. Two- and 3-dimensional CT imaging techniques have been utilized in the management of such cases on an individual basis [11].

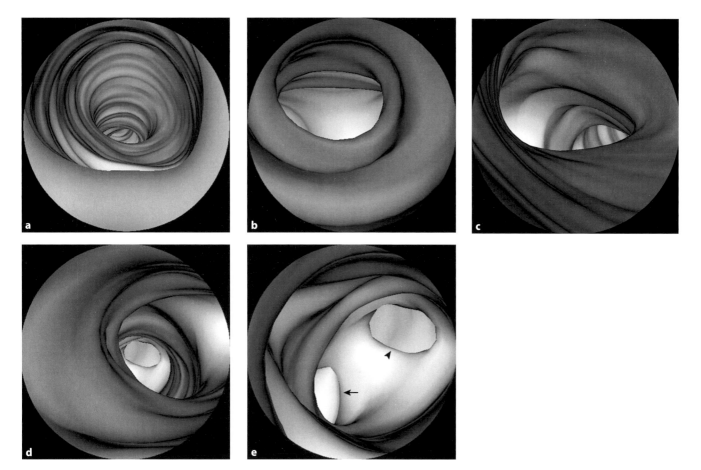

Fig. 4. VB image of the trachea and main bronchi of the patient presented in figure 1 (online suppl. video 1). **a** The tip of the virtual broncho-
scope is at the level of the normally sized extrathoracic portion. Progressively worsening stenosis of the tracheal lumen is demonstrated. **b** Image obtained immediately above the main carina at the level of maximal tracheal stenosis. **c** The tip of the virtual bronchoscope has 'crossed' the level of maximal tracheal stenosis and is entering the normally sized orifice of the left main bronchus. **d** The virtual bronchoscope has just entered the normally sized orifice of the right main bronchus. **e** The virtual bronchoscope has been advanced into the right main bronchus at the point of the take-off of the right upper lobe bronchus (arrowhead). The orifice of the bronchus intermedius is partially visualized (arrow).

Special Considerations

Technical and Patient Characteristics
The parameters used for the CT (e.g. kilovoltage peak, current-time product, pitch (table speed), detector collimation, field of view) determine the quality of images but also the degree of radiation that the patient receives (Appendix). In general, the better the image, the higher the radiation dose. Thus, one should always consider whether the information provided by improved resolution justifies the increase in the radiation dose. In recent years, various institutions that perform MDCT imaging in children have standardized low-dose protocols (adjusted to the child's weight and the

diagnostic question) that best address this conflict [5]. To obtain high-quality 3-dimensional images in children, it is necessary to use fast scan times (≤1 s) and lower collimation (0.625–0.75 mm for a 16-row, and 0.5–0.6 mm for a 64-row detector with a pitch of 1.0–1.5) that increase the radiation dose. In order to improve 3-dimensional imaging, when slice thickness exceeds 1 mm, the volumetric data are reconstructed using slice overlap of approximately 50% (Appendix).

High-resolution scanning is required for imaging short focal stenosis and small-airway disease, and for obtaining CT angiograms, e.g. to delineate cardiovascular anomalies or mediastinal masses. In CT angiograms, careful

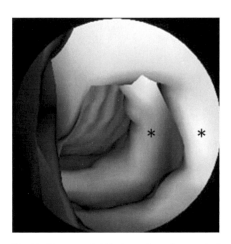

Fig. 5. Retrograde VB view of a unique spiral web (asterisks) winding down the distal trachea and proximal right main stem bronchus of a 13-year-old boy treated for 'uncontrolled asthma' since the age of 4 years (online suppl. video 2). The tip of the virtual bronchoscope is located above the main carina and turned 180°; thus, the lesion is visualized from below.

■Video

selection of dose, rate and timing of administration of the intravenous contrast medium is essential for the accurate imaging of the specific area of interest. In current practice, non-ionic low-osmolarity contrast material is used to minimize discomfort at the injection site and systemic side effects, such as nausea and vomiting. Intravenous contrast medium should be injected by a mechanical pump when a 22-gauge or larger cannula is in place, otherwise it should be administered manually. Although conventional HRCT achieves optimal resolution of lung parenchyma in diffuse interstitial or airway disease (including bronchiectasis) at relatively lower than MDCT radiation dosage, it does not provide volumetric data because sampling is not continuous. Therefore, true volumetric scanning can be selected for the initial diagnostic evaluation in such cases, while HRCT, at a lower radiation dose, can be used for patient follow-up [12].

In cooperating patients, scans are performed in suspended inspiration, ideally at total lung capacity. However, this is often not possible in young children. Children older than 6 years can be instructed to hold their breath, and scans are obtained in suspended inspiration although not always at total lung capacity. Children between 6 and 10–12 years usually require support in order to cooperate, while after the age of 12 years most children comply with the instructions used for adults. In sedated children and those under 6 years (with the exception of an unusually cooperative child), the examination is performed during quiet breathing. When investigating tracheobronchomalacia (TBM) or peripheral obstruction, usually 3–5 additional slices during expiration are obtained in order to reveal tracheobronchial collapse or air-trapping [5]. In young children in whom breath-holding is not possible, scans are obtained during quiet breathing in both left and right lateral decubitus positions [12]. When performing this manipulation, the dependent lung is compressed due to the increased compliance of the young child's chest, thus behaving as in the expiratory phase; conversely, the non-dependent lung behaves as in the inspiratory phase. Therefore, trapping can be visualized. On occasion, non-invasive controlled ventilation of infants – which takes advantage of the Hering-Breuer reflex similarly to infant pulmonary function testing – or general anaesthesia that provides complete control of breathing may be required.

Patient Handling and Sedation
As with any procedure, an effort should be made to prevent or minimize the discomfort that the patient may experience and ease the anxiety of the patients and their parents. The intravenous catheter, if required, should be placed beforehand. A resuscitation cart, wall oxygen and suction should be readily available as well as heating blankets or warming lamps for young infants. Staff should be familiar with techniques of immobilizing infants and young children while maintaining patient comfort and fulfilling imaging requirements. Radiation-sensitive organs such as the breasts and thyroid gland need to be protected, and a lead apron may be used to protect adjacent regions from scattered radiation. It should be remembered that protection may inadvertently increase the radiation dose when an automated dose-control protocol is in place because the CT tube can sense the decrease in radiation penetrating the patient and will automatically increase the emitted dose of radiation.

The fast scanning time of current MDCT scanners has dramatically reduced patient sedation requirements. Children over 3 years after becoming familiar with the environment usually cooperate and breathe calmly during the scan, while recently fed infants less than 3 months of age remain peaceful through the short duration of the examination. Children that require sedation or intravenous administration of contrast material should be fasted before the examination (2 h for clear liquids, 4 h for breast milk and 6 h for bottle milk or solids). Children from 4 months to 5 years can be sedated using the same precautions used for sedation during invasive procedures [13; chapter 2, this vol., pp. 22–29]. A quiet area for sleep should be available in the radiology department.

Anthracopoulos · Alexopoulou · Kagadis

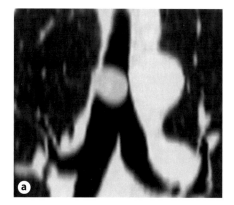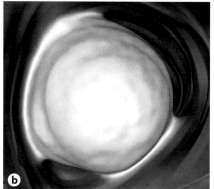

Fig. 6. a MPR image of an endotracheal hamartoma in a 16-year-old adolescent male who presented with a 6-month history of shortness of breath, wheezing and cough misdiagnosed and treated as asthma. **b** VB image demonstrating almost complete occlusion of the tracheal lumen by the hamartoma. The virtual bronchoscope was able to visualize the airway distally to the mass (images not shown).

Table 1. Advantages and disadvantages of VB as compared to FB in children

Advantages	Disadvantages
Non-invasive technique (but may require mild sedation of young uncooperative patients)	Relatively high radiation dose requirements
Accurate localization and evaluation of the extent and degree of airway stenosis – improved diagnostic confidence	Inability to distinguish mucus from 'true' obstruction or foreign body
Interactive evaluation of the volumetrically acquired data with simultaneous display of axial, coronal and sagittal views, MPRs and 3-dimensional externally and internally rendered reconstructions of the airways by using different algorithms without additional radiation or inconvenience to the patient	Inability to assess colour, vascularity and texture of airway mucosa or subtle mucosal lesions
	Inability to perform BAL or invasive procedures (but may have a complementary role in procedure planning)
Precise localization of extraluminal cause of airway compression through 'transparent' rendering of airway wall with simultaneous visualization of airway lumen and mediastinal structures	Restricted ability to adequately assess 'dynamic' airway abnormalities (i.e. tracheo-/bronchomalacia and vocal cord dysfunction) mainly due to high radiation dose requirements
Ability to rotate images in order to better define their spatial relationships	Limitations due to lack of patient cooperation (infants, young children, seriously ill patients)
Ability to 'cross' severe stenosis and evaluate airway geometry distally to the obstruction	Workload burden due to postprocessing of raw data
Improved planning of invasive procedures (mapping of abnormal structures and guidance of transbronchial biopsies, stent deployment, laser treatment, cryotherapy and endobronchial brachytherapy, surgical planning)	Cannot be performed at the bedside and requires potentially hazardous transport of seriously ill patients
Bronchoscopy training without risk for the patient	

BAL = Bronchoalveolar lavage.

Clinical Applications of 3-Dimensional Imaging in Paediatric Patients

Airway obstruction can be classified on the basis of its location (intrathoracic vs. extrathoracic, intraluminal vs. extraluminal) and its characteristics (diffuse vs. focal, fixed vs. dynamic). Combinations of these components may coexist and airway wall involvement may need to be assessed. The diagnostic process may include pulmonary function tests, FB and imaging studies. Chapters 10 and 12 of this volume [pp. 114–119 and 130–140] discuss the anatomical variations of the normal bronchial tree, and chapters 11 and 12 [this vol., pp. 120–129 and 130–140] describe the main congenital and acquired abnormalities of the upper and lower airways, respectively. Table 2 lists airway lesions the diagnosis and management of which may benefit from CT scanning, especially the newer MDCT imaging technology. A discussion of specific situations where 2- and 3-dimensional imaging can complement airway endoscopy is presented below.

Table 2. Disorders causing tracheobronchial airway compromise in children the diagnosis of which may be assisted by CT

Congenital

Intraluminal

Bronchial agenesis, aplasia, hypoplasia (including scimitar syndrome, horseshoe lung etc.)
Bronchial atresia (bronchocele ± foregut communication)
Tracheobronchial branching anomalies (bronchial isomerism, tracheal bronchus, cardiac bronchus, tracheal diverticulum)
Tracheo-oesophageal fistula (±oesophageal atresia)
Tracheal stenosis (focal, carrot-shaped trachea/complete tracheal rings)
Tracheal webs, cartilaginous sleeves, oesophageal remnants
Laryngotracheo-oesophageal cleft
Tracheo- and/or bronchomalacia (dynamic airway collapse)

Extraluminal

Foregut duplication cysts (i.e. bronchogenic cysts, enteric cysts/oesophageal atresia pouch, neurenteric cysts)
Sequestration spectrum (intra- or extralobar sequestration*, cystadenomatoid malformation, mixed lesion)
Cardiovascular malformations (vascular ring)

Infectious/inflammatory

Intraluminal

Bacterial tracheitis
Tuberculosis
Histoplasmosis
Relapsing polychondritis
Wegener granulomatosis
Bronchial inflammatory myofibroblastic tumour (inflammatory pseudotumour, plasma cell granuloma, fibrous histiocytoma)
Peripheral airway disease (CF and non-CF bronchiectasis, bronchopulmonary dysplasia, aspiration, constrictive or obliterative bronchiolitis, cryptogenic organizing pneumonia, follicular bronchiolitis, neuroendocrine cell hyperplasia of infancy, hypersensitivity pneumonitis)

Extraluminal

Neck abscess
Enlarged lymph nodes (tuberculosis, histoplasmosis, granulomatous disease)
Fibrosing mediastinitis (histoplasmosis, mucormycosis, blastomycosis, cryptococcosis, Behçet disease, methysergide use)

Neoplastic

Intraluminal

Capillary haemangioma
Papilloma
Neurofibroma
Hamartoma (chondroma)
Juvenile xanthogranuloma
Muco-epidermoid tumour
Bronchial carcinoid
Pleuropulmonary blastoma
Adenoid cystic carcinoma (cylindroma)
Malignant fibrous histiocytoma
Bronchogenic carcinoma
Metastatic (extremely rare)

Table 2. Continued

Extraluminal

Haemangioma
Lymphangioma
Lymphoma (Hodgkin, non-Hodgkin)
Germ cell tumours (e.g. various grades of teratoma, seminoma, embryonal carcinoma, choriosarcoma, yolk sac tumours and mixed type)
Ewing sarcoma
Rhabdomyosarcoma
Parenchymal tumours (rarely malignant)
Pulmonary nodules (usually benign)
Thymic tumours
Thyroid tumours
Metastatic (e.g. Wilms tumour, rhabdomyosarcoma, osteosarcoma, hepatoblastoma, peripheral neuroectodermal tumour, Askin tumour)

Other

Intraluminal

Vocal cord paralysis (unilateral, bilateral), vocal cord dysfunction
Foreign-body aspiration
Mucous plug
Postintubation/tracheostomy stricture, granuloma, malacia
Partial lung resection with bronchial anastomosis, lung transplantation
Acquired tracheo-/bronchomalacia (intubation, tracheostomy, extrinsic compression, trauma, infection, surgery)
Mucopolysaccharidosis

Extraluminal

Oesophageal foreign body

CF = Cystic fibrosis.
* Rarely cause airway compromise.

Tracheobronchial Stenosis/Atresia, Tracheo-Oesophageal Fistula, Branching Anomalies

MPRs and VRs are the most commonly utilized adjuncts to axial CT for elucidating fixed stenoses and complex structures, communicating the radiographic findings to clinicians, and planning the surgical approach (fig. 1–3, 6) [6, 14, 15]. In suspected *congenital* or *acquired tracheobronchial stenosis*, the CT may reveal parenchymal involvement (e.g. infiltrates) with or without airway disease and thus help to explain the clinical and/or chest X-ray (CXR) presentation or re-orient the investigation. MPRs and VRs help to describe *intraluminal lesions* (e.g. webs, haemangiomas, hamartomas, granulomas, papillomas; table 2) and aid the exact measurement of the calibre and extent of airway stenosis as well as the distance between the *oesophageal pouches* in *oesophageal atresia*

[16]. Axial CT is the imaging modality of choice for the confirmation of *congenital bronchial atresia* revealing the cylindrical mucoid impaction within the dilated bronchus distally to the atretic segment, which is associated with hyperlucency and decreased vascularity of the relevant lung segment (usually the apical or apicoposterior of the upper lobe). VB and external rendering can highlight the findings of axial images but do not usually add important diagnostic information [17]. Although MDCT usually performs well in the diagnosis of *tracheo-oesophageal fistulas* and VB can depict the tracheal ostium of the fistula, false-positive findings (as compared to FB) have been reported [18]. Visualization of *tracheal diverticuli* can be enhanced by MPR and external VR [14], while VB provides an excellent image quality of *tracheobronchial branching anomalies* [19].

Foreign-Body Aspiration

It has been proposed that low-dose MDCT with VB can serve as a first-line non-invasive examination to rule out suspected foreign-body aspiration in children [20]; the authors of the article correctly suggest that because a mucous plug or an alternative diagnosis (e.g. tumour), which cannot be differentiated from foreign body by this method, may be responsible for the presence of obstruction, a positive finding should prompt evaluation by conventional bronchoscopy in order to confirm the diagnosis and remove the foreign body. It should be noted, however, that conventional bronchoscopy was not performed in patients with normal MDCT findings in this study, and that foreign body was 'ruled out' by following the patients for 5–20 months. Thus, we believe that conventional bronchoscopy should remain the gold standard for diagnosis, and FB should be performed even in cases of low clinical suspicion [chapter 12, this vol., pp. 130–140].

Peripheral Airway Disease

HRCT is usually the method of choice for evaluating peripheral (small) airway disease. Airways as small as 1–2 mm in diameter with wall thicknesses of 0.2–0.3 mm – which by definition cannot be inspected by FB – can be visualized. Air-trapping, best seen on expiratory images, is the most common finding in peripheral airway disease, and it is the predominant finding in constrictive (obliterative) bronchiolitis. Ground-glass opacities predominate in *fibrosing bronchiolitis* and *neuroendocrine hyperplasia of infancy*. MPVRs provide excellent images of *bronchiectasis*, while use of the maximum intensity projection algorithm helps to better appreciate the relation between *peripheral nodules* and the relevant bronchus when planning transbronchial biopsy [5].

Dynamic Airway Compression

TBM can be conclusively diagnosed under direct real-time visualization of the airways during breathing manoeuvres (forced inspiration/expiration and coughing) [chapter 12, this vol., pp. 130–140]. However, patient cooperation during the procedure is important, and careful 'titration' of sedation is required.

Newer-technology high-resolution fast MDCT scanners provide a dynamic imaging tool to assess the airway. Although still somewhat limited in z-axis coverage, such scanners are able to completely 'sample' the entire airway during a single forced or coughing manoeuvre, or to at least obtain complete anatomical coverage with several acquisitions. Axial images are indispensable for the evaluation of TBM but they may underestimate the craniocaudad extent of disease. Therefore, 2- and 3-dimensional images,

including VB, can assist in mapping the exact location of malacia and its longitudinal extent as well as in grading the severity of collapse by obtaining exact measurements of airway diameters at end-inspiration and comparing them with those at end-expiration or during a forced expiration/cough manoeuvre. In addition, 3-dimensional renderings can provide a comprehensive assessment of tracheomalacia associated with mediastinal vascular malformations or non-vascular paratracheal masses.

This technique has been studied in infants [21] and children [22]. Children 5–6 years or older can usually be coached to perform successful paired end-inspiratory/end-expiratory or forced expiratory manoeuvres. Using 64-MDCT (or a scanner of more advanced generation), cine CT can also be performed during a coughing manoeuvre, especially when investigating focal airway malacia. Infants, preschoolers and non-cooperating older children require general anaesthesia and endotracheal intubation in order to achieve the breath-hold that is necessary for paired end-inspiratory/end-expiratory manoeuvres. End-inspiratory pressure in such cases should be maintained at 15–20 cm H_2O to avoid 'artificial' distension of the airway lumen. The recently introduced 320-MDCT shows great promise for the evaluation of TBM because it can cover the entire central airway of infants and young children in a single acquisition, thus offering excellent anatomical precision. Intravenous contrast medium is not necessary for routine assessment of TBM; however, it may prove very useful and should at least be considered in the settings of known or suspected vascular anomalies. As is the case for FB, the standard CT criterion for TBM is an at least 50% reduction in the cross-sectional luminal area of the trachea and/or bronchi during expiration as compared to end-inspiration [23]. However, since forced expiration and cough result in greater collapse of the large airways than the end-expiration manoeuvre, different threshold criteria may be more appropriate for different techniques (e.g. a 60 or 70% reduction in the luminal area with the coughing manoeuvre). The need for normative CT data for both manoeuvres in the paediatric population is obvious.

Despite the fact that drastic dose reduction is possible without significant negative influence on measurements of luminal dimensions, the radiation dose to the patient is still of concern in these studies. MRI is an attractive alternative for the evaluation of TBM, especially due to the lack of radiation exposure that permits repeated assessments. New fast cine MRI techniques provide acceptable contrast resolution and temporal resolution as low as 150 ms/slice, which yields multiple images during a forced manoeuvre. Therefore, MRI can demonstrate dynamic tracheal compression that varies with the respiratory cycle and integrate information regarding relationships of mediastinal structures [15].

Vascular Anomalies

The term 'vascular ring' in its broad sense encompasses aortic arch (e.g. double aortic arch, lesions associated with right or left aortic arch, anomalous innominate artery, cervical aortic arch) and pulmonary artery (e.g. pulmonary artery sling) anomalies in which the trachea and usually the oesophagus are completely or partially surrounded by vascular structures that are not necessarily patent. Vascular rings can cause compression (usually pulsating) of the trachea, bronchi and oesophagus. Pulsating airway compression may also be the result of congenital heart disease such as dilated pulmonary arteries, left atrial enlargement, massive cardiomegaly or aortopulmonary collaterals (typically tetralogy of Fallot and pulmonary atresia) [15, 24].

Apart from FB, a number of imaging studies is available for the diagnosis of vascular ring, and the imaging approach may vary according to the clinical setting [chapter 12, this vol., pp. 130–140]. Traditionally CXR and upper gastrointestinal study (barium swallow) are the initial imaging modalities used when vascular ring is suspected. The diagnostic accuracy of barium swallow is acceptable regarding tracheal compression but it does not adequately describe the anatomy of the vascular anomaly. Evaluation of the patient with echocardiography for associated congenital heart disease is of vital importance. It should be noted that when vascular abnormalities are present the narrowing of the tracheal lumen is not always due to malacia but can be due to complete tracheal rings that in up to 50% of cases are associated with an anomalous left pulmonary artery originating from the right pulmonary branch (ring-sling syndrome) [6].

MRI and MDCT, usually with contrast in order to depict the great vessels (MR angiography and MDCT angiography), are used interchangeably and occasionally together in the surgical planning of vascular ring. The intrinsic properties of MRI along with its 3-dimensional reconstruction capabilities and its ability superior to CT for the assessment of cardiac anatomy and physiology have made it, until recently, the standard imaging method (fig. 3b). However, the role of MDCT in evaluating tracheobronchial narrowing associated with mediastinal vascular anomalies in neonates and children has rapidly expanded in recent years. Indeed, MDCT is a much faster examination that usually places substantially fewer airway management demands upon patients with a compromised airway and provides exquisite detail of the lung parenchyma and central airways. Axial cuts, external VR of the airways and VB images help to visualize the airway beyond severe narrowing, reveal additional airway anomalies and further contribute to presurgical planning [6]. On the down side, MDCT does not usually provide adequate details of intracardiac defects and in a study of 12 children with various types of vascular ring contrast-enhanced 16-MDCT failed to detect 1 bronchoscopically proven tracheal stenosis due to innominate artery compression, which nevertheless did not require surgery [25].

The degree and craniocaudad extent of *coarctation of the aorta* can be precisely assessed by MPR and external VR. MDCT angiography with 3-dimensional rendering can be very useful for the detection and accurate delineation of other *complex congenital vascular anomalies*, such as proximal interruption of the pulmonary artery (associated with hypoplastic ipsilateral lung and enlarged contralateral pulmonary vessels), unilateral pulmonary agenesis, pulmonary vein stenosis, pulmonary varix (i.e. enlarged pulmonary vein without a large feeding artery or nidus), scimitar syndrome (hypogenetic lung syndrome), patent ductus arteriosus and pulmonary arteriovenous malformation [17].

Although not relevant to airway disease, the recent literature supports pulmonary MDCT angiography as the new reference standard for the diagnosis of *pulmonary emboli*. In a study using 16- and 64-MDCT angiography, successful visualization of 100% of segmental and 80% of subsegmental pulmonary arteries was achieved in 98 studies of children investigated for pulmonary embolism [26]. The need for careful attention to the protocol of contrast administration to the patient in order to prevent incomplete evaluation and misdiagnosis cannot be overemphasized [27].

Non-Vascular Mediastinal Masses

These are conveniently categorized for diagnostic purposes into anterior (approx. 45%), middle (approx. 20%) and posterior (approx. 35%) masses. Depending on their location and size, mediastinal masses may cause compression of the trachea and/or the main stem bronchi, thus creating the need for evaluation of the airways. Initial investigation typically involves anteroposterior (AP) and lateral CXR, which is usually followed by additional imaging studies that may include ultrasonography, CT or MRI. The potentially important role of MRI in evaluating non-vascular mediastinal and pulmonary masses – due to its superior soft tissue characterization as compared to other currently available imaging modalities – is limited by its disadvantages (previously described), especially in young children; however, the utility of MRI has been demonstrated particularly in the evaluation of posterior mediastinal neurogenic tumours and foregut duplication cysts with high attenuation on non-contrast CT [28].

Anterior mediastinal non-vascular masses are basically comprised (85%) of thymic enlargement, Hodgkin (typically in the first decade of life) and non-Hodgkin lymphoma (in both the first and second decades of life) and germ cell tumours (mostly benign, usually teratomas). Evaluation of the CXR by an experienced reviewer is usually sufficient to diagnose an enlarged thymus, but ultrasound (the unossified sternal and costal cartilages in the first year of life provide an adequate acoustic window), MRI (on occasion) and CT (hardly ever) may be performed to confirm the diagnosis. The diagnosis of lymphoma and germ cell tumours requires confirmation by CT or MRI, while positron emission tomography (PET) scanning has been proven valuable for initial staging of lymphomas and assessment of treatment response. Three-dimensional imaging enhances the perception of tumour anatomy, and hybrid ('fused') PET/CT imaging can combine functional and anatomical information, thus offering a complete evaluation of paediatric lymphoma [14, 28]. Perger et al. [29] have described an algorithm for the management of children with severe airway compromise due to compression by an anterior mediastinal mass, usually due to lymphoblastic lymphoma or Hodgkin disease.

Middle mediastinal non-vascular masses are mostly comprised of embryonic foregut malformations (i.e. bronchogenic, enteric and neurenteric cysts), lymphoma and lymphadenopathy of infectious or inflammatory aetiology (i.e. tuberculosis, histoplasmosis, granulomatous disease, sarcoidosis). When the lesions become large enough, symptoms may occur due to mass effect on adjacent mediastinal structures such as the central airways and the oesophagus [28, 29]. On CT the degree of attenuation of a bronchogenic cyst depends on the amount of its proteinaceous content. With intravenous contrast medium, a non-enhancing or minimally enhancing thin wall is typically seen and, in case of an air-fluid level or a thick wall, a superimposed infection should be considered [17]. Acutely inflamed lymph nodes can also show peripheral enhancement with low-attenuation centres or enhance homogeneously. Three-dimensional external rendering MDCT images accurately delineate these masses and may assist with surgical planning [14, 15].

The great majority (88%) of *posterior mediastinal non-vascular masses* is neurogenic in origin. These tumours are primarily derived from ganglion cells of the paravertebral sympathetic chain and do not impinge on the central airways. They include neuroblastoma (most common), ganglioneuroblastoma and ganglioneuroma, while the remaining are usually nerve sheath tumours such as schwannoma and neurofibroma. CT or MRI is usually necessary to confirm the diagnosis and evaluate the disease extent. MRI is probably the imaging method of choice due to its high sensitivity in detecting intraspinal extension without exposing the patient to radiation [28].

Non-Vascular Pulmonary Lesions
These include a wide spectrum of conditions such as congenital anomalies, neoplasms, inflammatory pseudotumour, infections and pseudomasses. Excluding neoplasms, these lesions do not usually affect the airways; however, they are briefly presented because MDCT with external 3-dimensional rendering is particularly useful in describing the anatomy of some of these lesions.

Congenital cystic adenomatoid malformation (CCAM) results from disorganized proliferation of the airways (usually the bronchioles) of unknown aetiology; the dysplastic airway communicates with the bronchial tree. There are 3 types of CCAM with distinct radiographic and pathological appearances (type 1: at least 1 cyst >2 cm in size; type 2: numerous small cysts with diameters 1–10 mm; type 3: solid in appearance with numerous microcysts). CT is very useful in the identification and characterization of CCAM, the evaluation of mass effect and the differentiation of CCAM from sequestration although there may be overlap between the two malformations (e.g. systemic arterial supply of CCAM). External VR images improve delineation of the malformation and assist in pre-operative evaluation [14, 15].

Pulmonary sequestration is a congenital malformation characterized by dysplastic non-functioning pulmonary tissue that is not normally connected to the tracheobronchial tree; its arterial supply comes from systemic vessels. Extralobar sequestration is contained in its own pleura, its venous drainage is in the systemic circulation (usually through the azygous and less commonly through the portal vein) and is often associated with other congenital malformations. Intralobar sequestration manifests itself within the lung (not contained in its own pleura), its venous drainage is typically in the inferior pulmonary vein, and it is associated with recurrent infections while coexistent congenital anomalies are quite rare; in fact, it is considered by certain experts as a secondary lesion due to recurrent infections that produce the aberrant systemic feeding vessels. CT imaging is integral to the management of sequestration. MDCT angiography with external VR offers 3-dimensional images that are particularly helpful in pre-operative planning by delineating the anomalous veins and therefore differentiating between extra- and intralobar sequestration, also in detecting the anomalous arterial vessels and thus avoiding potentially life-threatening haemorrhage during surgery [17, 30]. The area scanned should be extended to below the diaphragm in order to include feeding vessels that originate from the abdominal aorta [14].

Congenital lobar emphysema may appear in the newborn period as an opacity on CXR or CT owing to the retention of foetal lung fluid. As the fluid is cleared by the lymphatic circulation and replaced by air, the affected lobe becomes hyperlucent with a mass effect on adjacent lobes. CT is useful for diagnosing multilobar involvement and defining the anatomy; 3-dimensional imaging does not usually add important diagnostic information [17].

Pulmonary neoplasms are rare in children but should be considered in the differential diagnosis of a persistent abnormality on CXR. Most often they involve the large airways and present as airway obstruction. Primary airway neoplasms are usually benign although malignant lesions do occasionally occur (table 2). With the use of FB, the intraluminal and the mucosal components of the airway tumour can be identified, and biopsy can be performed but extraluminal extension of the mass cannot be assessed. Enhanced MDCT with external VR can demonstrate the extraluminal mass extent, configuration, homogeneous, heterogeneous or peripheral rim enhancement (depending on the vascularity of the tumour), while VB offers excellent images of intraluminal masses (fig. 6 and table 2) [15, 30]. This information is important when planning biopsy or assessing surgical resectability.

Pulmonary *inflammatory pseudotumour* (also termed bronchial inflammatory myofibroblastic tumour, plasma cell granuloma or fibrous histiocytoma) is a non-neoplastic reactive proliferative process histologically characterized by (myo)fibroblasts, histiocytes, lymphocytes and plasma cells. Affected children can be asymptomatic or quite ill. CT, including external VR images, shows a well-marginated mass with variable contrast enhancement and calcifications that is usually situated at the periphery of the lungs and typically (but not always) does *not* invade adjacent structures [30].

Pulmonary mass-like lesions of infectious cause include [30]: (a) *lung abscess*, which typically is a low-attenuation cystic structure on axial CT with an enhancing wall of variable thickness and border definition that depend on the degree of abscess maturity and inflammation of surrounding lung parenchyma; (b) *fungal infection* (invasive pulmonary aspergillosis), which occurs in immunocompromised children and appears on axial CT as ill-defined macronodules, often bilateral, with a 'halo' sign (ground-glass opacity due to alveolar haemorrhage surrounding the nodule), and possibly cavitation (the so-called air crescent sign that may represent either disease progression or a favourable response to treatment); (c) *hydatid (ecchinococcal) cyst*, which presents on axial CT as a cystic mass with homogeneous water density content, is indistinguishable from other pulmonary cysts and, when ruptured, may produce the 'water lily' sign (ruptured cyst membranes floating on the remaining fluid); (d) *round pneumonia* (more commonly seen in children), which may occasionally lead to CT imaging if the consolidation persists despite appropriate antibiotic treatment and the suspicion of an underlying abnormality is raised, and (e) *round atelectasis* (quite rare in children), in which even CT findings may not be able to resolve the diagnostic confusion.

Vocal Chord Paralysis and Vocal Cord Dysfunction
Laryngoscopy is the gold standard for evaluating vocal chord motion [chapter 11, this vol., pp. 120–129]. Fluoroscopy and ultrasound of the vocal chords are currently used as non-invasive diagnostic methods of vocal chord paralysis and vocal chord dysfunction [31]. Cine MRI, similarly to TBM, has been shown to adequately demonstrate vocal chord motion and its abnormalities [15]. Laryngeal CT reconstructed images during vowel phonation have been shown to effectively demonstrate functional changes in the larynx and to diagnose vocal chord paralysis in adult patients [32]. Although patient cooperation is important in order to achieve sustained phonation in these studies, given the ongoing advances in technology, such problems are expected to be overcome in the near future.

Radiation Exposure and Dose Reduction

Radiation Dose
The ionizing effect of X-rays in tissues may lead to permanent DNA alterations and carcinogenesis [33]. The risk of radiation-induced fatal cancer is considered to be 1:20,000 per millisievert (mSv) in adults. This risk is estimated to increase approximately 10-fold in children (between 1:1,000 and 1:10,000 depending on their age) who are considerably more sensitive to radiation. Indeed, children have a higher proportion of dividing cells, a wider window of opportunity to express radiation damage due to longer life expectancy and suffer higher organ doses as a result of their small size [34, 35]. Most available quantitative data on the risk of low-dose radiation-induced cancer and cancer fatality come from the atomic bomb survivors in Japan [36, 37]. Despite the obvious differences in uniformity of radiation exposure between A-bomb survivors and patients undergoing CT, most authorities consider it valid to extrapolate specific organ cancer risk calculated from the A-bomb low-dose exposure data to equivalent radiation exposure by CT.

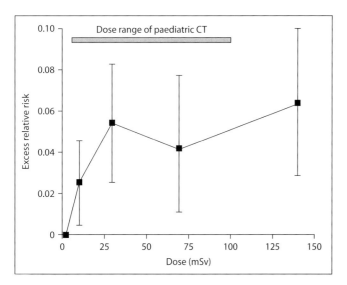

Fig. 7. Mean radiation-related additional relative risk and standard error for solid cancer mortality in Japanese A-bomb survivors of any age at exposure. The graph focuses on exposure to radiation doses relevant to those used in paediatric CT, especially when multiple examinations are performed (redrawn from Pierce et al. [36]).

Figure 7 illustrates that A-bomb radiation exposure within the range of effective doses delivered by paediatric CT increases fatal solid cancer mortality, especially when dose reduction is not implemented.

It is estimated that the mean annual background radiation dose is 2.6 mSv in the UK and 3 mSv in the USA, while the dose of a round-trip transatlantic flight is 0.1 mSv. In paediatric hospitals with carefully selected low-dose radiation protocols, the dose of an AP CXR ranges, depending on the child's size, from 0.00487 to 0.0176 mSv for children up to 44 kg. The radiation dose of a typical HRCT of the lungs is equivalent to approximately 45–90 AP CXRs and that of a thoracic 'combiscan' (CT angiography with use of intravenous contrast medium and concomitant high-quality imaging of lung parenchyma) to 100–220 AP CXRs, according to the size and sex of the patient [5, 12]. In a multiphase CT that involves 2–4 scans per study, the scanned area, depending on the machine settings, may receive a radiation dose as high as 15 mSv in the adult and 30 mSv in the neonate, while follow-up scanning is not unusual [34]. These doses are associated with a small, albeit distinct, increase in cancer risk that is important at a population level. There appears to be a linear dose-response relationship between radiation dose and solid cancer risk, and there is no evidence for a threshold.

The annual collective population radiation dose for diagnostic purposes has increased by a dramatic 750% over the last 20 years, while paediatric CT examinations have increased during the same period by about 800%. CT comprises today approximately 9–12% of all radiological examinations in the USA and UK and is responsible for 45–47% of the medical radiation dose; over 10% of the studies are conducted in children [35, 38]. It is estimated that the current use of CT accounts for 1.5–2.0% of all cancers in the USA [34].

Dose Reduction

The radiation dose in CT is considered to be a major issue by several national and international organizations and radiation protection boards [39]. Continuous communication between clinicians and radiologists is imperative in order to eliminate unnecessary examinations, take advantage of alternative imaging modalities and minimize patient exposure. The CT image quality is determined by image contrast and noise, which depend on scan parameters and patient size (i.e. radiation dose). At this time no large-scale long-term epidemiological data are available on cancer risk from CT, although at least one such study is under way [34]. In the meantime, adherence to the 'as low as reasonably achievable' (ALARA) principle must be observed [35, 39].

In CT, unlike film screen radiography, overexposure is not visually evident as it does not directly alter film quality. The operator makes the necessary computer adjustments, and therefore radiologists may remain unaware of the potential danger. CT demonstrates variations in delivered dose within the scan plane and along the z-axis. A number of CT-specific dose descriptors have been developed. The ones most commonly used are the weighted CT dose index ($CTDI_w$), the dose-length product and the effective dose [38]. The $CTDI_w$ provides a weighted average of the central and peripheral contributions to dose within the scan plane. The dose-length product descriptor takes into account the $CTDI_w$, the pitch and the scan length. Both $CTDI_w$ and dose-length product are readily displayed by the scanner and help to visualize the impact of scan parameters on patient dose. They are useful for quality control but they are not directly related to organ dose or risk. The effective dose is a more relevant descriptor that represents the weighted sum of organ doses resulting from the examination, while taking into account their radiation risk factors. The effective dose is difficult to calculate but complex mathematical patient models have been developed for its estimation. It is measured in millisieverts and it constitutes the best single parameter for quantifying the radiation that an individual receives during any radiographic examination. Therefore, it allows comparison of possible CT radiation effects to those of other radiation exposures. Selection of scanning parameters such as photon beam energy, tube current-scanning time product, beam collimation, pitch, field of view adjustment and dose modulation function affect the radiation dose administered to the patient (Appendix). In addition, careful patient preparation, patient size (smaller patients receive larger radiation doses), inherent tissue contrast (e.g. air-tissue contrast of the lung) and individual scanner design contribute to the radiation doses administered to particular organs. Last but not least, clinician-radiologist communication should consider alternative imaging modalities (e.g. sonogram or MRI), assure that the CT scan is necessary for diagnosis and minimize the number of scans required for the examination (e.g. precontrast scans are rarely needed during follow-up) [38].

There is always a trade-off between the quest for high-resolution low-noise imaging and the need for a low radiation dose administered to the patient. As CT scanners evolve, all major components such as X-ray filters, beam collimators and detectors are optimized, new features are implemented, and paediatric scanning protocols are updated in order to reduce the dose by adjusting the settings according to the characteristics of the patient, the scanned areas and the relevant clinical question.

Future Trends

CT is a powerful non-invasive tool for quantifying airway dimensions, and the rationale behind the strengths and the limitations of MDCT imaging of the lung has been addressed in previous sections. Although accurate and precise measurements in airways as small as 2 mm in diameter are currently possible, there is a need for deeper penetration into the bronchial tree and for reliable measurements in even smaller airways. Therefore, further advancements in CT-based measurement techniques will have important clinical implications: (a) thinner slices (cubic voxel scanners) will further improve resolution and reduce partial volume-averaging effects; (b) faster tube revolution speeds will achieve acquisition of the entire lung in shorter time periods; (c) refined automated (as opposed to manual) tracing systems will improve speed, reproducibility and accuracy, and will reduce subjectivity of measurements, and (d) improved skeletonization algorithms will facilitate the reconstruction of CT data orthogonal to the airway axis, thus reducing the effects of partial volume averaging and aiding navigation through the tracheobronchial tree.

The ability to combine functional with precise anatomical information by the merging of PET scan and 3-dimensional MDCT images (hybrid PET/CT imaging) in the case of paediatric lymphoma has already been mentioned. Another example of 'merging' of different techniques is the integration of CT and digital bronchoscopic images (colour bronchoscopy and fluorescence detection systems). By using highly sophisticated techniques, the coloured bronchoscopic picture is 'pasted' onto the VB image derived from MDCT, producing a virtual bronchoscopic image in true colour from which airway dimensions can be accurately measured and subtle mucosal colour changes can be assessed [40].

Until recently, despite the ability of MRI to provide functional information without ionizing radiation, its limited signal from the lung tissue and the longer – as compared to MDCT – acquisition time have limited its use in lung imaging. MRI with hyperpolarized helium that diffuses rapidly into the air spaces of the lungs can greatly improve the lung signal, thus resulting in high spatial and temporal resolution images of the airways and the alveolar spaces. Clinical studies in children with asthma and cystic fibrosis have been conducted, and a strong correlation has been shown between forced expiratory volume in 1 s and ventilation defects [41]. This technique, which is free from the harmful effects of ionizing radiation, may prove to be extremely useful in the follow-up of lung microstructure and function of these patients as well as those with chronic rejection of lung transplant or other chronic lung diseases. Recently, hyperpolarized xenon has emerged as the gas imaging agent of choice due to its improved ability to measure chemical diffusion, its unlimited supply in nature and its modest production costs [42]. Nevertheless, availability of these techniques is limited, and further research on their clinical applications and cost-effectiveness is required.

Future trends with respect to videobronchoscopy in paediatric patients, including endobronchial ultrasound and confocal fluorescent laser microscopy (alveoloscopy), are touched upon in chapter 4 of this volume [pp. 42–53]. Despite the great advancements in overcoming optical limitations such as distal and radial distortion that are inherent to the system, the 'holy grail' of real-time quantitative videobronchoscopy is still elusive. Newer technologies such as optical coherence tomography and the already mentioned confocal fluorescence endomicroscopy are light microscopy techniques with enhanced 'optical sectioning' (effective resolution in depth) that is beyond that of conventional microscopy. These technologies, recently presented in more detailed reviews [43, 44] and actively being researched [45], have made imaging of terminal airways and even alveoli possible and may hold an important future role in the assessment of small-airway remodelling.

Appendix

Glossary of Radiological Technical Terms

Collimation: The width of the radiation detectors in the scanner. It represents the z-axis dimension of the voxel and is often used interchangeably with the term 'slice thickness'. On the one hand, narrow collimation improves z-axis spatial resolution and decreases artefacts; however, a much larger number of narrow slices is required to cover a given anatomical area. Such coverage of the lung is impossible in one breath-hold by single-slice CT but has become feasible with the introduction of multirow detector arrays (MDCT). On the other hand, narrow collimation increases image noise; therefore an increase in kilovoltage peak and/or current-time product (in order to obtain a sufficient number of photons) may be required for compensation, which in turn increases radiation dose to the patient.

Current-(scan) time product (milliamperes × seconds): The tube current (milliamperes) represents the electron flux from the cathode to the anode of the X-ray tube and ultimately controls the number of photons generated. The tube current is an important determinant of image quality. Scan time (seconds) represents the time interval required for tube rotation during which the patient is being irradiated, also affecting the number of photons generated; the subsecond scan time that can be achieved by the newer scanners is important in order to minimize heart and/or breathing motion artefacts. The tube current-time product proportionally affects the radiation dose administered to the patient. By using the *dose modulation function*, the computer samples patient thickness along the z-axis and adjusts the radiation dose accordingly. However, operators should be aware that the time-current product is usually adjusted automatically according to the pitch in order to improve resolution; therefore, low current-time product selection may not translate to the expected dose reduction.

Detectors: Rows of radiation detectors (detector array), which vary in number from 1 (single detector) to tens or hundreds of rows (multidetector, i.e. 16-, 64-, 128-, 256- or 320-MDCT).

Field of view: The field within the gantry opening from which scan data are generated. The field of view should closely approximate the largest cross-sectional area to be scanned. Spatial resolution is improved by using a smaller field of view because as it decreases, the pixel size also decreases. An inappropriately large field of view results in wasted matrix space, loss of resolution and increased partial volume averaging.

Kilovoltage peak: Measure of the energy of the X-ray beam generated by the CT scanner tube (photon beam energy). Kilovoltage peak is selected by the operator; it is influenced by the filtration used for the scan, and it directly affects the radiation dose administered to the patient. In paediatric patients, kilovoltage peak should be adjusted according to the child's weight in order to minimize the radiation dose without compromising diagnostic image quality.

Matrix space: The field of view from a cross-sectional (2-dimensional) image is usually displayed upon a digital matrix of 512 × 512 pixels.

Misregistration: Failure to image portions of the lung due to differences in respiratory excursion when repeated breath-holds are required for total lung volume acquisition.

Partial volume averaging: The term refers to the inaccurate representation of scanned detail (e.g. airway wall thickness and lumen area) resulting from the inclusion of elements of different densities (e.g. airway wall and intraluminal air) into a single voxel. In such a case, the voxel's greyscale value reflects the mean weighted average of the different tissue densities. Partial volume averaging leads to overestimation of airway wall thickness and underestimation of airway lumen diameter; it increases as the angle that the airway crosses the scanned plane increases; this phenomenon becomes worse in the case of airways that run parallel to the scanned plane because then the probability of a voxel to contain a mixture of airway wall and air is further increased.

Pitch: The distance in millimetres that the examination table travels during a single revolution of the X-ray tube in helical CT. When this distance is divided by the collimation thickness (in millimetres) the outcome is termed 'pitch ratio', which is usually referred to simply as pitch, and represents an important technical parameter that is selected (along with kilovoltage peak, current-time product, collimation and anatomical coverage) prior to the initiation of scanning. A lower pitch (ratio) provides a higher z-axis resolution and fewer artefacts. In single-detector CT scanners, the higher the pitch (ratio), the lower the radiation dose due to the decrease in duration of exposure of the patient. However, this is not the case in MDCT, where the concept of pitch (ratio) is complex and is determined by beam collimation (a combination of all detector thicknesses) and table speed but is independent of gantry rotation time.

Pixel: Picture element, i.e. the voxel (square) surface that appears on the screen.

Postprocessing: Application of image reformatting techniques onto the raw CT data. These techniques include MPR (sagittal, coronal, oblique and curved), MPVR, SSD, external VR and VB.

Reconstruction interval: Image reconstruction is the conversion of raw data to an axial image (via complex mathematical algorithms). However, it is often 'loosely' used in the context of the various reformatting or 3-dimensional rendering techniques (e.g. MPR, MPVR, external VR and VB). The reconstruction interval is derived by dividing the pitch by the number of reconstructed images per tube revolution; the wider the reconstruction interval, the fewer the reconstructed images. The reconstruction interval is an important independent variable of a CT scan examination. Although it is selected prior to scanning, it can be manipulated retrospectively, i.e. during postprocessing. Reduction of the reconstruction interval results in improved spatial resolution along the z-axis. In addition, overlapping ≥50% of the reconstructed images results in reduced partial volume averaging and therefore improved density and volume measurement of small lesions as compared to 'contiguous' slicing. Such postprocessing of scan data is accomplished without further irradiation to the patient.

Volumetric data: In helical CT, the spiral movement of the beam in reference to the patient's longitudinal axis (z-axis) allows 'continuous' sampling of data from the scanned body region, which can be reconstructed at any position and along any plane of the scanned volume and thus constitute 'volumetric' information. This reconstruction is achieved through special interpolation algorithms that regulate the relative contribution of data to the final radiographic picture. To obtain high image quality in MPR and 3-dimensional rendering, voxels are required to be of cubic (or near cubic) shape (isotropic imaging). This has become possible with the newer-generation MDCT scanners that can acquire contiguous submillimetre slices of the entire lung in a single breath-hold, thus generating 'a true volumetric data set'. The differences in the images produced with the various 3-dimensional rendering techniques are the result of the different ways that voxels are selected, and their relative contribution is weighted.

Voxel: Volume element, i.e. the elemental oblong (ideally cube; isotropic imaging) that constitutes along with a multitude of other such cubes the irradiated (axial) slice of body tissues. In essence, a voxel is the 3-dimensional equivalent of a pixel that combines the pixel area (x- and y-axis) with the tomogram slice thickness (z-axis).

Terms such as MPR, MPVR, SSD, (external) VR and VB that are explained in the text are not included in the glossary.

References

1   Wood RE: Spelunking in the pediatric airways: explorations with the flexible fiberoptic bronchoscope. Pediatr Clin North Am 1984;31:785–799.

2   Ueno J, Murase T, Yoneda K, Tsujikawa T, Sakiyama S, Kondoh K: Three-dimensional imaging of thoracic diseases with multidetector row CT. J Med Invest 2004;51:163–170.

3   Kohl G: The evolution and state-of-the-art principles of multislice computed tomography. Proc Am Thorac Soc 2005;2:470–476.

4   Siegel MJ: Multiplanar and three-dimensional multi-detector row CT of thoracic vessels and airways in the pediatric population. Radiology 2003;229:641–650.

5   Papaioannou G, Young C, Owens CM: Multidetector row CT for imaging the pediatric tracheobroncheal tree. Pediatr Radiol 2007;37:515–529.

6   Kagadis GC, Panagiotopoulou EC, Priftis KN, Vaos G, Nikiforidis GC, Anthracopoulos MB: Preoperative evaluation of the trachea in a child with pulmonary artery sling using 3-dimensional computed tomographic imaging and virtual bronchoscopy. J Pediatr Surg 2007;42:E9–E13.

7   Sorantin E, Geiger B, Fotter R, Meyer H, Eber E: Virtual tracheobronchoscopy – how to compute and how to visualize; in Lemke HU, Vannier MW, Inamura K, Farman AG (eds): CAR '98 – Computer-Assisted Radiology and Surgery. Amsterdam, Elsevier, 1998, pp 124–128.

8   Kahn MF, Herzog C, Ackermann H, Wagner TO, Maataoui A, Harth M, Abolmaali ND, Jacobi V, Vogl TJ: Virtual endoscopy of the tracheo-bronchial system: sub-millimeter collimation with the 16-row multidetector scanner. Eur Radiol 2004;14:1400–1405.

9   Sorantin E, Geiger B, Lindbichler F, Eber E, Schimpl G: CT-based virtual tracheobronchoscopy in children – comparison with axial CT and multiplanar reconstruction: preliminary results. Pediatr Radiol 2002;32:8–15.

10 Yu KC, Gibbs JD, Graham MW, Higgins WE: Image-based reporting for bronchoscopy. J Digit Imaging 2010;23:39–50.

11 Antón-Pachero JL, Cabezalí D, Tejedor R, López M, Luna C, Comas JV, de Miguel E: The role of airway stenting in pediatric tracheobronchial obstruction. Eur J Cardiothorac Surg 2008;33:1069–1075.

12 Ramachandran N, Owens CM: Imaging of the airways with multidetector row computed tomography. Pediatr Respir Rev 2008;9:69–76.

13 Scottish Intercollegiate Guidelines Network (SIGN): Safe sedation of children undergoing diagnostic and therapeutic procedures: a national clinical guideline. www.sign.ac.uk/guidelines/fulltext/58/index.html (accessed February 6, 2010).

14 Yedururi S, Guillerman RP, Chung T, Braveman RM, Dishop MK, Giannoni CM, Krishnamurthy P: Multimodality imaging of tracheobronchial disorders in children. Radiographics 2008;28:e29.

15 Lee EY, Siegel MJ: Pediatric airway disorders: large airways; in Boiselle PM, Lynch DA (eds): CT of the Airways. Totowa, Humana Press, 2008, pp 351–379.

16 Lam WW, Tam PK, Chan FL, Chan KL, Cheng W: Esophageal atresia and tracheal stenosis: use of three-dimensional CT and virtual bronchoscopy in neonates, infants, and children. AJR Am J Roentgenol 2000;174:1009–1012.

17 Lee EY, Boiselle PM, Cleveland RH: Multidetector CT evaluation of congenital lung anomalies. Radiology 2008;247:632–648.

18 Heyer CM, Nuesslein TG, Jung D, Peters SA, Lemburg SP, Rieger CH, Nicholas V: Tracheobronchial anomalies and stenosis: detection with low-dose multidetector CT with virtual tracheobronchoscopy – comparison with flexible tracheobronchoscopy. Radiology 2007;242:542–549.

19 Heyer CM, Kagel T, Lemburg SP, Nicolas V, Rieger CH: Evaluation of tracheobronchial anomalies in children using low-dose multidetector CT: report of a 13-year-old boy with a tracheal bronchus and recurrent pulmonary infections. Pediatr Pulmonol 2004;38:168–173.

20 Adaletli I, Kurugoglu S, Ulus S, Ozer H, Elicevik M, Kantarci F, Mihmanli I, Akman C: Utilization of low-dose multidetector CT and virtual bronchoscopy in children with suspected foreign body aspiration. Pediatr Radiol 2007;37:33–40.

21 Lee EY, Mason KP, Zurakowski D, Waltz DA, Ralph A, Riaz F, Boiselle PM: MDCT assessment of tracheomalacia in symptomatic infants with mediastinal aortic vascular anomalies: preliminary technical experience. Pediatr Radiol 2008;38:82–88.

22 Lee EY, Zurakowski D, Waltz DA, Mason KP, Riaz F, Ralph A, Boiselle PM: MDCT evaluation of the prevalence of tracheomalacia in children with mediastinal aortic vascular anomalies. J Thorac Imaging 2008;23:258–265.

23 Lee EY, Boiselle PM: Tracheobronchomalacia in infants and children: multidetector CT evaluation. Radiology 2009;252:7–22.

24 McLaren CA, Elliot MJ, Roebuck DJ: Vascular compression of the airway in children. Pediatr Respir Rev 2008;9:85–94.

25 Honnef D, Wildberger JE, Das M, Hohl C, Mahnken AH, Barker M, Günther RW, Staatz G: Value of virtual tracheobronchoscopy from 16-slice multidetector-row spiral computed tomography for assessment of suspected tracheobronchial stenosis in children. Eur Radiol 2006;16:1684–1691.

26 Kritsaneepaiboon S, Lee EY, Zurakowski D, Strauss KJ, Boiselle PM: MDCT pulmonary angiography evaluation of pulmonary embolism in children: AJR Am J Roentgenol 2009;192:1246–1252.

27 Prabhu SP, Mahmood S, Sena L, Lee EY: MDCT evaluation of pulmonary embolism in children and young adults following a lateral tunnel Fontan procedure: optimizing contrast-enhancement techniques. Pediatr Radiol 2009;39:938–944.

28 Lee EY: Evaluation of non-vascular mediastinal masses in infants and children: an evidence-based practical approach. Pediatr Radiol 2009;39(suppl 2):S184–S190.

29 Perger L, Lee EY, Shamberger RC: Management of children and adolescents with a critical airway due to compression by an anterior mediastinal mass. J Pediatr Surg 2008;43:1990–1997.

30 Yikilmaz A, Lee EY: CT imaging of mass-like non-vascular pulmonary lesions in children. Pediatr Radiol 2007;37:1253–1263.

31 Jadcherla SR, Gupta A, Stoner E, Coley BD, Wiet GJ, Shaker R: Correlation of glottal closure using concurrent ultrasonography and nasolaryngoscopy in children: a novel approach to evaluate glottal status. Dysphagia 2006;21:75–81.

32 Kim BS, Ahn KJ, Park YH, Hahn ST: Usefulness of laryngeal phonation CT in the diagnosis of vocal cord paralysis. AJR Am J Roentgenol 2008;190:1376–1379.

33 Hall EJ: Radiation biology for pediatric radiologists. Pediatr Radiol 2009;39(suppl 1):S57–S64.

34 Brenner DJ, Hall EJ: Computed tomography – an increasing source of radiation exposure. N Engl J Med 2007;357:2277–2284.

35 National Cancer Institute: Radiation risks and pediatric computed tomography (CT): a guide for health care providers. US National Institutes of Health. http://www.cancer.gov/cancertopics/causes/radiation-risk-pediatric-CT (accessed February 6, 2010).

36 Pierce DA, Shimizu Y, Preston DL, Vaeth M, Mabuchi K: Studies of the mortality of atomic bomb survivors. Report 12, part I. Cancer: 1950–1990. Radiat Res 1996;146:1–27.

37 Preston DL, Ron E, Tokuoka S, Funamoto S, Nishi N, Soda M, Mabuchi K, Kodama K: Solid cancer incidence in atomic bomb survivors: 1958–1998. Radiat Res 2007;168:1–64.

38 Mazrani W, McHugh K, Marsden PJ: The radiation burden of radiological investigations. Arch Dis Child 2007;92:1127–1131.

39 Goske MJ, Applegate KE, Boylan J, Butler PF, Callaghan MJ, Coley BD, Farley S, Frush DP, Hernanz-Schulman M, Jaramillo D, Johnson ND, Kaste SC, Morrison G, Strauss KJ, Tuggle N: The 'image gently' campaign: increasing CT radiation dose awareness through a national education and awareness program. Pediatr Radiol 2008;38:265–269.

40 Suter MJ, Reinhardt JM, McLennan G: Integrated CT/bronchoscopy in the central airways: preliminary results. Acad Radiol 2008;15:786–798.

41 Fain SB, Korosec FR, Holmes JH, O'Halloran RL, Sorkness RL, Grist TM: Functional lung imaging using hyperpolarized gas MRI. J Magn Reson Imaging 2007;25:910–923.

42 Mata JF, Altes TA, Ruppert K, Mitzner W, Hagspiel KD, Patel B, Salerno M, Brookeman JR, de Lange EE, Tobias WA, Wang HT, Cates GD, Mugler JP: Evaluation of emphysema severity and progression in a rabbit model: comparison of hyperpolarized ^{3}He and ^{129}Xe diffusion MRI lung morphometry. J Appl Physiol 2007;102:1273–1280.

43 Williamson JP, James AL, Phillips MJ, Sampson DD, Hillman DR, Eastwood PR: Quantifying tracheobronchial tree dimensions: methods, limitations and emerging techniques. Eur Respir J 2009;34:42–55.

44 Wanner A: Twenty-fourth transatlantic airway conference: imaging pulmonary pathology and target molecular signatures. Proc Am Thorac Soc 2009;9:397–485.

45 Williamson JP, Armstrong JJ, McLaughlin RA, Noble PB, West AR, Becker S, Curatolo A, Noffsinger WJ, Mitchell HW, Phillips MJ, Sampson DD, Hillman DR, Eastwood PR: Measuring airway dimensions during bronchoscopy using anatomical optical coherence tomography. Eur Respir J 2010;35:34–41.

Michael B. Anthracopoulos
Respiratory Unit, Department of Paediatrics, University of Patras
GR–265 04 Rio, Patras (Greece)
Tel. +30 2610 999544, Fax +30 2610 994533, E-Mail manthra@otenet.gr

Anthracopoulos · Alexopoulou · Kagadis

Airway Anatomy and Abnormalities

Priftis KN, Anthracopoulos MB, Eber E, Koumbourlis AC, Wood RE (eds): Paediatric Bronchoscopy.
Prog Respir Res. Basel, Karger 2010, vol 38, pp 114–119

Normal Anatomy

Colin Wallis

Great Ormond Street Hospital for Children and Institute of Child Health, University College London, London, UK

Abstract

Knowledge of the normal anatomy of the airways in childhood is essential for any bronchoscopist undertaking paediatric studies. There are important anatomical differences that occur with growth, and normal variants need to be recognized. This chapter reviews the airway nomenclature and common variations encountered.

Copyright © 2010 S. Karger AG, Basel

Knowledge of the normal structure of the paediatric airway is a fundamental step for any bronchoscopist undertaking diagnostic or therapeutic procedures. A clear understanding of the anatomy comes from repeated examinations of the airway, preferably adopting the same 'route' on each exploratory journey, recognizing landmark configurations (online suppl. video 1) for orientation (the trachea and carina are the most obvious example) and returning to these recognizable landmarks when lost or confused [1–15]. Only when the normal configuration is intuitive and familiar can deviations and abnormalities be diagnosed.

For the purposes of this chapter, it is anticipated that the bronchoscopist is standing at the child's head and facing down the bronchial tree with the patient's right side on the right of the bonchoscopist.

Further, for the purposes of this chapter, the airway is conveniently divided into the upper airway, larynx, trachea and carina and the bronchial tree.

The Upper Airway

The opportunity to examine the upper airway (fig. 1) may not be possible if the child is intubated or anaesthetized via a laryngeal mask. Under sedation or with the use of a facial mask for anaesthesia, the flexible bronchoscope can be passed through the nose and will often run a course along the middle meatus (between the inferior and the middle turbinates) or the inferior meatus. Because the patient is lying supine, confusion can arise when first examining the nose as the anatomy is inverted from customary. The floor of the nose is superior in the bronchoscopist's view, and the roof of the nose is inferior. The turbinate should be smooth and uninflamed, and the course of the bronchoscope should be unobstructed by polyps or turbinate inflammation. The superior turbinate is rarely seen. Minor deviations of the septum may allow easier passage of the bronchoscope through one side than the other.

The orifices of the sinuses are rarely visible in children. The opening of the eustachian tube may be missed in the young child but is visible in the lateral wall of the nasopharynx in older children. Entering the nasopharynx, adenoidal tissue may be present in the posterior view. Adenoidal tissue can be normally abundant, especially in the preschool child and even normal adenoids may bleed on contact. Tonsillar tissue is best inspected via an oral approach. The next crucial landmark on the journey through the airways is the sight of the epiglottis and laryngeal opening. The uvula points to the epiglottis, the epiglottis leads into the larynx.

The Normal Larynx

The paediatric epiglottis has a more pronounced curvature (omega shaped) than the adult epiglottis. In the infant and young child the larynx (fig. 2) is positioned anteriorly and with growth in late childhood and adolescence adopts a more central and inferior position. The lower level of the cricoid cartilage is at the mid level of C_5 in the newborn and at the lower level of C_6 in adults. The larynx is best inspected

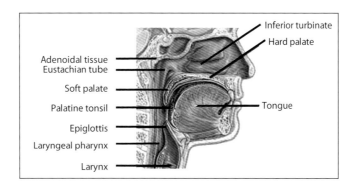

Fig. 1. The upper airway.

Inferior turbinate
Hard palate
Adenoidal tissue
Eustachian tube
Soft palate
Palatine tonsil
Tongue
Epiglottis
Laryngeal pharynx
Larynx

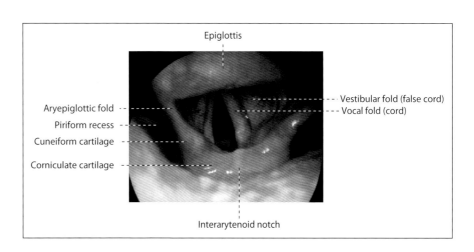

Fig. 2. The larynx.

Epiglottis
Vestibular fold (false cord)
Vocal fold (cord)
Aryepiglottic fold
Piriform recess
Cuneiform cartilage
Corniculate cartilage
Interarytenoid notch

during light anaesthesia with spontaneous breathing. The cords should move equally and meet centrally, and if the procedure is done under anaesthesia, inspection of the cords may best be left to the end and observed as the child awakens from the anaesthetic. A similar approach is advocated for inspection of malacia in the large airways.

The arytenoids are often more mobile during infancy and may contribute to a benign stridor that is common during the first months of life. Prolapsing of the arytenoids into the laryngeal inlet can be a normal finding during early infancy but if obstructive and clinically significant may require surgical intervention. In the child, the cuneiform and corniculate cartilages may not be discernable as separate structures. There should be no cleft in the posterior laryngeal wall. This can be difficult to see with the flexible bronchoscope which favours a view of the anterior structures, and if a type 1 laryngeal cleft is suspected, it is best examined by rigid instrumentation of the posterior wall to exclude a subtle fusion defect.

In children up to several years of age, the cricoid cartilage is the smallest cross-sectional area of the airway. During growth, the subglottis enlarges and the airway at the level of the cords becomes the narrowest section.

The Normal Trachea and Carina

The normal trachea is characterized by incomplete cartilaginous rings with an absent section posteriorly that is bridged by a softer pars membranacea (membranous trachea). The rings are more complete in the child extending to an arc of nearly 320°, but the ends of the tracheal cartilage 'rings' should not meet. Completely fused rings are not a normal variant. During childhood and adolescence, the width of the membranous trachea increases and the cartilage adopts a more C-shaped appearance. Adolescent females tend to preserve a round configuration, while males tend to have some sagittal widening and transverse narrowing.

The normal tracheal lumen is unobstructed and perceived bronchoscopically as straight without branches. Pulsation of the large vessels and right atrium abutting on the trachea and main bronchi may cause pulsatile deflections through the wall around the level of the carina but the lumen should not be obstructed or permanently distorted in the normal subject. The airway should maintain its integrity during quiet breathing with some minimal narrowing of the calibre due to inward bulging of the posterior membrane.

Abnormal malacia may be masked by rigid instrumentation or positive pressure ventilation.

The normal trachea has sparse secretions that are clear, light and frothy and are easily suctioned away. The mucosa is smooth throughout. The trachea consists of between 18 and 22 rings and enlarges in length and width with somatic growth. Like the larynx, the trachea is situated higher in infants with the upper level at the level of the 4th cervical vertebra. In adults the upper level descends to C_6–C_7.

Contrary to the numerous variations of lobar or segmental bronchial subdivisions, abnormal bronchi arising from the trachea or main bronchi are rare. A true tracheal bronchus is any bronchus originating from the trachea, usually within 2–6 cm of the carina. When the entire right upper lobe bronchus is displaced onto the tracheal bronchus it is also called a 'pig bronchus' and has a reported frequency of 0.2%. A prevalence of 0.1–2% for a right tracheal bronchus and 0.3–1% for a left tracheal bronchus has been found in bronchographic and bronchoscopic studies. A bridging bronchus is a displaced bronchus arising from the left main bronchus and crossing through the mediastinum to supply the right lower lobe. The principle of what constitutes a normal branching variant is that a normal variant should provide unobstructed airflow in inspiration and expiration to and from a normal lung structure distally with congruous blood supply and free mucociliary clearance of secretions into the proximal airway. A normal variant will always be asymptomatic and discovered incidentally.

The tracheal carina is a key landmark on the bronchoscopist's journey through the paediatric airway and should be instantly recognizable and a point of reference at times of disorientation. In the first 2 years of life, the carina is situated on the right of the midline and successively becomes more medial. It is a keel-shaped structure with a characteristic cartilaginous ring arrangement. The angle of the carina is more obtuse in infancy and early childhood. The carina adopts a more acute angle in adolescence and adulthood. This blunted appearance of the main carina in paediatrics is true of many of the other airway bifurcations.

The Bronchial Tree

The carina is the point of division into a left- and right-sided bronchial tree (fig. 3; table 1). There is remarkable consistency of the branching of the primary bronchial tree in humans although normal variants do occur especially at the subsegmental level. A full examination of the bronchial tree should be completed in all procedures if possible and should preferably follow a systematic route. An example of a normal examination is as follows from the carina.

The opening of the right main bronchus quickly comes into view when descending down the tracheal lumen. In newborns the right main stem bronchus is 4 times shorter than the left; at 3 years of age, it is one third, and in adolescents it is half the length of the left main bronchus. Having entered the right main bronchus, a turn of the bronchoscope tip towards the right side will bring the right upper lobe orifice into view with its trifurcation into an apical, posterior and anterior division. Withdrawing the bronchoscope, you enter the right bronchus intermedius. Three orifices will be noted. They are the right middle lobe anteriorly, right lower lobe straight down and its superior segment posteriorly across from the right middle lobe opening. The right middle lobe can be entered to reveal its bifurcation into the medial and lateral segments each with their bifurcation. Withdraw the bronchoscope again and advance towards the right lower lobe. The medial basal segment will branch off first along the medial side. At the distal end of the right bronchial tree, you will see the anterior, lateral and posterior basal segments clustered together and known by some as 'the 3 musketeers'.

Return to the carina.

The opening of the left main bronchus is slightly smaller than the right and adopts a longer course entering the upper division with a less acute angle than on the right. The upper division commonly bifurcates into an apicoposterior and anterior lobe. Withdraw the bronchoscope and enter the lingular segment of the left upper lobe with its division into a superior and inferior segment. On withdrawing the bronchoscope and directing further down the left main bronchus, the superior segment of the left lower lobe branches off posteriorly. Upon entering the left lower lobe, the 3 basal segments can be seen (anteromedial, lateral, posterior). Common normal variations on the left side include a separation of the apicoposterior branch of the left upper lobe into separate bronchial openings and individual bronchial openings of the anteromedial basal segment rather than a common carina.

Recognizable bronchial configurations are illustrated in figure 3.

Bronchial Nomenclature

The nomenclature used in this chapter adopts the recommendations of a consensus meeting at a congress of anatomists in the 1950s. Inevitably it was not universally accepted and led to

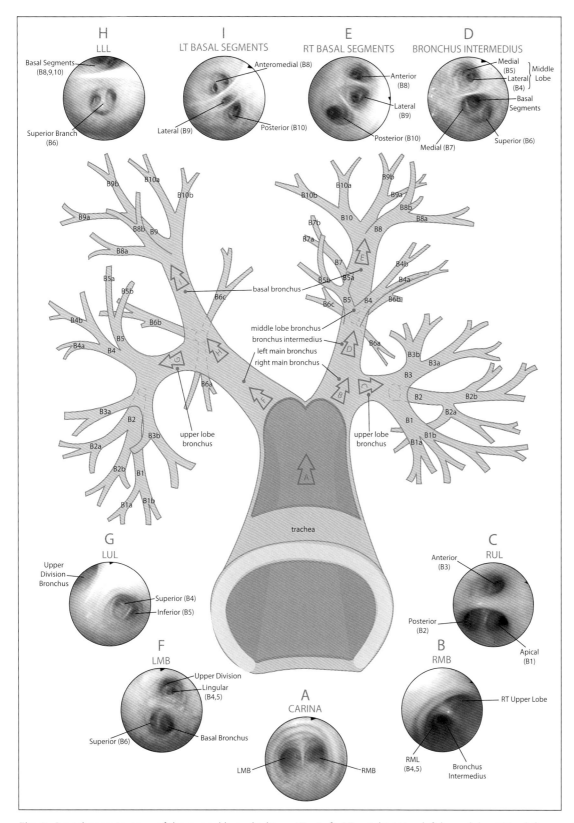

Fig. 3. Bronchoscopic views of the normal bronchial tree. LT = Left; RT = right; LLL = left lower lobe; LUL = left upper lobe; LMB = left main bronchus; RMB = right main bronchus; RML = right middle lobe; RUL = right upper lobe; for further explanations, see text.

Table 1. Anatomical nomenclature system and variations of the bronchi

Anatomical nomenclature	Numbering system	Further subdivision	Common variations
Right lung (right main bronchus)			
Upper lobe			
Apical	B1	a and b	may be absent or arise from B2 or B3
Posterior	B2	a and b	numbering swapped around in Boyden system
Anterior	B3	a and b	
Middle lobe			
Lateral	B4	a and b	may have a superior/inferior division similar to the lingula
Medial	B5	a and b	
Lower lobe			
Superior (apical)	B6	a, b and c	
Medial basal	B7	a and b	occasionally there is an additional accessory cardiac branch
Anterior basal	B8	a and b	the basal bronchi are the most variable divisions of the right lung
Lateral basal	B9	a and b	
Posterior basal	B10	a, b and c	
Left lung (left main bronchus)			
Upper lobe			
Apicoposterior	B1 + 2	a, b and c	may have a separate carina B1, B2
Anterior	B3	a, b and c	
Superior lingular	B4	a and b	
Inferior lingular	B5	a and b	
Lower lobe			
Superior (apical)	B6	a, b and c	
Anteromedial basal	B8	a and b	may have an additional medial bronchus B7 with a separate anterior branch B8
Lateral basal	B9	a and b	
Posterior basal	B10	a and b	may trifurcate into a, b and c

Note: the Boyden [4] surgical anatomical focus refers to the anterior and posterior segments of the upper lobe as B2 and B3. This nomenclature is not used by many bronchoscopists who prefer the Japanese system of Yamashita [15] using anterior as B3 and posterior as B2.

vigorous debate and correspondence. Although these terms are widely used by bronchoscopists, an alternative nomenclature still occurs. The term 'apical' is often used interchangeably for the superior segment of the lower lobes. Similarly the term 'dorsal' may be substituted for 'posterior'. Occasionally the lower lobe will be referenced as the inferior lobe.

Anatomists and radiologists have also devised a numbering system for the bronchial tree which allows for detailed isolation of specific subdivisions beyond the primary nomenclature. For example the superior segment of the upper lobe is labelled B1, and subsequent bifurcations are then given the label B1a and B1b with the facility for still further subdivision. Trifurcations, such as commonly occur in the anteromedial branch of the LLL or the posterior basal branches, are labelled a, b and c. Whereas there are some useful applications for this approach such as precise small tumour localization in adult oncology, the majority of paediatric bronchoscopy procedures rarely need identification beyond the anatomical descriptive nomenclature. Both systems are presented in table 1 for reference and are further illustrated in figure 3.

An accessory cardiac bronchus is a supernumerary bronchus from the inner wall of the right main bronchus or intermediate bronchus that progresses toward the pericardium (frequency 0.08%). Most accessory cardiac bronchi have a blind extremity, but imaging and anatomical studies have demonstrated that some develop into a series of small bronchioles, which may end in vestigial or rudimentary parenchymal tissue or even a ventilated lobule.

Anatomical variations are most commonly seen in the left upper lobe and in the arrangements of the basal bronchi in the lower lobes. Examples are listed in table 1. By definition, these normal variations are asymptomatic and discovered incidentally.

References

1 Adewale L: Anatomy and assessment of the pediatric airway. Paediatr Anaesth 2009;19(suppl 1): 1–8.
2 Baden W, Schaefer J, Kumpf M, Tzaribachev N, Pantalitschka T, Koitschev A, Ziemer G, Fuchs J, Hofbeck M: Comparison of imaging techniques in the diagnosis of bridging bronchus. Eur Respir J 2008;31:1125–1131.
3 Boyden EA, Clark SL, Danforth CH, Greulich WW, Corner GW: Committee on anatomical nomenclature. Science 1942;96:116.
4 Boyden EA: Segmental Anatomy of the Lungs. New York, McGraw-Hill, 1955.
5 Campos JH: Update on tracheobronchial anatomy and flexible fiberoptic bronchoscopy in thoracic anesthesia. Curr Opin Anaesthesiol 2009;22:4–10.
6 Dalal PG, Murray D, Messner AH, Feng A, McAllister J, Molter D: Pediatric laryngeal dimensions: an age-based analysis. Anesth Analg 2009;108:1475–1479.
7 Desir A, Ghaye B: Congenital abnormalities of intrathoracic airways. Radiol Clin North Am 2009;47:203–225.
8 Doolittle AM, Mair EA: Tracheal bronchus: classification, endoscopic analysis, and airway management. Otolaryngol Head Neck Surg 2002;126:240–243.
9 Edell E, Krier-Morrow D: Navigational bronchoscopy: overview of technology and practical considerations – new CPT codes effective 2010. Chest 2009, E-pub ahead of print.
10 Ghaye B, Szapiro D, Fanchamps JM, Dondelinger RF: Congenital bronchial abnormalities revisited. Radiographics. 2001;21:105–119.
11 Gonlugur U, Efeoglu T, Kaptanoglu M, Akkurt I: Major anatomical variations of the tracheobronchial tree: bronchoscopic observation. Anat Sci Int 2005;80:111–115.
12 Jackson CL, Huber JF: Correlated anatomy of the bronchial tree and lungs with a system of nomenclature. Dis Chest 1943;9:319–326.
13 Jafek BW, Carter DR: Endoscopic nomenclature for bronchopulmonary anatomy. Otolaryngol Head Neck Surg 1979;87:815–817.
14 Williamson JP, James AL, Phillips MJ, Sampson DD, Hillman DR, Eastwood PR: Quantifying tracheobronchial tree dimensions: methods, limitations and emerging techniques. Eur Respir J 2009;34:42–55.
15 Yamashita H: Roentgenologic Anatomy of the Lung, ed 1. Tokyo, Igaku-Shoin, 1978.

Dr. Colin Wallis, MD, FRCPCH, FCP, DCH
Respiratory Unit, Great Ormond Street Hospital for Children, Great Ormond Street Hospital
London WC1N 3JH (UK)
Tel. +44 207 405 9200, ext. 5453, Fax +44 207 813 8514, E-Mail c.wallis@ich.ucl.ac.uk

Chapter 11

Priftis KN, Anthracopoulos MB, Eber E, Koumbourlis AC, Wood RE (eds): Paediatric Bronchoscopy.
Prog Respir Res. Basel, Karger 2010, vol 38, pp 120–129

Congenital and Acquired Abnormalities of the Upper Airways

Ernst Eber

Respiratory and Allergic Disease Division, Department of Paediatrics and Adolescence Medicine, Medical University of Graz,
Graz, Austria

Abstract

Flexible airway endoscopy allows a detailed systematic inspection of the upper airways from the nose down to the thoracic inlet and is the ultimate diagnostic test for evaluation of upper airway obstruction (UAO). The dynamic view it provides is essential in diagnosing upper airway abnormalities such as pharyngeal collapse, laryngomalacia and vocal cord paralysis. Knowledge of growth, development and functional anatomy of the upper airways is important for the diagnostic competence of the endoscopist. This chapter presents a brief general discussion of UAO, respiratory noises and the indications for endoscopy with regard to the upper airways. The main focus is on the aetiology, frequency, endoscopic appearance and typical clinical presentation of important congenital and acquired abnormalities of the nose, pharynx and larynx. The nasopharyngeal lesions discussed include choanal stenosis and atresia, nasal masses, craniofacial abnormalities, adenotonsillar hypertrophy, pharyngeal collapse and base of the tongue masses. The laryngeal abnormalities described include laryngomalacia (infantile larynx), subglottic stenosis, subglottic oedema, vocal cord paralysis, haemangioma, cyst, papillomatosis, web, cleft and vocal cord dysfunction. A brief discussion of the reported associations between gastro-oesophageal reflux and upper airway disease is also included. Acute infections of the upper airway such as croup (viral laryngotracheobronchitis) and epiglottitis are only touched upon as they generally are not indications for flexible endoscopy unless symptoms are prolonged or endoscopic intubation is needed. Likewise, it is beyond the scope of this article to discuss treatment options of the various disorders.

Copyright © 2010 S. Karger AG, Basel

From a physiology-orientated perspective, the upper airways are the part of the air-conducting system extending from the nose to the thoracic inlet, and include the nasal cavity, the pharynx, the larynx and the extrathoracic part of the trachea. In addition, adjacent spaces such as the paranasal sinuses and the eustachian tubes are considered integral parts of the upper airways. This chapter will deal with the nose, pharynx and larynx; the trachea will be discussed in detail in chapter 12 [this vol., pp. 130–140].

Structural or functional abnormalities of the upper airways can greatly affect their main functions, i.e. respiration, protection of the lower respiratory tract and phonation. Details on the normal anatomy of the upper airways (in particular with regard to location, size, configuration and tissue consistency of the larynx) are given in the previous chapter 10 [this vol., pp. 114–119]. Obviously, knowledge of the embryonic and fetal development of the upper airways will enhance the understanding of congenital abnormalities in this area; however, a review of upper airway development is beyond the scope of this chapter, and the reader is referred to the relevant literature.

Congenital and acquired abnormalities of the upper airways commonly result in airway obstruction. Many infants with *upper airway obstruction* (UAO) have significant feeding problems that can lead to failure to thrive and often to recurrent aspiration with the potential for immediate and long-term damage to the lung parenchyma.

The causes and prevalence of UAO differ substantially between newborns and older children. In the newborn period and in early infancy, UAO is relatively rare and almost always the result of congenital abnormalities. In contrast, in childhood UAO is much more frequent and usually of infectious origin as in the case of viral croup (acute laryngotracheobronchitis).

In an effort to overcome the obstruction, patients with UAO generate high negative intrathoracic pressures; with increasing negative pleural pressures, dynamic collapse of the soft extrathoracic airways occurs, further worsening UAO and thus feeding a vicious cycle. UAO may be life-threatening; thus, early and accurate diagnosis and treatment are essential.

Respiratory Noises

Snoring is an inspiratory noise of irregular quality and usually results from partial obstruction of the oropharynx during sleep. The noise is due to vibrations of the uvula, soft palate and tongue, and may be heard in children without obvious respiratory abnormalities or disease. When the obstruction is severe, snoring may be interspersed with periods of apnoea. The most common causes for snoring with or without obstructive apnoea are pharyngeal collapse, adenotonsillar hypertrophy and congenital malformations of the palate, tongue, maxilla and mandible.

Stridor is often the most prominent symptom of UAO. It is a variably pitched respiratory sound, caused by tissue vibration from airflow of increased turbulence and velocity passing through a narrowed segment of the large airways. Usually, stridor is indicative of substantial narrowing or obstruction of the larynx or (extrathoracic) trachea; on occasion, it may be produced by an oesophageal lesion (especially a foreign body). Stridor is predominantly an inspiratory sound; however, in some infants with subglottic lesions (particularly if there is involvement of the upper trachea as well), a soft expiratory element may be noted. Biphasic stridor suggests severe, fixed airway obstruction that may be localized anywhere from the level of the glottis to the midtracheal region. In neonates, the most common causes of biphasic stridor are vocal cord paralysis and subglottic stenosis [1]. In general, the intensity of the stridor is directly related to the degree of airway obstruction. However, a sudden decrease in intensity signifies decreased air movement due to worsening of the obstruction. Conversely, when the obstruction is relatively mild, the breathing may be quiet at rest, but stridor may develop with increased activity (e.g. crying) due to the increased velocity of airflow.

Hoarseness with or without stridor suggests an abnormality of the vocal cords. If present at or shortly after birth, it suggests either a structural (e.g. laryngeal web) or a functional abnormality (e.g. vocal cord paralysis). Intermittent hoarseness of varying degree is most often due to oedema, whereas progressive hoarseness could be due to vocal cord lesions such as nodules or papillomas. Hoarseness associated with a high-pitched inspiratory stridor suggests narrowing of the glottis. A *muffled voice* associated with a low-pitched stridor

but no hoarseness suggests a supraglottic process such as epiglottitis (supraglottitis), whereas a weak voice accompanied by a high-pitched inspiratory stridor but no hoarseness can result from a subglottic obstruction.

Indications for Flexible Airway Endoscopy

Stridor is one of the most common indications for diagnostic airway endoscopy in infants and children [2–7], and endoscopy has a very high diagnostic yield in patients with stridor [4, 5, 8–11]. Children with stridor should be examined while they are stridulous, as the vibrating structures should then always be visible [3, 12]. In many cases, 'negative' findings are as important as 'positive' ones. The documentation of laryngomalacia and the exclusion of other causes of stridor in an infant usually alleviate parental anxiety and may prevent further diagnostic evaluation. In general, flexible endoscopes are passed through the nose. This transnasal approach allows the examination of the upper airways in detail, and leaves the head and neck in a neutral position so that the dynamics of the pharynx and larynx can be observed without distortion.

Although the clinical features are quite often suggestive of the type of the airway abnormality present in a newborn, an endoscopic examination is usually necessary to confirm the diagnosis and guide management. Similarly, infants with persistent stridor should be investigated endoscopically to establish a precise diagnosis so that appropriate treatment can be planned and an accurate prognosis can be given to the parents. Direct examination of the airways is indicated in virtually all infants with persistent stridor, especially when it is progressive or associated with hoarseness, apnoeas, difficulty in feeding or growth retardation as well as when there are any unusual features. Sometimes it appears difficult to decide whether to perform endoscopy in an infant who develops stridor at the age of few weeks or months. In infants and children with viral croup, endoscopy is rarely indicated unless there are unusual features.

Even when the primary indication for the procedure involves the upper airway, a strong case can be made for performing endoscopy of the lower airways as well, because upper airway lesions are frequently associated with lower airway lesions. Several series have demonstrated that in up to a quarter of children with persistent stridor concomitant lower airway abnormalities or two or more synchronous airway lesions may be detected [2, 10, 11, 13, 14]. However, as both the population and the indications for bronchoscopy vary greatly among centres, insufficient information exists on the frequency of concomitant abnormalities [7].

One exception to the inspection of the lower airways is the detection of a lesion causing significant upper airway obstruction. In such a case, the passage of the bronchoscope beyond the point of obstruction may cause additional oedema that may create a truly critical airway. In adults and older children, it may be possible to prevent this problem by using a smaller bronchoscope. However, this is often not an option for young infants due to their naturally small-sized airway.

Other indications for endoscopic evaluation may be *abnormal crying* or *hoarseness* (with or without stridor) persisting for longer than 2 weeks. Possible endoscopic findings include vocal cord paralysis and laryngeal papillomatosis. Unless mild sedation is used, the diagnosis of vocal cord paralysis, particularly of the unilateral form, may be difficult to establish.

Children with *atypical croup*, characterized by prolonged symptoms (longer than 2 weeks), lack of response to treatment or an age less than 6 months should also be investigated by flexible endoscopy. In addition, children with recurrent croup (commonly defined as more than 2 episodes of croup-like symptoms such as hoarseness, barking cough and inspiratory stridor) should be assessed by airway endoscopy, especially if there were episodes of severe or prolonged stridor. While children with recurrent croup less than 3 years of age are more likely to have an airway abnormality (e.g. a subglottic stenosis that favours the development of stridor with respiratory infections) found, diagnostic airway endoscopy should also be considered in older children [15].

When a patient with *vocal cord dysfunction* (VCD) is symptomatic, the diagnosis can be confirmed by visualization of the paradoxical inspiratory narrowing of the anterior portion of the vocal cords during inspiration.

Flexible endoscopy has also proved to be a useful method for assessing patients with postextubation stridor. While some infants or children fail immediately and require re-intubation, in others it may take many hours to develop UAO. Thus, in some patients initial endoscopic findings may be normal due to temporary stenting by the endotracheal tube and development of oedema at a later time.

Abnormalities of the Nasopharyngeal Airway

Choanal Stenosis and Atresia

Choanal atresia is the most common congenital abnormality of the nose, with bony occlusion of the airway in most cases and membranous obstruction in some. The incidence is approximately 1 in 7,000 live births [16]. Bilateral choanal atresia or choanal stenosis may cause severe respiratory difficulties immediately after birth. Unilateral lesions are twice as common as bilateral ones and are often not detected until later in childhood. Some children present with feeding difficulties and persistent rhinorrhoea, especially if the patent nostril is occluded during intercurrent infections. Diagnosis is confirmed by passing a flexible endoscope through the nose to assess the choanae. Computed tomography is often necessary in order to delineate the exact site of obstruction and also whether it is bony or membranous. Choanal atresia is frequently associated with other abnormalities; the most common and most serious of these is the CHARGE association (coloboma of the eye, heart defect, atresia of the choanae, retarded growth or development, genital hypoplasia and ear anomalies or deafness) [17].

Nasal Masses

Congenital mass lesions in the nasal passages are rare but can be of major significance both functionally and pathologically. These lesions vary from cystic masses (e.g. dermoid cysts, meningoceles) to more solid lesions such as haemangiomas, neurofibromas and gliomas [18]. Encephaloceles and gliomas are commonly associated with midline defects such as cleft palate [16]. Polyps in a neonate should be considered an encephalocele or a glioma until a definitive diagnosis is established.

Craniofacial Abnormalities

The *Pierre Robin sequence* consists of micrognathia, glossoptosis and cleft palate, resulting in obstruction of the pharyngeal airway. The severity of airway obstruction is very variable; in some cases it is mild with little intervention required, while in others airway support is needed to prevent chronic or recurrent severe hypoxia and the development of cor pulmonale. As the mandible grows forward with age, particularly during the first 6 months of life, airway and feeding problems gradually resolve. The Pierre Robin sequence can occur in isolation or can be associated with other congenital malformations (e.g. *Stickler syndrome*) [16].

A number of syndromic craniofacial abnormalities can affect the patency of the nose and the pharynx. These dysmorphic syndromes are typically characterized by mandibular or maxillary hypoplasia and include *craniofacial dysostosis (Crouzon syndrome)*, *mandibulofacial dysostosis (Treacher Collins syndrome)* and *acrocephalosyndactyly (Apert syndrome)* [16, 18].

Several abnormalities such as a narrowed nasopharynx with associated adenotonsillar hypertrophy, midface hypoplasia and hypertrophy of the tongue can cause airway compromise in children with *Down syndrome (trisomy 21)*.

An enlarged tongue may be relative or true macroglossia; the latter is the case in patients with *Beckwith-Wiedemann syndrome (exomphalos-macroglossia-gigantism syndrome)* [16].

Adenoidal/Adenotonsillar Hypertrophy
Adenoidal hypertrophy is a common finding in children; in some, it can cause complete nasal airway obstruction, and this observation may serve as a criterion for adenoidectomy. Enlarged adenoids, together with enlarged tonsils, are a common cause of obstructive sleep apnoea in children. Adenotonsillar hypertrophy may further aggravate airway obstruction in patients with pharyngeal collapse.

Pharyngeal Collapse
Increased pharyngeal collapsibility may be due to reductions in pharyngeal neuromuscular activity and/or anatomical narrowing of the airway by pharyngeal structures. Complete airway obstruction at the level of the oropharynx during inspiration is usually accompanied by laryngomalacia or other concomitant airway abnormalities, and generalized hypotonia is a frequently associated systemic finding [19, 20]. Dynamic events in the airway are influenced by its muscle tone at the time of the examination; thus, the degree of sedation is of importance.

Base of Tongue Masses
Cysts or mass lesions arising from the dorsal surface of the tongue are rare but may cause significant airway obstruction, usually with associated feeding difficulties. As some cysts vary in size with time, symptoms may be intermittent. Differential diagnosis includes lingual thyroid, thyroglossal duct cyst, mucus retention cyst (fig. 1; online suppl. video 1) and others [16].

Abnormalities of the Larynx

Laryngomalacia (Infantile Larynx)
Laryngomalacia is a usually benign, self-limited disorder; it is the most common congenital laryngeal anomaly (50–75%) and the most common cause of persistent stridor in children (approx. 60%) [21]. The term 'laryngomalacia' suggests that the cartilage of the larynx is abnormally soft, but there is no good evidence supporting this hypothesis [22]. Thus, whether laryngomalacia is primarily an anatomical abnormality or whether it is due to delayed neuromuscular development is controversial. Laryngomalacia is frequently associated with other airway lesions and with gastro-oesophageal reflux, and infants with laryngomalacia

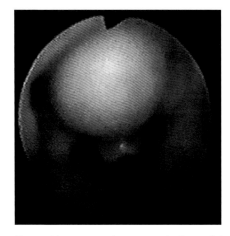

Fig. 1. Mucus retention cyst at the base of the tongue.

may have episodes of micro-aspiration [23–25]. The natural history of laryngomalacia is characterized by an onset of inspiratory stridor usually within the first 4–6 weeks of life; cry and cough are normal. The stridor varies considerably with posture and airflow, is loudest with increased ventilation (e.g. crying, agitation, feeding) and worsens during intercurrent respiratory tract infections. Some patients will have increasing symptoms during the first few months of life but thereafter stridor tends to resolve with time. Depending on the form of laryngomalacia, stridor may persist for the first year of life or even up to several years. Treatment (i.e. surgery) is only rarely needed.

Laryngoscopy demonstrates supraglottic collapse, i.e. prolapse of the epiglottis and/or the aryepiglottic folds and/or arytenoids during inspiration into the glottis (fig. 2; online suppl. video 2). The state of consciousness of the patient may be critical in the examination of the larynx; some children are stridulous only when crying, others only when they are asleep. Topical anaesthesia can potentially exaggerate the findings associated with laryngomalacia; thus, the larynx should be examined before applying topical anaesthesia [26].

According to Holinger [21], 5 types of laryngomalacia (2 or more may occur simultaneously) can be distinguished (table 1). Others have suggested alternative classifications [27, 28].

Subglottic Stenosis
Congenital subglottic stenosis is a common cause of stridor in infants [21] and may be seen in 2 forms. The more common form, membranous subglottic stenosis, is characterized by thickening of the soft tissues in the subglottic area which results in bilateral symmetrical narrowing of the subglottic space (fig. 3). Thus, the endoscopic appearance may

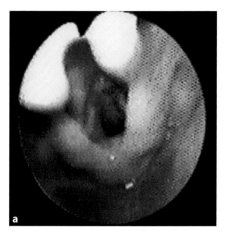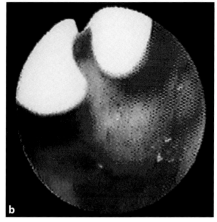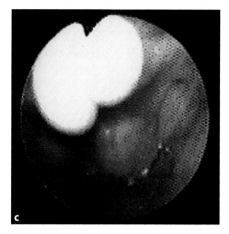

Fig. 2. Laryngomalacia (infantile larynx). **a** Patent airway during expiration. **b** Prolapse of arytenoids and aryepiglottic folds into the glottis during midinspiration. **c** Prolapse of arytenoids and aryepiglottic folds and folding of epiglottis along its long axis ('floppy epiglottis') at end-inspiration, resulting in complete obstruction of the larynx.

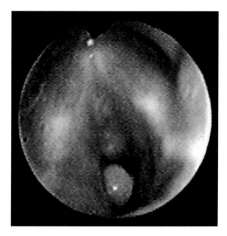

Fig. 3. Acquired subglottic stenosis (subglottic cyst) on the basis of congenital subglottic stenosis (membranous form).

Table 1. Types of laryngomalacia according to Holinger [21]

Type 1	Inward collapse of the aryepiglottic folds, primarily the cuneiform cartilages which are often enlarged
Type 2	Long, tubular epiglottis (a pathological exaggeration of the normal omega shape)
Type 3	Anterior, medial collapse of the arytenoid cartilages
Type 4	Posterior inspiratory displacement of the epiglottis against the posterior pharyngeal wall or inferior collapse to the vocal cords
Type 5	Short aryepiglottic folds

resemble acute subglottic oedema. Cartilaginous subglottic stenosis is due to a malformation of the cricoid cartilage, resulting in circumferential stenosis of variable appearance (e.g. normal shape but small size; abnormal shape). In children with a normal-appearing but small larynx, the diagnosis of subglottic stenosis may be difficult. Children with subglottic stenosis may have a wide range of problems, from severe respiratory distress at birth to the development of inspiratory or biphasic stridor within the first few months of life; patients with the latter usually present with recurrent or atypical croup [29]. Signs and symptoms clearly depend on the grade of the stenosis; Myer et al. [30] proposed a grading system for subglottic stenosis based on endotracheal tube sizes (table 2).

Acquired subglottic stenosis is more common than the congenital forms and is the result of airway trauma (mostly iatrogenic such as prolonged endotracheal intubation or tracheostomy). In infants and children, the most vulnerable part of the airway is the cricoid cartilage. The endoscopic appearance is usually irregular (not symmetrical). In some children, the stenosis may resemble a congenital web, in others ulcerations, granulation tissue or subglottic cysts may be seen (fig. 3) [31, 32]. The symptoms of acquired subglottic stenosis are similar to those of congenital stenosis; with involvement of the glottis, hoarseness or aphonia may occur. Extubation failure may be the initial clinical presentation of subglottic stenosis.

Subglottic Oedema
Subglottic oedema may be caused by infection (croup, bacterial laryngotracheitis), allergy or trauma (e.g. thermal injury; laryngeal foreign body; iatrogenic – endotracheal

Table 2. Grading system for subglottic stenoses according to Myer et al. [30]

Grade I	Up to 50% obstruction of the lumen
Grade II	51–70% obstruction of the lumen
Grade III	More than 71% obstruction of the lumen (any detectable lumen)
Grade IV	No detectable lumen

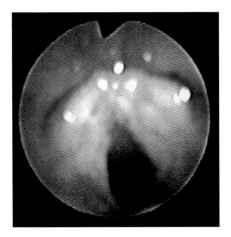

Fig. 4. Subglottic oedema after endotracheal intubation.

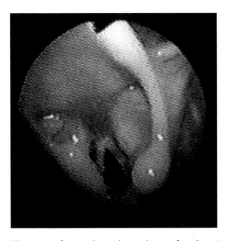

Fig. 5. Left vocal cord paralysis after ligation of a patent ductus arteriosus.

intubation, rigid bronchoscopy). In fact, subglottic oedema is the most common complication of rigid bronchoscopy. Endoscopically, the subglottic space appears swollen and symmetrically narrowed with the glottic shape preserved (fig. 4); sometimes the airway is slit-like, and the mucosa may appear inflamed. Subglottic oedema is often combined with supraglottic oedema.

Vocal Cord Paralysis
Unilateral vocal cord paralysis may result from traumatic delivery or thoracic surgery and most often affects the left side (fig. 5; online suppl. video 3). Bilateral paralysis may be due to birth trauma or an associated severe malformation of the central nervous system resulting in raised intracranial pressure (e.g. Arnold-Chiari malformation) [33]. While the rare adductor paralysis ('open glottis') is characterized by aphonia and aspiration, the more common abductor paralysis ('closed glottis') may present with hoarseness, stridor and respiratory distress (bilateral paralysis) or may be asymptomatic (unilateral paralysis). The diagnosis of unilateral vocal cord paralysis may be difficult to establish; the movement of the vocal cords and the arytenoids can only be fully evaluated when the patient is awake or under light sedation. As return of vocal cord function after general anaesthesia may not be symmetrical and is not predictable, examination of vocal cord movement is not recommended at the conclusion of general anaesthesia. If adequate visualization of the vocal cords is not possible with a flexible endoscope (e.g. due to large arytenoids), rigid laryngoscopy may provide anatomic details of the posterior aspects of the larynx.

Haemangioma
Haemangiomas represent the most common tumours in infancy but are an uncommon cause of stridor in infants. They may occur in the supraglottic (not so common) or subglottic (more common) space. Most subglottic haemangiomas are located unilaterally with or without posterior extension,

and some infants with laryngeal haemangiomas also have cutaneous haemangiomas [34]. The lesions often show rapid growth until 6–10 months, with involution usually beginning at approximately 18 months. In the first 3 months of life, affected infants present with insidiously or abruptly developing (biphasic) stridor, often as recurrent or atypical croup. Endoscopic recognition may be difficult as the lesion may be covered with normal epithelium; usually, haemangiomas present as an asymmetrical subglottic mass (fig. 6).

Laryngeal Cyst
Supraglottic cysts, commonly located at the aryepiglottic folds or at the epiglottis, are usually congenital (fig. 7; online suppl. video 4). In contrast, subglottic cysts are usually acquired as a result of airway trauma (e.g. intubation). The appearance of cysts varies widely: while some are covered by

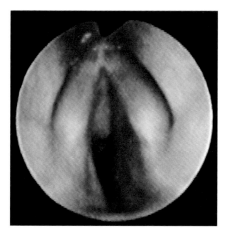

Fig. 6. Right-sided subglottic haemangioma in an infant presenting with atypical croup.

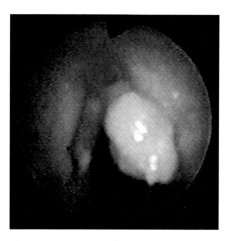

Fig. 8. Laryngeal papillomatosis.

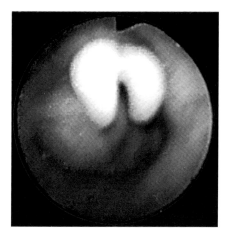

Fig. 7. Laryngeal cyst arising from the left false vocal cord, and bifid epiglottis.

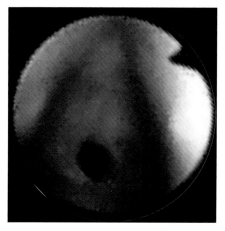

Fig. 9. Subglottic web in an infant with Down syndrome.

thin mucosa and are easy to recognize, others appear as a submucosal mass. A *laryngocele* is a rare special form of a laryngeal cyst, which originates from the laryngeal ventricle, consists of an air-filled saccule and may be difficult to diagnose endoscopically [21]. Infants commonly present with stridor, hoarseness, weak cry or aphonia, and sometimes feeding difficulties.

Laryngeal Papillomatosis
Laryngeal papillomatosis is a rare disease but the most common benign neoplasm of the larynx beyond infancy. It is caused by human papillomavirus types 6 and 11, and is characterized by proliferation of squamous papillomas [35]. Its clinical course is unpredictable; spontaneous regression is possible, but papillomatosis tends to recur and spread

throughout the respiratory tract and thus may be associated with significant morbidity and mortality. The vocal cord is usually the first and predominant site of the lesions, which typically appear as multiple, sessile or pedunculated, irregular and friable masses (fig. 8; online suppl. video 5). Presenting symptoms are usually hoarseness and stridor, less commonly cough or respiratory distress.

Laryngeal Web
Congenital laryngeal webs are uncommon. They are usually encountered at the level of the glottis, but supraglottic and subglottic webs may also occur (fig. 9). The webs may be complete or incomplete, and vary in thickness. Several types of glottic webs may be distinguished, according to their extension. An acquired lesion is usually named 'synechia'. Symptoms range

Table 3. Classification system for laryngeal clefts according to Benjamin and Inglis [37]

Type 1	Supraglottic interarytenoid cleft that extends inferiorly no further than the vocal cord level
Type 2	Cleft with extension below the vocal cord level (cricoid cartilage partially involved)
Type 3	Cleft that extends through the cricoid cartilage with or without extension into the cervical trachea
Type 4	Cleft with extension into the thoracic trachea (may extend as far as the carina)

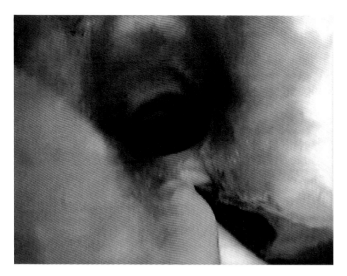

Fig. 10. Type 2 laryngeal cleft extending inferiorly to – but not through – the cricoid plate; nasogastric tube in the oesophagus.

from hoarseness and aphonia to (biphasic) stridor and respiratory distress [21].

Laryngeal Cleft

A congenital posterior laryngeal cleft, characterized by a deficient separation between larynx and hypopharynx in the midline, is a rare lesion; in severe cases, it may extend inferiorly into the trachea. Laryngeal clefts may be familial and may be associated with other anomalies of the trachea or the oesophagus and with multiple congenital anomalies of other organ systems [21, 36]. Depending on the extension, several types of clefts can be distinguished (table 3; fig. 10; online suppl. video 6) [37]. A type 1 cleft (interarytenoid cleft) extending to the level just above the posterior cricoid cartilage may be more common than previously thought and should be suspected in all infants with laryngomalacia [38]. With feeding, aspiration occurs and causes cyanosis, coughing and choking; stridor results from laryngeal collapse. Diagnosis requires a high index of suspicion; nevertheless, a cleft may be difficult to diagnose with a flexible instrument, as manipulation of the posterior commissure may be necessary to detect the cleft. Thus, rigid bronchoscopy is ideal for the documentation of pathology of the posterior glottis, subglottis and trachea [39].

Bifid epiglottis and anterior cleft of the larynx are very rare congenital abnormalities; while a bifid epiglottis is often associated with other malformations (fig. 7), an anterior cleft appears to be an isolated defect [21].

Vocal Cord Dysfunction

VCD is characterized by paradoxical adduction of the vocal cords during inspiration or during both inspiration and expiration. The resulting symptoms and signs are abrupt onset of dyspnoea, throat or chest tightness, inspiratory or biphasic stridor or wheezing, and cough; thus, VCD is most often

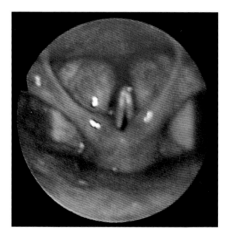

Fig. 11. VCD with paradoxical adduction of the vocal cords during inspiration.

confused with asthma. In addition, associations between VCD and both asthma and gastro-oesophageal reflux have repeatedly been described as well as exercise and physical activity as well-known triggers of acute episodes [40]. The duration of attacks can vary from a few minutes to days. Important clues in the differential diagnosis to asthma are a predominantly inspiratory dyspnoea, an absence of symptoms at night, an absence of oxygen desaturation, no (or only a marginal) response to bronchodilator therapy and no deterioration after discontinuation of asthma medication, and the inspiratory limb of the maximal flow-volume curve showing variable flattening suggestive of extrathoracic airway obstruction in symptomatic patients [41]. Diagnosis is often difficult and may be confirmed by laryngoscopy without sedation during an acute episode of VCD which shows adduction of the anterior portion of the vocal cords, with only a narrow chink left for respiration (fig. 11). A normal laryngoscopy during a symptom-free interval does not exclude the diagnosis.

Gastro-Oesophageal Reflux and Upper Airway Disease

In infants and children, gastro-oesophageal reflux has been associated with many respiratory signs and symptoms (including hoarseness, chronic cough, stridor and wheeze), and otorhinolaryngological disease manifestations such as chronic rhinitis, chronic sinusitis, otitis media, chronic laryngitis, recurrent croup, laryngomalacia, subglottic stenosis, laryngeal papillomatosis, VCD and vocal cord granulomas [23, 24, 35, 40, 42, 43]. However, proof of these associations is sparse. While gastro-oesophageal reflux should be considered a possible cause of upper airway lesions in children, a causal relationship between reflux and an airway lesion is very difficult to confirm. Reflux may be the cause of such a lesion, an exacerbating factor (and thus may compromise surgical repair or conservative treatment) or may simply coexist with an airway lesion.

Typical endoscopic findings include granular changes to the epiglottis, erythema and oedema of the mucous membrane overlying the arytenoid cartilages and the posterior wall of the glottis ('posterior laryngitis'), mucosal cobblestoning, vocal cord nodules, ulcers and granulation tissue, and subglottic stenosis [42, 43].

References

1 Mancuso RF: Stridor in neonates. Pediatr Clin North Am 1996;43:1339–1356.
2 Wood RE: Spelunking in the pediatric airways: explorations with the flexible fiberoptic bronchoscope. Pediatr Clin North Am 1984;31:785–799.
3 Eber E, Zach M: Flexible fiberoptic bronchoscopy in pediatrics – an analysis of 420 examinations. Wien Klin Wochenschr 1995;107:246–251.
4 Godfrey S, Avital A, Maayan C, Rotschild M, Springer C: Yield from flexible bronchoscopy in children. Pediatr Pulmonol 1997;23:261–269.
5 Barbato A, Magarotto M, Crivellaro M, Novello A Jr, Cracco A, de Blic J, Scheinmann P, Warner JO, Zach M: Use of the paediatric bronchoscope, flexible and rigid, in 51 European centres. Eur Respir J 1997;10:1761–1766.
6 Nicolai T: Pediatric bronchoscopy. Pediatr Pulmonol 2001;31:150–164.
7 Midulla F, de Blic J, Barbato A, Bush A, Eber E, Kotecha S, Haxby E, Moretti C, Pohunek P, Ratjen F: Flexible endoscopy of paediatric airways. Eur Respir J 2003;22:698–708.
8 Wood RE: The diagnostic effectiveness of the flexible bronchoscope in children. Pediatr Pulmonol 1985;1:188–192.
9 Lis G, Szczerbinski T, Cichocka-Jarosz E: Congenital stridor. Pediatr Pulmonol 1995;20:220–224.
10 Eber E, Zach M: Flexible fiberoptic endoscopy in children with upper airway obstruction. Monatsschr Kinderheilkd 1996;144:43–47.
11 Zoumalan R, Maddalozzo J, Holinger LD: Etiology of stridor in infants. Ann Otol Rhinol Laryngol 2007;116:329–334.
12 Wood RE: Pitfalls in the use of the flexible bronchoscope in pediatric patients. Chest 1990;97:199–203.

13 Gonzalez C, Reilly JS, Bluestone CD: Synchronous airway lesions in infancy. Ann Otol Rhinol Laryngol 1987;96:77–80.
14 Masters IB, Chang AB, Patterson L, Wainwright C, Buntain H, Dean BW, Francis PW: Series of laryngomalacia, tracheomalacia, and bronchomalacia disorders and their associations with other conditions in children. Pediatr Pulmonol 2002;34:189–195.
15 Chun R, Preciado DA, Zalzal GH, Shah RK: Utility of bronchoscopy for recurrent croup. Ann Otol Rhinol Laryngol 2009;118:495–499.
16 Lusk RP: Nasal and pharyngeal lesions; in Holinger LD, Lusk RP, Greene CG (eds): Pediatric Laryngology and Bronchoesophagology. Philadelphia, Lippincott-Raven, 1997, pp 117–135.
17 Morgan D, Bailey M, Phelps P, Bellman S, Grace A, Wyse R: Ear-nose-throat abnormalities in the CHARGE association. Arch Otolaryngol Head Neck Surg 1993;119:49–54.
18 Dinwiddie R: Congenital upper airway obstruction. Paediatr Respir Rev 2004;5:17–24.
19 Shatz A, Goldberg S, Picard E, Kerem E: Pharyngeal wall collapse and multiple synchronous airway lesions. Ann Otol Rhinol Laryngol 2004;113:483–487.
20 Goldberg S, Shatz A, Picard E, Wexler I, Schwartz S, Swed E, Zilber L, Kerem E: Endoscopic findings in children with obstructive sleep apnea: effects of age and hypotonia. Pediatr Pulmonol 2005;40:205–210.
21 Holinger LD: Congenital laryngeal anomalies; in Holinger LD, Lusk RP, Greene CG (eds): Pediatric Laryngology and Bronchoesophagology. Philadelphia, Lippincott-Raven, 1997, pp 137–164.
22 Chandra RK, Gerber ME, Holinger LD: Histological insight into the pathogenesis of severe laryngomalacia. Int J Pediatr Otorhinolaryngol 2001;61:31–38.

23 Bibi H, Khvolis E, Shoseyov D, Ohaly M, Dor DB, London D, Ater D: The prevalence of gastroesophageal reflux in children with tracheomalacia and laryngomalacia. Chest 2001;119:409–413.
24 Midulla F, Guidi R, Tancredi G, Quattrucci S, Ratjen F, Bottero S, Vestiti K, Francalanci P, Cutrera R: Microaspiration in infants with laryngomalacia. Laryngoscope 2004;114:1592–1596.
25 Dickson JM, Richter GT, Meinzen-Derr J, Rutter MJ, Thompson DM: Secondary airway lesions in infants with laryngomalacia. Ann Otol Rhinol Laryngol 2009;118:37–43.
26 Nielson DW, Ku PL, Egger M: Topical lidocaine exaggerates laryngomalacia during flexible bronchoscopy. Am J Respir Crit Care Med 2000;161:147–151.
27 Shah UK, Wetmore RF: Laryngomalacia: a proposed classification form. Int J Pediatr Otorhinolaryngol 1998;46:21–26.
28 Olney DR, Greinwald JH Jr, Smith RJH, Bauman NM: Laryngomalacia and its treatment. Laryngoscope 1999;109:1770–1775.
29 Schroeder JW Jr, Holinger LD: Congenital laryngeal stenosis. Otolaryngol Clin North Am 2008;41:865–875.
30 Myer CM 3rd, O'Connor DM, Cotton RT: Proposed grading system for subglottic stenosis based on endotracheal tube sizes. Ann Otol Rhinol Laryngol 1994;103:319–323.
31 Benjamin B: Prolonged intubation injuries of the larynx: endoscopic diagnosis, classification, and treatment. Ann Otol Rhinol Laryngol Suppl 1993;160:1–15.
32 Downing GJ, Hayen LK, Kilbride HW: Acquired subglottic cysts in the low-birth-weight infant: Characteristics, treatment, outcome. Am J Dis Child 1993;147:971–974.

33 Holinger PC, Holinger LD, Reichert TJ, Holinger PH: Respiratory obstruction and apnea in infants with bilateral abductor vocal cord paralysis, meningomyelocele, hydrocephalus, and Arnold-Chiari malformation. J Pediatr 1978;92:368–373.

34 Rahbar R, Nicollas R, Roger G, Triglia J-M, Garabedian E-N, McGill TJ, Healy GB: The biology and management of subglottic hemangioma: past, present, future. Laryngoscope 2004;114:1880–1891.

35 Derkay CS, Wiatrak B: Recurrent respiratory papillomatosis: a review. Laryngoscope 2008;118:1236–1247.

36 Pezzettigotta SM, Leboulanger N, Roger G, Denoyelle F, Garabédian EN: Laryngeal cleft. Otolaryngol Clin North Am 2008;41:913–933.

37 Benjamin B, Inglis A: Minor congenital laryngeal clefts: diagnosis and classification. Ann Otol Rhinol Laryngol 1989;98:417–420.

38 Van der Doef HP, Yntema JB, van den Hoogen FJ, Marres HA: Clinical aspects of type 1 posterior laryngeal clefts: literature review and a report of 31 patients. Laryngoscope 2007;117:859–863.

39 Eber E: Evaluation of the upper airway. Paediatr Respir Rev 2004;5:9–16.

40 Noyes BE, Kemp JS: Vocal cord dysfunction in children. Paediatr Respir Rev 2007;8:155–163.

41 King CS, Moores LK: Clinical asthma syndromes and important asthma mimics. Respir Care 2008;53:568–580.

42 Yellon RF, Goldberg H: Update on gastroesophageal reflux disease in pediatric airway disorders. Am J Med 2001;111(suppl 8A):78S–84S.

43 Hoa M, Kingsley EL, Coticchia JM: Correlating the clinical course of recurrent croup with endoscopic findings: a retrospective observational study. Ann Otol Rhinol Laryngol 2008;117:464–469.

Univ.-Prof. Dr. Ernst Eber
Klinische Abteilung für Pulmonologie/Allergologie, Universitätsklinik für Kinder- und Jugendheilkunde
Medizinische Universität Graz
Auenbruggerplatz 34
A–8036 Graz (Austria)
Tel. +43 316 385 12620, Fax +43 316 385 14621, E-Mail ernst.eber@medunigraz.at

Chapter 12

Priftis KN, Anthracopoulos MB, Eber E, Koumbourlis AC, Wood RE (eds): Paediatric Bronchoscopy.
Prog Respir Res. Basel, Karger 2010, vol 38, pp 130–140

Congenital and Acquired Abnormalities of the Lower Airways

Petr Pohunek[a] · Ruben Boogaard[b] · Peter Merkus[c]

[a]Division of Paediatric Respiratory Diseases and Bronchology, Paediatric Department, Charles University, 2nd Medical Faculty, University Hospital Motol, Prague, Czech Republic; [b]Department of Paediatrics, Division of Respiratory Medicine, Erasmus University Medical Centre, Sophia Children's Hospital, Rotterdam, and [c]Department of Paediatrics, Division of Respiratory Medicine, Children's Hospital, Radboud University Medical Centre, Nijmegen, the Netherlands

Abstract

Bronchoscopy provides a unique technical possibility to visualize the airways, document pathological lesions and collect relevant biological material directly from the lower airways. Diagnostic flexible bronchoscopy performed under sedation or general anaesthesia with preserved spontaneous breathing and coughing reflex also allows for a proper diagnosis of dynamic changes of the airway patency and the correlation of the bronchoscopic findings with clinical symptoms and physiological measurements. With the advancement of modern flexible instruments, it has become possible to perform certain therapeutic procedures, such as dilatation of the airways, targeted removal of intrabronchial material and, in specific limited instances, to also remove an aspirated foreign body. The functional examination of paediatric lower airways requires a lot of experience, as some of the pathologies involved are rather rare and the differentiation between normal variation and true pathology is not always easy.

Copyright © 2010 S. Karger AG, Basel

Bronchoscopy provides a unique opportunity to examine the morphology of the lower airways and also some of the functional aspects, such as stability or instability of the airway wall during changes of intrathoracic pressure throughout the breathing cycle. In order to observe the variations of airway patency during breathing, bronchoscopy is preferably conducted while preserving spontaneous breathing. Within this context, it is also necessary to understand the differences between rigid and flexible bronchoscopy. While rigid bronchoscopy allows better manipulation and interventions in the lower airways, it is generally performed under general anaesthesia with muscle relaxation and positive pressure ventilation. Therefore it is not possible to properly appreciate

the stability of the airways and the mechanics of breathing. On the other hand, flexible bronchoscopy always obstructs the airway lumen to some degree and may therefore increase the pressure gradients and enhance this variation. The decision whether the rigid or the flexible instrument should be used depends mainly on the goal of the procedure. For diagnostic evaluation of the lower airways including sampling of various materials, the vast majority of centres use flexible bronchoscopy with the procedures performed under conscious or deep sedation, but always trying to preserve spontaneous ventilation.

Interpretation and classification of many findings in the airways are largely subjective, though there is some consensus on how to describe the most common abnormalities. Attempts have been made to quantify macroscopic abnormalities, but these all have their limitations, and no international guidelines or properly performed studies exist that clearly describe how to interpret and classify structural abnormalities of the bronchial tree and quantify their contribution to clinical respiratory pathology.

In this chapter, we try to describe the main congenital and acquired abnormalities of the lower airways as they appear during bronchoscopy.

Major Congenital Abnormalities

Agenesis/Aplasia of the Lung

Agenesis of one lung is a major defect that is apparently a consequence of arrested signalling during the development of the airways in the first weeks of fetal life. No clear causal factors have been identified so far. Often, this defect is associated with other congenital defects, such as tracheo-oesophageal fistula or arterial sling [1–3]. There have been attempts to differentiate between agenesis (complete absence of the lung) and aplasia (at least some detectable rudimentary structures of the undeveloped lung) but from a clinical point of view this differentiation is irrelevant. Indeed, in most patients with non-developed lung a rudimentary stump of the main bronchus can be found. In patients with one lung missing, bronchoscopy usually reveals some deviation of the trachea; however, this is more visible with imaging techniques than with bronchoscopy. At the main carina, the rudimentary bronchus can be found, and the remaining bronchial tree is significantly rotated (clockwise with agenesis of the right lung, anticlockwise with agenesis of the left lung). Various airway complications have been described, mainly due to compression by the surrounding vessels [4]. In some of these patients, this anomaly may be associated with hypoplasia of the remaining bronchial tree. This may be appreciated during bronchoscopy comparing the limited accessibility of the airways with paediatric bronchoscopes to the usual situation in normal children.

Abnormal Branching of the Bronchial Tree
Branching of the bronchial tree is rather variable in humans. Usually, the central airways follow the usual pattern that is typical of humans. The more we proceed into the peripheral airways, the greater variability we may find. It is very important but sometimes also very difficult to distinguish between variability and pathology. Most of the 'variant' bronchi are normally patent and supply normal lung parenchyma, therefore they do not represent any clinically relevant pathology. However, some of the abnormally branching bronchi can be partially obstructed or can supply abnormal pulmonary tissue. This is often the case with the tracheal bronchus. A tracheal bronchus originates from the right lateral wall of the trachea above the level of the main carina and courses to the right (fig. 1). In most cases, this bronchus supplies the apical segment of the right upper lobe. In such situations there is usually an additional orifice at the usual position of the right upper lobe bronchus, which usually has only 2 visible segmental branches. Less frequently, the tracheal bronchus is associated with other anomalies, such as stenosis of the right main stem bronchus, or supplies additional, dysplastic pulmonary tissue [5, 6]. In such situations there is usually a normal bronchus for the right upper lobe in the usual position with the usual pattern of 3 segmental branches. A tracheal bronchus can complicate airway management in intubated

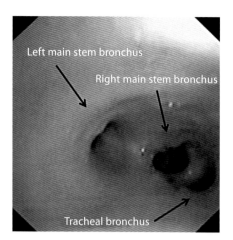

Fig. 1. Tracheal bronchus originating from the trachea above the main carina.

children as the endotracheal tube can obstruct the orifice and lead to atelectasis [7].

Very rarely, a separate bronchus for the apical segment of the left upper lobe can be seen originating from the left main stem bronchus.

Tracheo-Oesophageal Fistula
Tracheo-oesophageal fistula (TOF) is a pathological connection between trachea and oesophagus, mostly associated with oesophageal atresia. While oesophageal atresia and the possibility of surgical anastomosis mostly determine the overall prognosis of an affected child, TOF may be responsible for considerable morbidity, long-term respiratory symptoms or severe sequelae. These are mostly associated with often severe tracheomalacia which interferes with normal airway clearance, leads to retention of mucus and development of chronic bronchitis. The most frequent type of distal fistula (also described as type Vogt 3B fistula) should be easily diagnosed based on the presence of oesophageal atresia and radiographically documented aeration of the gastrointestinal tract. Bronchoscopy remains useful for documenting the exact position of the fistula and also for detecting potentially associated abnormalities, such as tracheomalacia (fig. 2, 3). Tracheoscopy-assisted repair of TOF has been described as a useful method that facilitates surgical management [8]. The clinical presentation of H-type fistula is more subtle, and its detection may be delayed in the absence of oesophageal atresia; such patients may suffer from recurrent aspirations for long periods of time. In many cases the H-type fistula is associated with significant tracheomalacia. These patients may suffer from long-term symptoms, mainly barking cough, recurrent and protracted

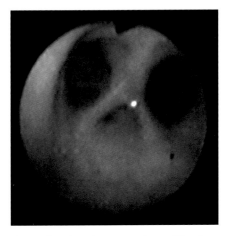
Fig. 2. Distal tracheo-oesophageal fistula.

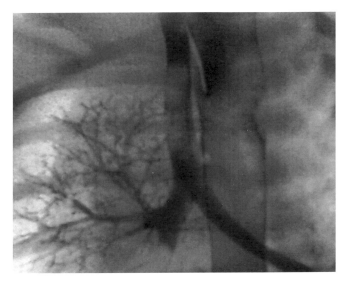
Fig. 4. Contrast imaging of a tracheo-oesophageal fistula.

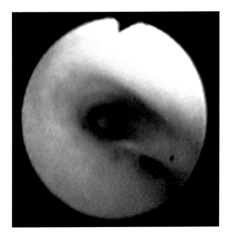
Fig. 3. H-type fistula associated with tracheomalacia.

contrast medium via the working channel (fig. 4). Presence of contrast medium in the oesophagus is diagnostic in this case. It is also possible to inject dye (e.g. methylene blue, indigo carmine) into the fistula and then look for the presence of the dye in the oesophagus. There have been attempts to bronchoscopically close the TOF using various biological glues, cauterization or mechanical abrasion. These methods generally had variable short- and long-term effects [10, 11]. Surgical resection of the TOF remains the only reliable solution. Recurrence of TOF has been described even in children with successfully closed and dissected fistulas; this should be respected in the diagnostic approach in children with continuing symptoms [12].

Tracheomalacia and Bronchomalacia

General Concept
In tracheomalacia, a weakness of the trachea is present, due to a reduction or atrophy of the longitudinal elastic fibres of the pars membranacea or due to impaired cartilage integrity. The airway at the site of a malacia is therefore more susceptible to collapse or dynamic compression. Tracheomalacia mostly affects the intrathoracic part of the trachea, therefore tracheal narrowing or collapse is most prominent during (forced) expiration or coughing when intrathoracic pressure exceeds the intraluminal pressure. Bronchomalacia is less frequent than tracheomalacia and occurs in association with tracheomalacia or independently.

tracheitis and bronchitis as well as exercise limitation [9]. Bronchoscopic assessment of the tracheal patency during spontaneous breathing and coughing can be very helpful in determining the severity of tracheomalacia and guiding the therapeutic approach. It is important to exclude duplicity of the TOF in children with continuing symptoms. In patients with suspected TOF, rigid bronchoscopy has been recommended as with the rigid bronchoscope the posterior tracheal wall can be partly distended and visualized better than with the flexible bronchoscope. By rotating the flexible bronchoscope by 180° and carefully examining the posterior wall with the bronchoscope in the anterior flexion, the disadvantage of flexible bronchoscopy can be eliminated and detailed visualization of the posterior tracheal wall be achieved. It may also be very useful to insert a thin bronchoscope into a suspected fistula under fluoroscopy and inject

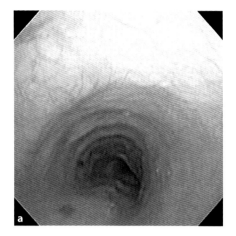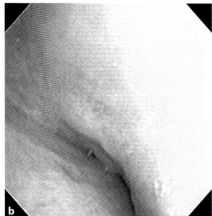

Fig. 5. Bronchoscopic appearance of tracheomalacia during inspiration (**a**) and expiration (**b**).

Strict criteria to diagnose tracheomalacia or bronchomalacia are not available. A rather subjective criterion that has been used in the literature is an observed ratio of cartilage to muscle of less than 3:1 [13], and abnormal collapsibility during cough or quiet breathing (fig. 5). Several methods have been described that aim to quantify the airway diameter and the severity of airway malacia [14, 15], but they are not widely used at present. Objective assessment of the size of the airways and exact measurement of the patency of stenotic or collapsing airways are not easy to accomplish during flexible bronchoscopy as there is always some radial distortion caused by the properties of the optical system. Thus, in flexible bronchoscopy the size of the central parts of the picture cannot be directly compared to the size of the structures at the periphery of the picture. Further, the distance of the bronchoscope from a stenotic area is not easily appreciable from the standard bronchoscopic image. Several methods have been described that allow for measurement of the airway size using bronchoscopic image recording. One of these methods uses a laser probe inserted into the working channel of a bronchoscope for distance measurements. A computer program is used to correct the distortion and to measure the size of the lumen [16]. Another recently described method used in adults with central airway obstruction is morphometric bronchoscopy, a special software processing method of bronchoscopic digital images. This allows to measure airway lumen diameter and thus to objectively quantify the degree of airway narrowing [17]. In everyday practice, such methods are usually not readily available or easily employed. For an approximate estimation of the airway size during routine bronchoscopy, a comparison of the size of the lumen to the known size of some bronchoscopy instrument, such as biopsy forceps, can be used.

Diagnosis of Intrathoracic Airway Malacia

As mentioned before, variable airway narrowing is only visible when spontaneous breathing is maintained, because it may only occur during forced expiration. In cooperative children, airway narrowing or major collapse may be expected based on properly performed pulmonary function tests; however, bronchoscopy is the only readily available method that can exactly locate the site of malacia and distinguish between tracheo- and bronchomalacia.

Based on percentages between 15 and 57% of observed airway malacia in paediatric bronchoscopy series [18–20], various authors concluded that airway malacia is more prevalent than previously thought. No population incidence studies are available, but one study estimated that the prevalence of airway malacia at birth was at least 1 in 2,100 children [9]. Airway malacia can be classified as primary or secondary (table 1). Congenital airway malacia can be further subdivided into isolated or part of a syndrome. Acquired airway malacia is typically caused by degeneration of normal cartilaginous support, mainly due to external compression of the airway. There is a male predominance of airway malacia disorders, and bronchomalacia is more common on the left than on the right side [9, 19]. A conclusive classification of a particular case cannot be made from bronchoscopy alone and without proper analysis of all other clinical findings as well.

Consequences of Airway Malacia

Airway malacia interferes with mucociliary clearance, alters the coughing pattern and may therefore lead to retention of airway secretions and development of chronic airway infection. In cases with severe malacia, complete closure of the airways may be observed with opposite

Table 1. Classification of paediatric airway malacia and associated diseases [13, 21–24]

Primary
Normal infants
Prematurity

Congenital cartilage abnormalities
    Dyschondroplasia/chondromalacia/chondrodysplasia
    Polychondritis
    Ehlers-Danlos syndrome

Congenital abnormalities associated with airway malacia
Oesophageal atresia and/or tracheo-oesophageal fistula

Conditions/syndromes associated with
airway malacia, e.g.:
    Down syndrome
    DiGeorge syndrome
    Larsen syndrome
    Mucopolysaccharidosis

Secondary
Prolonged intubation, tracheotomy
Severe tracheobronchitis
External compression

Vascular malformation, e.g.:
    Anomalous innominate artery
    Double aortic arch
    Anomalous left pulmonary artery
    Right aortic arch
    Aberrant right subclavian artery

Cardiac   Left atrium enlargement/hypertrophy

Skeletal
    Scoliosis
    Pectus excavatum

Tumours, intra- and extrathoracic masses including lymphadenopathy and metastasis
Congenital cysts
Infection, abscess
Post-traumatic

Table 2. Clinical features of paediatric airway malacia

Barking cough
Chronic wet cough
Stridor
Recurrent wheeze
Recurrent lower airways infection
Dyspnoea/shortness of breath
Reduced exercise tolerance
Retractions
Pectus excavatum
Dysphagia/regurgitation
Difficult to wean from mechanical ventilation
Apparent life-threatening event ('dying spell')
Sudden death

Characteristic Symptoms and Lung Function

There is a wide range of signs and symptoms and severity of symptoms in patients with airway malacia (table 2). Severe airway malacia is usually detected in the neonatal period when children present with ventilator dependency or acute severe obstructive episodes with cyanosis. Airway malacia associated with specific syndromes or congenital heart disease may be detected in early life because of selective screening of some patients as listed in table 1 [21, 25]. Children with mild airway malacia often present after the neonatal period with non-specific symptoms, such as rattling, wheeze, stridor, exercise intolerance, barking cough and recurrent lower airway infections. Because of the similarity in symptoms, the poor response to standard asthma treatment and the irreversible nature of the airway obstruction, isolated airway malacia may be misdiagnosed as severe persistent or 'difficult' asthma [26, 27].

One of the symptoms that has traditionally been linked to airway malacia in children is a typical cough sound, often described as 'brassy', 'barking' or 'seal-like' [22, 23], but this may be absent in up to half of the patients [9]. This typical cough sound is probably caused by vibration of the opposing airway walls during coughing. All the signs and symptoms of airway malacia become more marked when a child's respiratory efforts increase, such as during crying, feeding, coughing and – in older children – with exercise. Due to these activities, intrathoracic pressure increases until the extraluminal exceeds the intraluminal pressure, causing the trachea to collapse.

One of the most serious symptoms of patients with severe airway malacia is the so-called reflex apnoea (also known as 'dying spells' or 'apnoeic spells').

airway walls touching during coughing or with increased intrathoracic pressure (fig. 5; online suppl. video 1). This may lead to continuous irritation of airway wall mucosa and contribute to prolonged or persistent airway infections.

Video

Treatment Options for Airway Malacia

Respiratory symptoms in simple airway malacia without external compression or associated anomalies resolve spontaneously in many children in the first years of life; thus, conservative therapy is preferred. Management of children with airway malacia is pragmatic, as no evidence-based guidelines on treatment exist. The therapeutic approach is focused on treatment or prevention of lower airway infections and improvement of mucociliary clearance using physiotherapy, including the use of positive expiratory pressure devices. In patients with bronchoscopically identified localized lobar or segmental airway collapse, physiotherapy should be modified and techniques requiring less intrathoracic pressure as well as modified coughing techniques should be used.

For infants and children with severe, life-threatening symptoms, continuous positive airway pressure may be useful [28]. In some patients, tracheostomy and long-term mechanical ventilation [20, 29] may be the only remaining therapeutic option before tracheal surgery. Airway stenting is rarely used in children because of the high risk of complications. In some situations, aortopexy may be used.

Stenosis of the Airways

Tracheomalacia or bronchomalacia are frequently misinterpreted as airway stenosis. However, it should be understood that the impairment of tracheal patency in malacia is variable and highly dependent on intrathoracic pressures during breathing or coughing. On the other hand, stenosis represents fixed reduction of the airway lumen that may also have some additional variable component during breathing. There are several types of congenital stenosis that result from abnormal development of the airways. Fixed reduction of the airway lumen can also occur as a result of local endotracheal or endobronchial injury, or severe inflammation.

Congenital Airway Stenosis
A congenital stenosis of the airway may have several causes. From a pathogenetic point of view, it is always the result of a developmental defect of the airway wall during bronchogenesis (5th to 16th gestational week). The clinical presentation is variable and depends on the location of airway stenosis, its severity and potentially associated anomalies.

A typical example of tracheal stenosis is complete tracheal rings. In this condition one or more of the cartilaginous rings that support the tracheal wall do not have the typical posterior division and form a complete ring. This may be missed in young children whose airway mucosa is thicker than that of the older ones and the contours of the tracheal rings are poorly visible. Also, in young children the degree of stenosis is usually rather mild, and it is only with growth that the complete ring appears progressively smaller as compared to the normally developing tracheal cartilages [30]. Thus, the defect may become increasingly clinically relevant. It is very important to observe the contours of tracheal cartilages during the passage of the bronchoscope through the trachea. In some patients insignificant anomalies may be visualized, such as bridging of the rings. These are of no clinical relevance provided that the cartilages are properly separated in their posterior aspect.

Some cases of congenital airway stenosis may cause severe respiratory symptoms, compromising ventilation. It is crucial to properly evaluate the anatomy of the whole tracheobronchial tree as the quality and development of the airways beyond the stenosis ultimately determine the management and prognosis. In some cases it is possible to pass smaller bronchoscopes (2.2 or 2.9 mm in diameter) beyond the stenosis and examine the distal parts of the bronchial tree. However, even a gentle manipulation within the stenosis may cause swelling and closure of the stenotic segment and result in respiratory failure; even mechanical ventilation may be very difficult in such situations. Alternatively, imaging techniques, such as CT and 3-dimensional reconstruction or bronchography with targeted application of the contrast material via a flexible bronchoscope may be used to depict the extent of the stenosis and the quality of the distal airways, and to provide information for medical decision-making [chapter 9, this vol., pp. 95–112]. Management of such severe stenoses remains mainly surgical.

Acquired Airway Stenosis
Even a developmentally normal airway wall can react to single or recurrent injury or severe inflammatory changes with scarring and deformities. The most frequent cause of acquired tracheal stenosis is tracheal intubation. Postintubation stenosis mostly develops in the subglottic space in the area of physiological cricoid narrowing. However, even with no apparent injury during intubation, the tracheal wall can be irritated and inflamed, and together with formation of granulation tissue and scarring the tracheal lumen can become severely narrowed [31]. This occurs more often in long-term tracheostomy than in laryngotracheal intubation. The risk of tracheal or bronchial stenosis also depends on the quality of airway management. Inappropriate aggressive suctioning often leads to formation of granulation tissue in the airways and may even result in permanent narrowing (fig. 6; online suppl. video 2). A very frequent cause of air- ∎Video

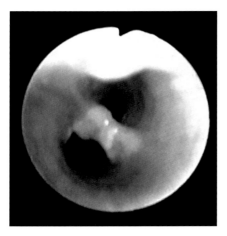

Fig. 6. Granulation tissue as a reaction to suction trauma.

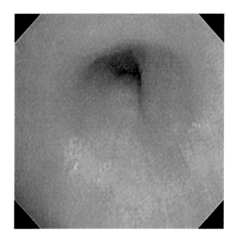

Fig. 8. Compression of the distal trachea by a right aortic arch.

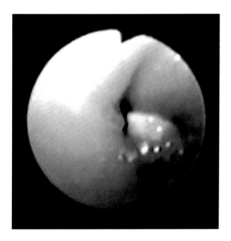

Fig. 7. Chronic foreign body embedded in granulation tissue.

way stenosis is a chronic foreign body. If the aspirated foreign body is not removed immediately, the airway wall always reacts to some degree depending on the type of the foreign material. Most foreign bodies are rather quickly embedded in granulation tissue (fig. 7). This may resolve spontaneously after removal of the foreign body; however, with long-term retained foreign bodies, some degree of permanent narrowing of the airway may develop [32].

Vascular Compression of the Airways

The intimate contact of the airways, heart and intrathoracic vessels may occasionally lead to pathological interactions resulting in compression of the airways and airway obstruction. In some of these disorders, the endoscopic appearance

is typical, while in others the compressing vascular structure cannot be reliably identified by bronchoscopy. Treatment will be based on the severity of respiratory symptoms, exercise limitation and burden of respiratory infections. These may not always have a clear relationship with the degree of airway compression. Surgical correction is often conducted to optimize airway development and growth.

Several types of vascular rings can be found with various vessels involved. Most of them result in compression of the distal part of the trachea and commonly involve also the orifices of the main stem bronchi. Rings involving systemic arteries have pronounced pulsations, while in rings involving pulmonary arteries pulsation may be less obvious. Although the shape of tracheal or bronchial obstruction may be strongly suggestive of the vessels involved, in most cases it is still necessary to confirm the anatomical situation by CT or MR angiography [chapter 9, this vol., pp. 95–112].

Right-Sided and Double Aortic Arch
A right-sided aortic arch can be suspected from a plain chest X-ray where the shape of the mediastinal shadow is altered lacking the normal left aortic arch and showing the descending aorta on the right margin of the mediastinum. At bronchoscopy, it has a rather typical appearance with compression or indentation of the right wall of the distal trachea, commonly involving the orifice of the right main stem bronchus and sometimes the orifice of the right upper lobe bronchus (fig. 8; online suppl. video 3). The shape of the narrowing depends on the obstructing anatomical structures. Commonly the ligamentum arteriosum is involved together with the Kommerell diverticulum, causing significant obstruction [33].

A double aortic arch may cause obstruction of the distal trachea and the left main stem bronchus.

Pulmonary Sling and Enlarged Heart

Compression by a pulmonary sling may have less pronounced pulsations due to lower than systemic systolic pressure. Typically, the distal trachea is obstructed by external pressure on both anterior and posterior walls. Mainly in young children, compression by the left pulmonary artery may be observed. As the left pulmonary artery runs around the anterior and upper wall of the left main stem bronchus and continues its course towards the left upper lobe bronchus, the shape of such an obstruction is also quite typical, forming a drop-like deformity of the bronchus with the narrowest part directed towards the medial wall. The left main stem bronchus can also be compressed by heart enlargement, mainly in children with congenital heart disease. In such cases the left main stem bronchus may be completely closed with markedly impaired ventilation and retention of mucus. Not rarely such a situation leads to either severe hyperinflation or complete atelectasis of the whole left lung. Careful passage of the bronchoscope through the stenosis excludes other anomalies and may help to improve ventilation by suctioning of the retained mucus.

Anomalous Innominate Artery

The innominate artery (truncus brachiocephalicus) is the common trunk that originates from the aorta and branches into the carotid and subclavian arteries on the right side. While this is a normal structure, it may in some individuals originate from the aorta more distally than usual, thus winding around the distal third of the trachea and causing more or less pronounced compression. As this is otherwise a normal vessel, its abnormal course is not apparent on echocardiography where it appears normal. On bronchoscopy, an impression by the innominate artery may be an incidental finding with no clinical implication; in other cases, it may cause significant compression that is associated with tracheomalacia, tracheal coughing and retention of mucus. This compression is also more or less typical, mostly running across the distal third of the anterior wall from its left lower to the right upper portion of the trachea (fig. 9). Patients with severe compression are at higher risk of bleeding during long-term intubation in intensive-care units or when tracheostomy is performed [34–36].

Anomalies of the Subclavian Arteries

In some individuals the right subclavian artery does not originate from the innominate artery but directly from the aortic arch. In order to get to its predestined position, it

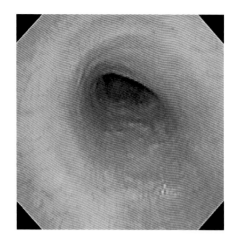

Fig. 9. Compression of the distal trachea by the innominate artery.

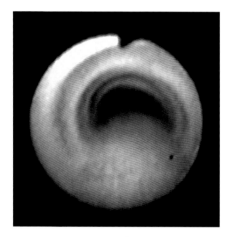

Fig. 10. Compression of the trachea by an arteria lusoria.

usually passes behind the oesophagus or between the oesophagus and the trachea (also called arteria lusoria). This anomaly may be associated with swallowing difficulties with compression of the posterior wall of the trachea and may often result in significant narrowing with visible pulsation (fig. 10; online suppl. video 4). Clinically it may be associated with protracted barking cough, mainly with viral respiratory infections. In some patients an aneurysm can develop in this artery with increased compression of the oesophagus (dysphagia lusoria). Therefore, such vessels should be carefully depicted by appropriate imaging techniques and surgically corrected. A left subclavian artery running from the right in some patients with right-sided aortic arch may cause a similar bronchoscopic appearance.

Intrinsic Lesions of the Bronchial Tree

Inflammation and Mucus Secretion

One of the main indications for diagnostic bronchoscopy in children is chronic respiratory symptoms, including productive cough associated with or following respiratory infections. Therefore evaluation of the quality and appearance of the bronchial mucosa is one of the important tasks for paediatric bronchoscopists. The appearance of bronchial mucosa should always be evaluated immediately after entering the airways with the bronchoscope. It should be noted that this is the original appearance of bronchial mucosa, prior to any iatrogenic irritation, swelling and hyperaemia that can be caused even by very gentle bronchoscopy performed by an experienced endoscopist. The bronchoscopic report should mention the colour and thickness of the bronchial mucosal layer, appearance of the cartilaginous rings, vascular markings and other potential abnormalities, such as prominent intra-/subepithelial lymphatic tissue. Increased secretions of different quality, variable thickness and viscosity of mucus, and mucus plugs can be visualized. Mucus plugs may be associated with impaired regional ventilation and can be removed in most instances by using gentle suctioning and attaching the mucus plug to the suction channel of the instrument and carefully withdrawing the bronchoscope while suctioning. Severe cases of intraluminal obstruction due to casts of acellular debris may also be encountered in plastic bronchitis patients [chapter 14, this vol., pp. 149–155]. In some situations, biopsy forceps can be used in an attempt to grab and withdraw the plug. In case of an unsuccessful attempt to unplug the airways, the use of mucolytics may be effective in facilitating detachment of the plugs from the segmental/subsegmental bronchi.

Severe mucopurulent secretions, often associated with mucus plugs and regional ventilation defects are frequently observed in cystic fibrosis patients (fig. 11). A similar endobronchial pathology can be seen in primary ciliary dyskinesia, chronic aspiration and immunodeficiencies.

Endobronchial Haemorrhage

Bleeding into the airways occurs very rarely in children, and it is mostly associated with severe destruction of pulmonary parenchyma or the airway wall, such as abscess-forming pneumonia, severe bronchiectasis and trauma or more diffuse intrapulmonary bleeding. If bronchoscopy is performed soon after the haemorrhagic episode, often there is still some blood present in the airways, and blood traces on the airway wall may direct toward the lesion. In severer bleeding, even small amounts of coagulated blood can form mucohaemorrhagic

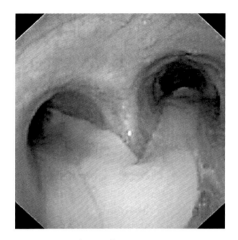

Fig. 11. Purulent inflammation in a patient with cystic fibrosis.

plugs and seal the site of bleeding. Any attempt to remove such mucohaemorrhagic plugs should be considered with caution as removal of the coagulum may lead to recurrence of the haemorrhage. It is better to wait at least 24 h and give the coagulum the opportunity to mature and retract before attempting to remove it. Examination of the bronchoalveolar lavage may show haemosiderin-laden macrophages, thus suggesting previous episodes of intrapulmonary bleeding. Based on the colour of the lavage fluid from different parts of the lungs, one can suspect the bleeding site. In non-resolving bleeding, local epinephrine or cold saline can be applied. In emergency situations, such as recurrence of bleeding during bronchoscopy, mechanical closure of the airways by the tip of the bronchoscope or by a balloon is a quicker and more effective means of managing haemorrhage than administration of vaso-active medication. By stabilizing the patient, time is gained to determine the optimal treatment.

Endobronchial Tumours

While tumours of the lung or bronchial tree are the most frequent indication for bronchoscopy in adults, in children this is an extremely rare situation. This is the reason why in children these conditions sometimes escape diagnosis for long periods of time. Pulmonary parenchymal masses in children are most often of benign nature. Such lesions can be inflammatory or infectious processes and include septic emboli, haematomas or localized reactive processes. Other causes comprise granulomatous inflammatory reaction (fungal, mycobacterial, parasitic) or local presentation of systemic diseases (sarcoidosis, vasculitis). Neoplastic lesions of the lung parenchyma are in most cases of metastatic origin with the primary lesion affecting other organs.

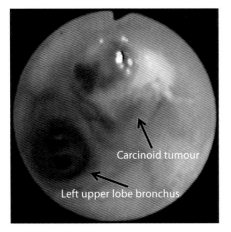

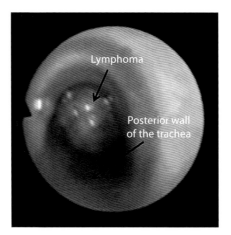

Fig. 12. Occlusion of the left lingular and left lower lobar bronchus by a carcinoid tumour.

Fig. 13. Obstruction of the distal trachea by a lymphoma.

Such lesions are hardly accessible by a bronchoscope, and diagnosis is mostly confirmed by open lung biopsy or videothoracoscopic parenchymal biopsy. On the other hand, endobronchial tumours are usually well accessible via the bronchial tree, and bronchoscopy in such cases is a very useful diagnostic procedure.

Endobronchial tumours mostly present with non-specific respiratory symptoms, such as cough. They may present with secondary signs, mainly atelectasis or non-resolving infiltration due to the closure of one or more segmental bronchi. The most frequent endobronchial tumour in children is a bronchial adenoma, in most cases a carcinoid [37]. This tumour of neuroendocrine origin has rarely any metabolic activity in children, and therefore it is usually the tumour-induced obstruction of the airways that leads to diagnosis. A carcinoid presents endobronchially mostly as a round or irregularly shaped multilobulated mass (fig. 12; online suppl. video 5). Its colour is usually slightly darker than that of the normal surrounding mucosa.

Bronchoscopy can help in the diagnosis by detection of the tumour and providing biopsy samples for histological diagnosis. A carcinoid grows both intraluminally and extrabronchially, and therefore it is not possible to remove this tumour using a bronchoscopic approach. Indeed, the larger part of the tumour usually lies beyond the mucosa, extra- and intramurally, and thus only surgical resection can remove the whole mass [38]. A carcinoid tends to be a very vascularized tumour, and a bronchial biopsy should be attempted with great caution and only in a setting ready to handle sudden bleeding. Haemangiomas can also occur within the lung parenchyma and the tracheobronchial tree with some risk of haemorrhagic complications.

Another relatively frequent endobronchial tumour is lymphoma. Various presentations of tumorous growth can be found endobronchially, ranging from disperse lymphatic infiltration presenting as nodular infiltration of the bronchial wall to solid, rapidly growing masses that can quickly lead to stenosis or complete occlusion of the airways with corresponding development of clinical symptoms and radiographic signs (fig. 13; online suppl. video 6). In lymphoma the tissue biopsy is usually diagnostic, and in most cases the tumour gradually disappears with appropriate oncological treatment.

Many other endobronchial tumours have been described in children, such as chondroma, hamartoma, mucous gland adenoma, but also muco-epidermal carcinoma, adenoid cystic carcinoma and squamous cell carcinoma. However, these are extremely rare and their detailed description is beyond the scope of this chapter.

Differential diagnosis of endobronchial tumours should also include inflammatory pseudotumours and granulation tissue that can easily develop with chronic irritation of the bronchial wall. Thorough bronchoscopic evaluation and biopsy of the lesion usually provide a definitive diagnosis.

Acknowledgement

The bronchoscopy laboratory of P.P. has been supported by the Research Project of the Ministry of Health of the Czech Republic – No. MZ0FNM2005. The work of R.B. and P.M. has been supported by an unrestricted research grant from Roche, the Netherlands.

References

1 Menon MP, Singla R, Chhabra SK: A case of agenesis of right lung with other rare congenital anomalies. Indian J Chest Dis Allied Sci 1987;29:98–102.
2 Munro HM, Sorbello AM, Nykanen DG: Severe stenosis of a long tracheal segment, with agenesis of the right lung and left pulmonary arterial sling. Cardiol Young 2006;16:89–91.
3 Surendran N: Agenesis of right lung with esophageal atresia and distal tracheoesophageal fistula. Saudi Med J 2000;21:302–303.
4 Chou AK, Huang SC, Chen SJ, Huang PM, Wang JK, Wu MH, Chen YS, Chang CI, Chiu IS, Wu ET: Unilateral lung agenesis – detrimental roles of surrounding vessels. Pediatr Pulmonol 2007; 42:242–248.
5 Doolittle AM, Mair EA: Tracheal bronchus: classification, endoscopic analysis, and airway management. Otolaryngol Head Neck Surg 2002;126:240–243.
6 Elmaci TT, Guler N, Aydogan U, Onursal E: Infantile lobar emphysema and tracheal bronchus in a patient with congenital heart disease. J Pediatr Surg 2001;36:1596–1598.
7 O'Sullivan BP, Frassica JJ, Rayder SM: Tracheal bronchus: a cause of prolonged atelectasis in intubated children. Chest 1998;113:537–540.
8 Deanovic D, Gerber AC, Dodge-Khatami A, Dillier CM, Meuli M, Weiss M: Tracheoscopy assisted repair of tracheo-esophageal fistula (TARTEF): a 10-year experience. Paediatr Anaesth 2007;17:557–562.
9 Boogaard R, Huijsmans SH, Pijnenburg MW, Tiddens HA, de Jongste JC, Merkus PJ: Tracheomalacia and bronchomalacia in children: incidence and patient characteristics. Chest 2005;128:3391–3397.
10 Jones C, Laurence BH, Faulkner KW, Cullingford GL: Closure of a benign broncho-oesophageal fistula by endoscopic injection of bovine collagen, cyanoacrylate glue and Gelfoam. Aust NZ J Surg 1996;66:53–55.
11 Willetts IE, Dudley NE, Tam PK: Endoscopic treatment of recurrent tracheo-oesophageal fistulae: long-term results. Pediatr Surg Int 1998;13:256–258.
12 Kafrouni G, Baick CH, Woolley MM: Recurrent tracheoesophageal fistula: a diagnostic problem. Surgery 1970;68:889–894.
13 Benjamin B: Tracheomalacia in infants and children. Ann Otol Rhinol Laryngol 1984;93:438–442.
14 Masters IB, Eastburn MM, Wootton R, Ware RS, Francis PW, Zimmerman PV, Chang AB: A new method for objective identification and measurement of airway lumen in paediatric flexible videobronchoscopy. Thorax 2005;60:652–658.

15 Rozycki HJ, Van Houten ML, Elliott GR: Quantitative assessment of intrathoracic airway collapse in infants and children with tracheobronchomalacia. Pediatr Pulmonol 1996;21:241–245.
16 Dörffel W, Fietze I, Hentschel D, Liebetruth J, Rückert Y, Rogalla P, Wernecke K-D, Baumann G, Witt C: A new bronchoscopic method to measure airway size. Eur Respir J 1999;14:783–788.
17 Murgu S, Colt H: Morphometric bronchoscopy in adults with central airway obstruction: case illustrations and review of the literature. Laryngoscope 2009;119:1318–1324.
18 Finder JD: Primary bronchomalacia in infants and children. J Pediatr 1997;130:59–66.
19 Chang AB, Boyce NC, Masters IB, Torzillo PJ, Masel JP: Bronchoscopic findings in children with non-cystic fibrosis chronic suppurative lung disease. Thorax 2002;57:935–938.
20 Jacobs IN, Wetmore RF, Tom LW, Handler SD, Potsic WP: Tracheobronchomalacia in children. Arch Otolaryngol Head Neck Surg 1994;120:154–158.
21 Austin J, Ali T: Tracheomalacia and bronchomalacia in children: pathophysiology, assessment, treatment and anaesthesia management. Paediatr Anaesth 2003;13:3–11.
22 McNamara VM, Crabbe DC: Tracheomalacia. Paediatr Respir Rev 2004;5:147–154.
23 Mair EA, Parsons DS: Pediatric tracheobronchomalacia and major airway collapse. Ann Otol Rhinol Laryngol 1992;101:300–309.
24 Carden KA, Boiselle PM, Waltz DA, Ernst A: Tracheomalacia and tracheobronchomalacia in children and adults: an in-depth review. Chest 2005; 127:984–1005.
25 Lee SL, Cheung YF, Leung MP, Ng YK, Tsoi NS: Airway obstruction in children with congenital heart disease: assessment by flexible bronchoscopy. Pediatr Pulmonol 2002;34:304–311.
26 Cohn JR: Localized bronchomalacia presenting as worsening asthma. Ann Allergy 1985;54:222–223.
27 Chung KF, Godard P, Adelroth E, Ayres J, Barnes N, Barnes P, Bel E, Burney P, Chanez P, Connett G, Corrigan C, de Blic J, Fabbri L, Holgate ST, Ind P, Joos G, Kerstjens H, Leuenberger P, Lofdahl CG, McKenzie S, Magnussen H, Postma D, Saetta M, Salmeron S, Sterk P: Difficult/therapy-resistant asthma: the need for an integrated approach to define clinical phenotypes, evaluate risk factors, understand pathophysiology and find novel therapies. ERS Task Force on Difficult/Therapy-Resistant Asthma. European Respiratory Society. Eur Respir J 1999;13:1198–1208.

28 Davis S, Jones M, Kisling J, Angelicchio C, Tepper RS: Effect of continuous positive airway pressure on forced expiratory flows in infants with tracheomalacia. Am J Respir Crit Care Med 1998; 158:148–152.
29 Altman KW, Wetmore RF, Marsh RR: Congenital airway abnormalities requiring tracheotomy: a profile of 56 patients and their diagnoses over a 9 year period. Int J Pediatr Otorhinolaryngol 1997; 41:199–206.
30 Faust RA, Stroh B, Rimell F: The near complete tracheal ring deformity. Int J Pediatr Otorhinolaryngol 1998;45:171–176.
31 De S, De S: Post intubation tracheal stenosis. Indian J Crit Care Med 2008;12:194–197.
32 Bugmann P, Birraux J, Barrazzone C, Fior A, Le Coultre C: Severe bronchial synechia after removal of a long-standing bronchial foreign body: a case report to support control bronchoscopy. J Pediatr Surg 2003;38:E14.
33 Morel V, Corbineau H, Lecoz A, Verhoye JP, Heautot JF, Bassen R, Delaval P, Desrues B: Two cases of 'asthma' revealing a diverticulum of Kommerell. Respiration 2002;69:456–460.
34 Chittithavorn V, Rergkliang C, Chetpaophan A, Vasinanukorn P: Tracheo-innominate artery fistula in children with high-lying innominate artery. Asian Cardiovasc Thorac Ann 2006;14:514–516.
35 Thorp A, Hurt TL, Kim TY, Brown L: Tracheoinnominate artery fistula: a rare and often fatal complication of indwelling tracheostomy tubes. Pediatr Emerg Care 2005;21:763–766.
36 Siobal M, Kallet RH, Kraemer R, Jonson E, Lemons D, Young D, Campbell AR, Schecter W, Tang J: Tracheal-innominate artery fistula caused by the endotracheal tube tip: case report and investigation of a fatal complication of prolonged intubation. Respir Care 2001;46:1012–1018.
37 Fauroux B, Aynie V, Larroquet M, Boccon-Gibod L, Ducou le Pointe H, Tamalet A, Clement A: Carcinoid and mucoepidermoid bronchial tumours in children. Eur J Pediatr 2005;164:748–752.
38 Rea F, Rizzardi G, Zuin A, Marulli G, Nicotra S, Bulf R, Schiavon M, Sartori F: Outcome and surgical strategy in bronchial carcinoid tumors: single institution experience with 252 patients. Eur J Cardiothorac Surg 2007;31:186–191.

Prof. Petr Pohunek, MD, PhD, FCCP
Head, Division of Respiratory Diseases, Paediatric Department, Charles University Prague
University Hospital Motol, V Uvalu 84
CZ–15006 Prague 5 (Czech Republic)
Tel. +420 224 432 012, Fax +420 224 432 020, E-Mail petr.pohunek@LFMotol.cuni.cz

Flexible Bronchoscopy in Specific Clinical Conditions

Priftis KN, Anthracopoulos MB, Eber E, Koumbourlis AC, Wood RE (eds): Paediatric Bronchoscopy.
Prog Respir Res. Basel, Karger 2010, vol 38, pp 142–148

Bronchial Asthma

Angelo Barbato[a] · Federica Bertuola[a] · Lorena Moreno[a] ·
Deborah Snijders[a] · Samuela Bugin[a] · Simonetta Baraldo[b] ·
Graziella Turato[b]

Departments of [a]Paediatrics and [b]Cardiac, Thoracic and Vascular Sciences, University of Padova, Padova, Italy

Abstract

In children with difficult asthma or in asthmatic patients with over-lapping disease, flexible bronchoscopy permits the examination of the morphology and the dynamics of the upper and lower airways. Moreover, it allows additional procedures to be performed. These include bronchoalveolar lavage (BAL) and endobronchial biopsy that help to complete the diagnostic evaluation and complement the findings with information from more peripheral airways. The study of the BAL fluid and bronchial mucosal biopsy have recently begun to contribute to a better understanding of the pathophysiology of asthma in children. In this chapter, we present the knowledge accumulated by the application of these bronchoscopic techniques in asthmatic children and briefly discuss their future prospects.

Copyright © 2010 S. Karger AG, Basel

Asthma is a heterogeneous condition with different phenotypes and clinical expressions [1, 2]. The airway inflammatory response involves eosinophils, mast cells and activated T lymphocytes and is associated with structural alterations of the bronchial wall. These changes consist of desquamation of bronchial epithelial cells, reticular basement membrane (RBM) thickening, angiogenesis and increased smooth muscle mass [3, 4]. The molecular mechanisms responsible for the recruitment and activation of inflammatory cells are still only partially understood, particularly in the first years of life. In fact, in preschool children, wheezing is most commonly caused by recurrent viral infections, therefore complicating the diagnosis of asthma in this age group. In these cases, flexible bronchoscopy (FB) with bronchoalveolar lavage (BAL) and endobronchial biopsy (EBB) can be used to elucidate the inflammatory processes in an attempt to identify different wheezing/asthma phenotypes.

Airway Inflammation in Wheezing Disorders

Several different patterns of wheezing have been described in children, which include: (a) transient wheeze, i.e. children who wheeze during the first years of life but usually not after the age of 3; (b) non-atopic wheeze, which is triggered mainly by viral infections, and (c) atopic wheeze, which is considered by many authorities to represent persistent asthma [1, 5–9]. It has recently been suggested by the ERS Task Force [2] that the use of terms such as 'transient', 'late-onset' and 'persistent wheeze' be limited to longitudinal cohort studies as they can only be applied retrospectively and therefore are not clinically useful. The same task force avoids the use of the term 'asthma' for preschoolers and, for clinical purposes, suggests the classification of wheezing into episodic (viral) wheeze, which manifests only in association with coryzal symptoms, and multiple-trigger wheeze; however, even this classification is being debated, and the wheezing phenotypes may change over time [10].

Most preschool children with wheeze will be symptom free by the time they reach school age, whereas only a minority remain symptomatic, develop persistent wheeze and are ultimately diagnosed as asthmatics. Atopy is generally believed to be a crucial determinant in the future development of persistent asthma [5, 6], although the relationship between wheezing and allergic sensitization in the first years of life is still controversial [7].

Airflow limitation in early infancy (at 1 month of age) is another factor associated with persistent wheezing at 11 years, and this association is independent of the effect of airway hyperresponsiveness and atopy in childhood [3]. This has been confirmed by the results of a number of studies

[4–8], which have demonstrated that poor airway function shortly after birth (at 2–3 months of age) is a risk factor for airflow obstruction in teenagers and young adults (at 11, 16 and 22 years of age). These findings suggest that airway changes typical of asthma start early in life and therefore highlight the need for better knowledge of the pathogenetic mechanisms in young children.

Due to the difficulties in obtaining pulmonary function measurements and bronchoscopic samples in the preschool age group, the mechanisms associated with the early reduction of lung function are not well understood in these patients. BAL and EBB have proven to be useful tools in gaining insight into the structural and inflammatory changes of the bronchial wall of asthmatic children. However, ethical concerns restrict the application of such invasive methods for the identification and monitoring of airway inflammation and remodelling to patients who fulfil clear clinical indications [11, 12].

Bronchoscopy and Asthma

Bronchoscopy is not routine in the diagnosis and follow-up of asthmatic children; it is recommended only in patients with difficult asthma or those with overlapping complications [13].

Although diagnostic bronchoscopy is an invasive procedure, it is safe when performed by an experienced team [chapter 2, this vol., pp. 22–29]. In experienced hands, the rigid bronchoscope [chapter 8, this vol., pp. 83–94] has been found to be as safe as the flexible one [14], but it is infrequently used in paediatric pulmonary centres. Nevertheless, rigid bronchoscopy does not come without limitations such as its inability to evaluate the stability of the tracheobronchial wall, which can only be achieved during spontaneous breathing and/or coughing during FB while using a less invasive sedation protocol [15; chapters 2 and 12, this vol., pp. 22–29 and 130–140]. It should be noted that some authors recommend the use of inhaled bronchodilating agents before FB for patients with asthma undergoing bronchoscopy in order to prevent bronchospasm during the procedure [16]. A possible complication of FB, in asthmatic just as in other patients, is minimal local bleeding after EBB, which resolves within 1–3 min. Transient fever may also be observed in these children after FB with BAL whether followed or not by EBB [16]. In many paediatric pulmonary centres, BAL and EBB are performed routinely in children with asthma, provided that the aforementioned indications and precautions are observed.

Bronchoalveolar Lavage Specimens

The examination of BAL fluid (BALF) in an inflammatory disease of the airways such as asthma can provide useful information regarding the pattern (e.g. total cellularity, differential cell count) and the immunological activity of the inflammation [17; chapter 3, this vol., pp. 30–41]. Following inspection of the bronchial tree and before obtaining biopsy specimens, BAL is usually performed in the right middle lobe with wedging of the bronchoscope into the lobar bronchus [18]. In the diagnostic evaluation of children with asthma, the first aliquot of the BALF, which represents the 'bronchial wash', is analysed and compared with the 2 aliquots that follow and represent the 'bronchoalveolar wash'. In general, the bronchial wash is used only for cultures as this aliquot contains a lower number of cells, also characterized by lower viability, and a higher percentage of neutrophils as compared to the other aliquots [19].

Several inflammatory cells and mediators have been detected in the BALF of asthmatic children. The inflammatory changes entail the recruitment of leucocytes, including neutrophils and eosinophils [20–26]. The recruitment of neutrophils has been associated with the release of interleukin (IL) 8, a potent neutrophil attractant [21], while eosinophils are considered to be the primary cause of tissue damage due to the release of toxic proteases, lipid mediators, cytokines and oxygen free radicals [27]. The various BALF cellular profiles reported in representative studies performed in asthmatic children are presented in table 1 [20, 22–24, 28–31].

The increased numbers of eosinophils, leucocytes and mast cell products observed in these patients, mostly children with multitrigger or persistent asthma, correlated with bronchial hyperresponsiveness [24–27, 30–32]. Therefore, some authors have proposed that an increase in the activation of pro-inflammatory cells and an increase in the expression of their mediators may serve as a marker for the development of asthma [33, 34]. Although some difference between transient or viral-infection-associated wheeze and multitrigger wheeze (persistent asthma) has been reported in mediators of eosinophilic and neutrophilic inflammation, the evidence is limited and the extensive overlap of measurements does not permit a clear distinction among wheezing phenotypes. For such a distinction, a much better understanding of the pathophysiology of wheezing disorders in children that will hopefully result in the discovery of more discriminative markers is necessary.

Table 1. Cellular profiles (n × 10³/ml) in the BALF of asthmatic children

	Patients n	Total cells	Ep.	AM	PMN	Ly.	Eo.
Ferguson and Wong[1] [28], 1989	22	144	/ (/)	113 (78.5)	18 (12.5)	5 (3.5)	7.7 (5.3)
Hein et al.[1] [29], 1991	17	176	/ (/)	148 (84)	5.9 (3.4)	5.1 (2.9)	16.1 (9.1)
Ferguson et al.[1] [24], 1992	15	2,300	/ (/)	713 (31)	/ (/)	128 (5.6)	110 (4.8)
Stevenson et al.[2] [20], 1997	52	83	11.7 (14.1)	59 (71.3)	2.9 (3.5)	1.2 (1.4)	9.1 (1.1)
Marguet et al.[2] [23], 1999	14	521	80 (15)	342 (65.6)	16 (3)	29 (5.5)	13 (2.5)
Barbato et al.[2] [22], 2001	13	1,314	5 (0.38)	714 (54.3)	80 (6)	75 (5.7)	0 (0)
Najafi et al.[2] [30], 2003	21	177	59 (/)	62 (39)	92 (39)	22 (12)	4 (3)
Snijders et al.[2] [31], 2010	91	167	/ (/)	/ (/)	19 (10)	/ (/)	0 (0)

Figures in parentheses indicate percentages. AM = Alveolar macrophages; Eo. = eosinophils; Ep. = epithelial cells; Ly. = lymphocytes; PMN = neutrophils; / = not reported.
[1] Mean values.
[2] Median values.

In this context, it has been reported that BALF eosinophilia and eosinophil cationic protein levels may be more prominent in asthmatic patients with atopy as compared to non-atopic ones [20, 25]; however, other studies found a similar pattern of inflammation in both atopic and non-atopic groups of asthmatic children [31]. Other authors have also found similar eosinophilia and eosinophil cationic protein levels in children with asthma, in those with viral-infection-associated wheeze and in non-asthmatic controls [21]. Mediators of neutrophilic inflammation such as IL-8 and tumour necrosis factor α may play a more important role in viral-infection-associated wheeze [21, 23] and acute exacerbations of asthma [35].

Because viral infections are an important trigger in asthma exacerbations, BALF analysis with PCR-based detection of the most frequent viruses (e.g. rhinovirus, adenovirus, respiratory syncytial virus) may also prove to be helpful [36]. Moreover, BALF from asthmatic patients should be cultured for bacteria, including *Mycoplasma pneumoniae* [37] and *Chlamydia* sp. [38].

Bronchial Biopsies in Asthmatic Children

Mucosal EBB is the main diagnostic technique for the evaluation of the pathological processes in the bronchial mucosa in children [39; chapter 4, this vol., pp. 42–53]. It allows the evaluation of cellularity, the pattern and type of inflammation, and provides evidence of the structural changes that may occur during the process of airway remodelling. In children, EBB during FB adds only 2–3 min to the duration of the procedure [40] (online suppl. video 1).

Technical Issues

In theory, EBB can be performed in children of any age; however, a size 1.2-mm working channel limits the size of the forceps that can be used and thus the quality of the biopsy. The best results are obtained using a flexible bronchoscope with a working channel of at least 2 mm in diameter and adequate forceps size (i.e. diameter ≥1.8 mm). The samples are shaken from the tip of the flexible bronchoscope, immediately plunged into a 10% formaldehyde solution and sent to the laboratory. The presence of a pathology technician when performing the procedure to directly check the size of the specimen is probably useful as it will help to minimize the number of the required specimens.

The basic processing of EBB samples includes standard haematoxylin-eosin staining and staining for collagen to assess main structural changes and the degree of remodelling. The thickness of the subepithelial basement membrane can be measured using various techniques [41]. Specific immunohistological staining of different cells (e.g. the anti-eosinophil cationic protein EG-2 antibody for eosinophils, an anti-elastase antibody for neutrophils and the antitryptase AA1 antibody for mast cells) improves the evaluation of the cellular profile of the inflammation [42]. Monoclonal antibodies against interleukins (e.g. IL-4, IL-5, IL-8 and IL-13) and growth factors (granulocyte-macrophage colony-stimulating factor, transforming growth factor β, basic fibroblast growth factor) can be used. In addition, viral pathogens can be detected in the bronchial epithelial cells with in situ hybridization by using appropriate molecular probes [43].

Airway Inflammation and EBB
The collection of bronchial biopsies from children with asthma and carefully chosen paediatric controls is of fundamental importance in order to evaluate the development of structural changes of the disease and to establish their relation, if any, to airway inflammation. Eosinophilic inflammatory infiltrate associated with thickening of the RBM, epithelial shedding and neo-angiogenesis are characteristic changes in asthma that have been widely described in adults [44] but have scarcely been investigated until recently in children [45, 46].

The observation that thickening of the RBM in asthmatic children is associated with epithelial desquamation and increased vascularization supports the hypothesis that disordered epithelial-mesenchymal signalling may play a fundamental role in bronchial asthma, not only in severe, but also in mild-to-moderate disease. In fact, exposure to allergens can cause damage of the epithelium, thus resulting in airway remodelling via the release of mitotic and fibrogenic growth factors, thereby promote angiogenesis and thickening of the RBM [47, 48]. It is of particular importance that all these cellular events can be activated also in children with non-atopic asthma, in whom a specific IgE response against allergens cannot be demonstrated and the wheezing episodes are induced by viral infections [49].

Pathological Changes Related to Disease Severity
The first study that investigated biopsy specimens in asthmatic children was performed by Cutz et al. [50], who described prominent eosinophilia in the specimens of 2 children with well-controlled asthma. Conversely, Cokuğraş et al. [51] reported eosinophilic inflammation in only 1 out of 10 children with moderate asthma. However, in these studies only a qualitative analysis was performed, and a control group of non-asthmatic children was not included. Subsequently, Payne et al. [46, 52], in quantitative well-controlled studies, demonstrated that children with difficult asthma had a thickened RBM in the absence of prominent

eosinophilia. However, the children studied were not typical of the majority of children with asthma, but rather represented the severest end of the disease severity spectrum (i.e. asthmatic children with persistent symptoms despite maximal steroid therapy). Conversely, eosinophilic inflammation was definitely present in children with mild-to-moderate disease, in whom the disease severity was not influenced by high doses of inhaled or even orally administered corticosteroids [45]. It is of interest that early detection of airway eosinophilia in these patients was associated with extensive remodelling of the airway wall, i.e. not only RBM thickening, but also epithelial loss, increased smooth muscle mass and angiogenesis (fig. 1) [53–55]. These structural changes appear early in the preschool age, but they are not present at birth, since RBM thickening was not demonstrated in wheezing infants up to the age of 26 months [56]; nevertheless, this latter issue needs further confirmation since, so far, only one study has examined the airway pathology of wheezing infants.

Pathological Changes Related to Atopy
Atopy is generally considered to be a crucial determinant for the persistence of wheezing in children and for the development of asthma. Indeed, certain data suggest that in atopic children wheezing persists into adulthood, whereas in non-atopic children it appears to resolve in adolescence [8]. Such data support the concept that airway pathology differs in these two groups of wheezers. However, recent studies have demonstrated that the BALF cytology of atopic and non-atopic children with wheezing responsive to bronchodilators is of a similar nature (i.e. active eosinophilic response) [31]; furthermore, it has been shown that the airway pathology of both groups of childhood wheezers does not differ from that observed in adult asthmatics [57]. Therefore, all the characteristic pathological features of asthma, including RBM thickening, marked epithelial loss, angiogenesis, eosinophilia and upregulation of IL-4 and IL-5, have been observed in both atopic and non-atopic children [42]. Taken together, these findings indicate that when asthmatic symptoms occur, airway pathology is typical of asthma irrespective of the presence of atopy.

Future Trends

It is anticipated that in the immediate future biopsies will become an essential tool in the exploration of the interactions among airway epithelial cells, fibroblasts, smooth

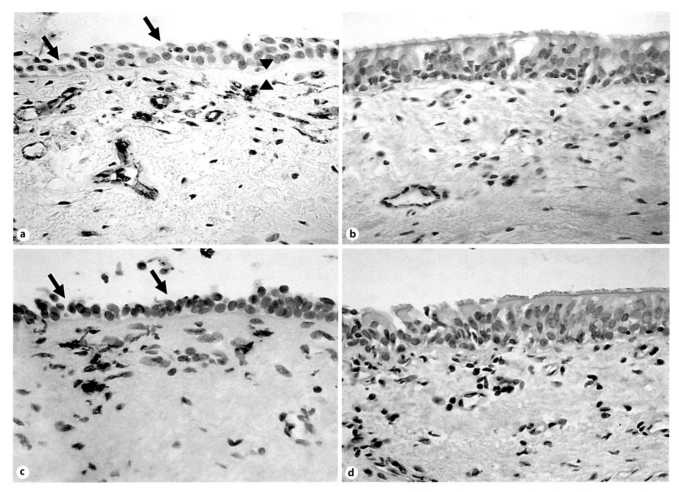

Fig. 1. Bronchial biopsy sections from a child with asthma (**a** and **c**) and a control child (**b** and **d**). An increased number of subepithelial vessels (**a**, brown) and eosinophils (**c**, red) are demonstrated in the child with asthma. The arrows indicate loss of epithelial cells (**a** and **c**), while the arrowheads indicate RBM thickening (**a**). Immunostaining with monoclonal antibody anti-CD31 (**a** and **b**) and anti-EG2 (**c** and **d**). Original magnification ×630. Reproduced with permission from Barbato et al. [55].

muscle, endothelial and inflammatory cells in chronic lung diseases such as asthma. The expansion of our knowledge on these cellular mechanisms is crucial for the understanding of the pathogenesis of asthma and will assist in the targeting of novel drug treatments.

The efforts of future studies should probably focus on younger children (less than 1–2 years of age) in whom the available data are scarce. Indeed, to date, it remains unclear at which point during the natural history of the disease airway remodelling begins, and the same is true for the potential association between remodelling and the inflammatory process. The investigation of the origins of remodelling will be greatly augmented by the cooperation among centres with experience in this type of research that will share common protocols in well-planned multicentre studies. The performance of BAL and EBB in young children with asthma offers the unique opportunity to directly investigate the inflammatory and remodelling processes early in the natural history of the disease. It is important that these investigations are complemented with less invasive techniques such as induced sputum, exhaled nitric oxide and exhaled breath condensate collection [58]. The development of non-invasive markers of disease activity based on sound pathological data is crucial as the follow-up of such patients via serial bronchoscopies is not feasible due to practical reasons and ethical concerns.

References

1 Martinez FD: Development of wheezing disorders and asthma in preschool children. Pediatrics 2002;109:362–367.
2 Brand PL, Baraldi E, Bisgaard H, Boner AL, Castro-Rodriguez JA, Custovic A, de Blic J, de Jongste JC, Eber E, Everard ML, Frey U, Gappa M, Garcia-Marcos L, Grigg J, Lenney W, Le Souëf P, McKenzie S, Merkus PJ, Midulla F, Paton JY, Piacentini G, Pohunek P, Rossi GA, Seddon P, Silverman M, Sly PD, Stick S, Valiulis A, van Aalderen WM, Wildhaber JH, Wennergren G, Wilson N, Zivkovic Z, Bush A: Definition, assessment and treatment of wheezing disorders in preschool children: an evidence-based approach. Eur Respir J 2008;32:1096–1110.
3 Turner SW, Palmer LJ, Rye PJ, Gibson NA, Judge PK, Cox M, Young S, Goldblatt J, Landau LI, Le Souëf PN: The relationship between infant airway function, childhood airway responsiveness, and asthma. Am J Respir Crit Care Med 2004; 169:921–927.
4 Stern DA, Morgan WJ, Wright AL, Guerra S, Martinez FD: Poor airway function in early infancy and lung function by age 22 years: a nonselective longitudinal cohort study. Lancet 2007;370:758–764.
5 Guilbert TW, Morgan WJ, Zeiger RS, Bacharier LB, Boehmer SJ, Krawiec M, Larsen G, Lemanske RF, Liu A, Mauger DT, Sorkness C, Szefler SJ, Strunk RC, Taussig LM, Martinez FD: Atopic characteristics of children with recurrent wheezing at high risk for the development of childhood asthma. J Allergy Clin Immunol 2004;114:1282–1287.
6 Sears MR, Greene JM, Willan AR, Wiecek EM, Taylor DR, Flannery EM, Cowan JO, Herbison GP, Silva PA, Poulton R: A longitudinal, population-based cohort study of childhood asthma followed to adulthood. N Engl J Med 2003;349: 1414–1422.
7 Saglani S, Bush A: The early-life origins of asthma. Curr Opin Allergy Clin Immunol 2007;7: 83–90.
8 Stein RT, Martinez FD: Asthma phenotypes in childhood: lessons from an epidemiological approach. Paediatr Respir Rev 2004;5:155–161.
9 Lowe LA, Simpson A, Woodcock A, Morris J, Murray CS, Custovic A: Wheeze phenotypes and lung function in preschool children. Am J Respir Crit Care Med 2005;171:231–237.
10 Handoyo S, Rosenwasser LJ: Asthma phenotypes. Curr Allergy Asthma Rep 2009;9:439–445.
11 McIntosh N, Bates P, Brykczynska G, Dunstan G, Goldman A, Harvey D, Larcher V, McCrae D, McKinnon A, Patton M, Saunders J, Shelley P: Guidelines for the ethical conduct of medical research involving children. Royal College of Paediatrics, Child Health: Ethics Advisory Committee. Arch Dis Child 2000;82:177–182.
12 Payne D: The ethics of bronchoscopic research in children. Allergy 2007;62:577–578.
13 Payne D, McKenzie SA, Stacey S, Misra D, Haxby E, Bush A: Safety and ethics of bronchoscopy and endobronchial biopsy in difficult asthma. Arch Dis Child 2001;84:423–426.
14 Lindahl H, Rintala R, Malinen L, Leijala M, Sairanen H: Bronchoscopy during the first month of life. J Pediatr Surg 1992;27:548–550.
15 Paspatis GA, Charoniti A, Manolaraki M, Vardas E, Papanikolaou N, Anastasiadou A, Gritzali A: Synergistic sedation with oral midazolam as a premedication and intravenous propofol versus intravenous propofol alone in upper gastrointestinal endoscopies in children: a prospective, randomized study. J Pediatr Gastroenterol Nutr 2006;43:195–199.
16 De Blic J, Marchac V, Scheinmann P: Complications of flexible bronchoscopy in children: prospective study of 1,328 procedures. Eur Respir J 2002;20:1271–1276.
17 De Blic J, Midulla F, Barbato A, Clement A, Dab I, Eber E, Green C, Grigg J, Kotecha S, Kurland G, Pohunek P, Ratjen F, Rossi G: Bronchoalveolar lavage in children. ERS Task Force on bronchoalveolar lavage in children. European Respiratory Society. Eur Respir J 2000;15:217–231.
18 Midulla F, de Blic J, Barbato A, Bush A, Eber E, Kotecha S, Haxby E, Moretti C, Pohunek P, Ratjen F, ERS Task Force: Flexible endoscopy of paediatric airways. Eur Respir J 2003;22:698–708.
19 Pohunek P, Pokorna H, Striz I: Comparison of cell profiles in separately evaluated fractions of bronchoalveolar lavage (BAL) fluid in children. Thorax 1996;51:615–618.
20 Stevenson EC, Turner G, Hearey LG: Bronchoalveolar lavage findings suggest two different forms of childhood asthma. Clin Exp Allergy 1997;9:1027–1035.
21 Marguet C, Dean TP, Basuyau JP, Warner JO: Eosinophil cationic protein and interleukin 8 levels in bronchial lavage fluid from children with asthma and infantile wheeze. Pediatr Allergy Immunol 2001;12:27–33.
22 Barbato A, Panizzolo C, Gheno M, Sainati L, Favero E, Faggian D, Giusti F, Pesscolderungg L, La Rosa M: Bronchoalveolar lavage in asthmatic children: evidence of neutrophil activation in mild-to-moderate persistent asthma. Pediatr Allergy Immunol 2001;12:73–77.
23 Marguet C, Jouen-Boedes F, Dean TP, Warner JO: Bronchoalveolar cell profiles in children with asthma, infantile wheeze, chronic cough or cystic fibrosis. Am J Respir Crit Care Med 1999; 159:1533–1540.
24 Ferguson AC, Whitelaw M, Brown H: Correlation of bronchial eosinophil and mast cell activation with bronchial hyperresponsiveness in children with asthma. J Allergy Clin Immunol 1992;90: 609–613.
25 Ennis M, Turner G, Schock BC, Stevenson EC, Brown V, Fitch PS, Heaney LG, Taylor R, Shields MD: Inflammatory mediators in bronchoalveolar lavage samples from children with and without asthma. Clin Exp Allergy 1999;29:362–366.
26 Krawiec ME, Westcott JY, Chu HW, Balzar S, Trudeau JB, Schwartz LB, Wenzel SE: Persistent wheezing in very young children is associated with lower respiratory inflammation. Am J Respir Crit Care Med 2001;163:1338–1343.
27 Rojas-Ramos E, Avalos AF, Pérez-Fernandez L, Cuevas-Schacht F, Valencia-Maqueda E, Terán LM: Role of the chemokines RANTES, monocyte chemotactic proteins-3 and -4, and eotaxins-1 and -2 in childhood asthma. Eur Respir J 2003; 22:310–316.
28 Ferguson AC, Wong FV: Bronchial hyperresponsiveness in asthmatic children: correlation with macrophages and eosinophils in broncholavage fluid. Chest 1989;96:988–991.
29 Hein J, Martens E, Bauer I, Dörfling P, Brock J, Gümlzow HU, Breuel K, Rudolph I: Die bronchoalveoläre Lavage (BAL): eine diagnostische Methode bei chronischen unspezifischen bronchopulmonalen Erkrankungen im Kindesalter? Z Erkr Atmungsorgane 1991;176:7–20.
30 Najafi N, Demanet C, Dab I, De Waele M, Malfroot A: Differential cytology of bronchoalveolar lavage fluid in asthmatic children. Pediatr Pulmonol 2003;35:302–308.
31 Snijders D, Agostini S, Bertuola F, Panizzolo C, Baraldo S, Turato G, Faggian D, Plebani M, Saetta M, Barbato A: Markers of eosinophilic and neutrophilic inflammation in bronchoalveolar lavage of asthmatic and atopic children. Allergy 2010, E-pub ahead of print.
32 Bousquet J, Chanez P, Lacoste JY, Enander I, Venge P, Peterson C, Ahlstedt S, Michel FB, Godard P: Indirect evidence of bronchial inflammation assessed by titration of inflammatory mediators in BAL fluid of patients with asthma. J Allergy Clin Immunol 1991;88:649–660.
33 Warner JO, Marguet C, Rao R, Roche WR, Pohunek P: Inflammatory mechanisms in childhood asthma. Clin Exp Allergy 1998;28(suppl 5): 71–75.
34 Von Ungern-Sternberg BS, Sly PD, Loh RK, Isidoro A, Habre W: Value of eosinophil cationic protein and tryptase levels in bronchoalveolar lavage fluid for predicting lung function impairment in anaesthetised, asthmatic children. Anaesthesia 2006;61:1149–1154.
35 Norzila MZ, Fakes K, Henry RL, Simpson J, Gibson PG: Interleukin-8 secretion and neutrophil recruitment accompanies induced sputum eosinophil activation in children with acute asthma. Am J Respir Crit Care Med 2000;161:769–774.
36 Hayden FG: Rhinovirus and the lower respiratory tract. Rev Med Virol 2004;14:17–31.
37 Biscardi S, Lorrot M, Marc E, Moulin F, Boutonnat-Faucher B, Heilbronner C, Iniguez JL, Chaussain M, Nicand E, Raymond J, Gendrel D: *Mycoplasma pneumoniae* and asthma in children. Clin Infect Dis 2004;38:1341–1346.
38 Webley WC, Salva PS, Andrzejewski C, Cirino F, West CA, Tilahun Y, Stuart ES: The bronchial lavage of pediatric patients with asthma contains infectious *Chlamydia*. Am J Respir Crit Care Med 2005;171:1083–1088.

39 Regamey N, Balfour-Lynn I, Rosenthal M, Hogg C, Bush A, Davies JC: Time required to obtain endobronchial biopsies in children during fiberoptic bronchoscopy. Pediatr Pulmonol 2009;44:76–79.

40 Bush A, Pohunek P: Brush biopsy and mucosal biopsy. Am J Respir Crit Care Med 2000;162:18–22.

41 Jeffery P, Holgate S, Wenzel S: Methods for the assessment of endobronchial biopsies in clinical research: application to studies of pathogenesis and the effects of treatment. Am J Respir Crit Care Med 2003;168:S1–S17.

42 Turato G, Barbato A, Baraldo S, Zanin ME, Bazzan E, Lokar-Oliani K, Calabrese F, Panizzolo C, Snijders D, Maestrelli P, Zuin R, Fabbri LM, Saetta M: Non atopic children with multitrigger wheezing have airway pathology comparable to atopic asthma. Am J Respir Crit Care Med 2008;178:476–482.

43 Malmström K, Pitkäranta A, Carpen O, Pelkonen A, Malmberg LP, Turpeinen M, Kajosaari M, Sarna S, Lindahl H, Haahtela T, Mäkelä MJ: Human rhinovirus in bronchial epithelium of infants with recurrent respiratory symptoms. J Allergy Clin Immunol 2006;118:591–596.

44 Jeffery PK: Remodelling in asthma and chronic obstructive lung disease. Am J Respir Crit Care Med 2001;164:28–38.

45 Barbato A, Turato G, Baraldo S, Bazzan E, Calabrese F, Tura M, Zuin R, Beghe B, Maestrelli P, Fabbri LM, Saetta M: Airway inflammation in childhood asthma. Am J Respir Crit Care Med 2003;168:798–803.

46 Payne DN, Rogers AV, Ädelroth E, Bandi V, Guntupalli KK, Bush A, Jeffery PK: Early thickening of the reticular basement membrane in children with difficult asthma. Am J Respir Crit Care Med 2003;167:78–82.

47 Holgate ST, Holloway J, Wilson S, Bucchieri F, Puddicombe S, Davies DE: Epithelial-mesenchymal communication in the pathogenesis of chronic asthma. Proc Am Thorac Soc 2004;1:93–98.

48 Holgate ST, Davies DE, Puddicombe S, Richter A, Lackie P, Lordan J, Howarth P: Mechanisms of airway epithelial damage epithelial-mesenchymal interactions in the pathogenesis of asthma. Eur J Respir 2003;22:S24–S29.

49 Martinez FD: Respiratory syncytial virus bronchiolitis and the pathogenesis of childhood asthma. Pediatr Infect Dis J 2003;22:S76–S82.

50 Cutz E, Levison H, Cooper DM: Ultrastructure in airways in children with asthma. Histopathology 1978;2:407–421.

51 Cokuğraş H, Akçakaya N, Seçkin I, Camcioğlu Y, Sarimurat N, Aksoy F: Ultrastructural examination of bronchial biopsy specimens from children with moderate asthma. Thorax 2001;56:25–29.

52 Payne DN, Qiu Y, Zhu J, Peachey L, Scallan M, Bush A, Jeffery PK: Airway inflammation in children with difficult asthma: relationships with airflow limitation and persistent symptoms. Thorax 2004;59:862–869.

53 Saglani S, Payne DN, Zhu J, Wang Z, Nicholson AG, Bush A, Jeffery PK: Early detection of airway wall remodeling and eosinophilic inflammation in preschool wheezers. Am J Respir Crit Care Med 2007;176:858–864.

54 Regamey N, Ochs M, Hilliard TN, Mühlfeld C, Cornish N, Fleming L, Saglani S, Alton EW, Bush A, Jeffery PK, Davies JC: Increased airway smooth muscle mass in children with asthma, cystic fibrosis, and non-cystic fibrosis bronchiectasis. Am J Respir Crit Care Med 2008; 177:837–843.

55 Barbato A, Turato G, Baraldo S, Bazzan E, Calabrese F, Panizzolo C, Zanin ME, Zuin R, Maestrelli P, Fabbri LM, Saetta M: Epithelial damage and angiogenesis in the airways of children with asthma. Am J Respir Crit Care Med 2006;174: 975–981.

56 Saglani S, Malmström K, Pelkonen AS, Malmberg LP, Lindahl H, Kajosaari M, Turpeinen M, Rogers AV, Payne DN, Bush A, Haahtela T, Mäkelä MJ, Jeffery PK: Airway remodeling and inflammation in symptomatic infants with reversible airflow obstruction. Am J Respir Crit Care Med 2005;171:722–727.

57 Amin K, Lúdvíksdóttir D, Janson C, Nettelbladt O, Björnsson E, Roomans GM, Boman G, Sevéus L, Venge P: Inflammation and structural changes in the airways of patients with atopic and nonatopic asthma. BHR Group. Am J Respir Crit Care Med 2000;162:2295–2301.

58 Robroeks CM, van de Kant KD, Jöbsis Q, Hendriks HJ, van Gent R, Wouters EF, Damoiseaux JG, Bast A, Wodzig WK, Dompeling E: Exhaled nitric oxide and biomarkers in exhaled breath condensate indicate the presence, severity and control of childhood asthma. Clin Exp Allergy 2007;37:1303–1311.

Prof. Angelo Barbato
Dipartimento di Pediatria, Università degli Studi di Padova
Via Giustiniani, 3
IT–35128 Padova (Italy)
Tel. +39 049 821 3505, Fax +39 049 821 3509, E-Mail barbato@pediatria.unipd.it

Priftis KN, Anthracopoulos MB, Eber E, Koumbourlis AC, Wood RE (eds): Paediatric Bronchoscopy.
Prog Respir Res. Basel, Karger 2010, vol 38, pp 149–155

Atelectasis, Middle Lobe Syndrome and Plastic Bronchitis

Kostas N. Priftis[a] · Bruce Rubin[b]

[a]Department of Allergy-Pneumonology, Penteli Children's Hospital, Athens, Greece; [b]Department of Pediatrics, Virginia Commonwealth University Medical Center, Richmond, Va., USA

Abstract

Atelectasis can result from obstruction of bronchial airflow, compression of the lung or surfactant dysfunction. Middle lobe (ML) or lingula atelectasis in children is often due to asthma and usually resolves spontaneously, but in cases of more extended or prolonged atelectasis, bronchoscopy provides clinically useful information. Bronchoscopy allows direct airway inspection or potential pathogenic micro-organism isolation, whereas repeated lavage may be beneficial for mucus plug removal; foreign-body removal is therapeutic and may be even life saving. The anatomy of the ML bronchus creates conditions for poor secretion drainage, resulting in impaired ventilation and eventually alveolar collapse; repeated episodes of infection, inflammation and obstruction may eventually lead to bronchiectasis. Plastic bronchitis is characterized by the formation of large gelatinous or rigid branching airway casts. These casts are larger and more cohesive than those seen in ordinary mucus plugging; removal of central casts should be attempted before medical therapy to mobilize the casts.

Atelectasis is a common finding in children that usually produces few symptoms and resolves quickly. However, atelectasis due to significant obstruction of a large airway can produce cough, fever and respiratory distress. In most children, the diagnosis can be made by radiographic imaging alone, but symptoms and imaging findings may be nonspecific, and laboratory tests are rarely helpful in establishing the cause of atelectasis [1]. Most cases of middle lobe (ML) or lingula atelectasis in children have been thought to be due to asthma in association with secretory hyperresponsiveness and these usually resolve spontaneously, but in cases of more extended or prolonged atelectasis or ML syndrome (MLS), bronchoscopy can be both diagnostic and therapeutic. For

example, plastic bronchitis is a condition in which large bronchial casts with rubber-like consistency develop in the tracheobronchial tree and cause airway obstruction; the treatment of choice is endoscopic extraction. The purpose of this chapter is to present up-to-date information regarding the role of bronchoscopy in children with atelectasis, MLS and plastic bronchitis.

Atelectasis

The term 'atelectasis' describes incomplete expansion or complete collapse of part of the lung parenchyma [2]. Atelectasis can result from obstruction of bronchial airflow, compression of the lung or surfactant dysfunction. Segmental, lobar or whole-lung collapse is associated with absorption of air in the alveoli. The developing lung is particularly predisposed to atelectasis once airway obstruction develops. In early childhood, the airways are smaller and more collapsible, the chest wall is more compliant, and the collateral ventilation through bronchiole-alveolar pores (the canaliculi of Lambert) is not completely developed [1, 2].

History and clinical examination are insensitive to detect atelectasis. The clinical manifestations depend on the underlying cause, the degree of volume loss within the lung, and how quickly volume loss develops. A slowly developing atelectasis of a lobe may produce no symptoms. Most children with atelectasis that occurs during the course of common diseases, such as asthma or infection, do not have many symptoms unless the obstructed area is large [1].

Classification

Obstructive Atelectasis

Obstructive atelectasis is the most common type and results from absorption of gas from the alveoli when communication between the alveoli and major airways is obstructed. Intrabronchial obstruction can be exogenous, as in foreign-body aspiration or recurrent aspiration of either gastric or oral contents due to a swallowing disorder, or endogenous, as is the case with tumours, mucus plugging or tracheo- or bronchomalacia.

Compression of Bronchi or Parenchyma

Compression atelectasis is caused by the inability to expand the lung due to any space-occupying lesion of the thorax: (a) tumours, cysts, enlarged lymph nodes, cardiomegaly or a vascular ring may compress the adjacent bronchi or parenchyma; (b) increased intrapleural pressure as with chylothorax, haemothorax, pneumothorax, and (c) chest wall defects and neuromuscular diseases may, directly or indirectly, result in alveolar hypoventilation and alveolar collapse.

Surfactant Deficiency or Dysfunction

Surfactant dysfunction has been reported in respiratory distress of the preterm newborn with inadequate surfactant production and in babies with meconium aspiration and surfactant destruction [3]. There is also surfactant breakdown in older patients with pneumonia and severe dysfunction in patients with the acute respiratory distress syndrome. Surfactant dysfunction causes increased alveolar surface tension as well as failure to maintain small airway patency.

Bronchoscopy for the Diagnosis of Atelectasis

Flexible bronchoscopy (FB) allows direct airway inspection and thus differentiation between obstructive and non-obstructive types of atelectasis and definition of the nature of obstruction when it occurs. Atelectasis is the second most frequent radiological sign of foreign-body aspiration in children after localized air-trapping, with fairly good diagnostic sensitivity, but low specificity [4]. In atelectasis caused by foreign-body aspiration, bronchoscopy is required for definitive diagnosis and identification of the type of foreign body and its integrity. In a series of 2,165 children with foreign-body aspiration, atelectasis and pneumonia (n = 362) were more commonly seen in patients with delayed diagnosis; however, only 15.7% of all foreign bodies were radio-opaque, and much fewer were opaque in children with delayed diagnosis [5]. By performing bronchoscopy, the presence of an endobronchial mass can often be

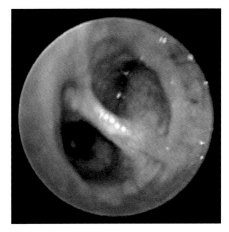

Fig. 1. Total occlusion of the subsegmental medial basal bronchus (B7) of the right lower lobe after prolonged atelectasis.

confirmed. In a case series of 17 children with carcinoid or muco-epidermoid tumours, 12 presented with evidence of bronchial obstruction. FB confirmed the presence of a bronchial tumour in all cases, and endobronchial biopsies were diagnostic in 11 of 12 cases [6].

Extrinsic or intrinsic bronchial obstruction may lead to loss of integrity of the bronchial wall cartilage, and bronchiectasis with bronchial collapse may occur. Consequently, bronchial obstruction could be either the cause or the result of atelectasis [7; chapter 12, this vol., pp. 130–140] (fig. 1, 2; online suppl. video 1). A typical example is children with heart disease and vascular anomalies who are at increased risk of airway obstruction and atelectasis. In these children, FB can be both diagnostic and often therapeutic [8, 9]. In a study of 72 patients (mean age 21 months) with acquired and congenital heart disease (CHD), most underwent FB assessment for atelectasis (35%), pneumonia (14%) or stridor (14%). Airway malacia was the most common finding, primarily left main bronchus malacia (24%) with the second most common finding being stenosis by extrinsic compression, again mostly of the left main bronchus [8].

Chronic atelectasis of any aetiology can become a nidus of chronic purulent infection with bronchial wall damage leading to bronchiectasis. Isolation of pathogenic micro-organisms by FB and protected specimen brush or lavage can help to direct appropriate antibiotic therapy [chapter 15, this vol., pp. 156–172]. Bronchoscopic bronchoalveolar lavage (BAL) allows direct sampling of the involved lobe [10].

Value of Bronchoscopy in the Treatment of Atelectasis

In an attempt to re-inflate an atelectatic lobe, repeated 'therapeutic' small-volume lavage is sometimes used although a

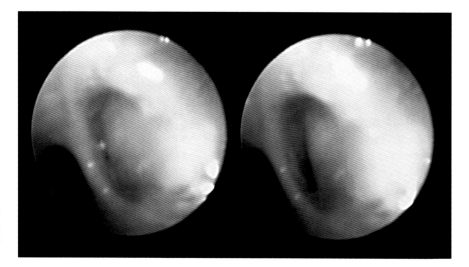

Fig. 2. Near total occlusion of the subsegmental medial basal bronchus (B7) of the right lower lobe in an 8-year-old girl with chronic wet cough (online suppl. video 1).

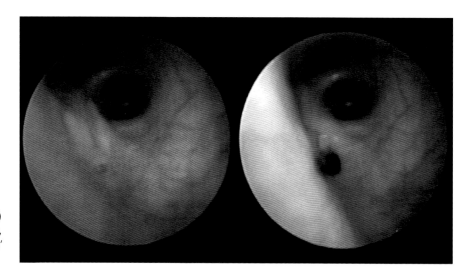

Fig. 3. Superior segmental bronchus (B6) with thick, tenacious purulent mucus plug, before and after repeated 'therapeutic' small-volume lavages.

benefit has not been clearly established (fig. 3). In pneumonia, if secretions completely occlude the airway and cannot be cleaned by coughing, suctioning or physical therapy, rigid bronchoscopy has been effective as a therapeutic procedure. In a study of 33 Taiwanese children with atelectasis caused by pneumonia, rigid bronchoscopy with lung lavage for removal of the mucus plugs or foreign bodies was performed. Twenty-one (64%) children had significant improvement in either oxygen saturation or chest radiography within 72 h [11]. Obviously, removing a foreign body obstructing the airway by using a bronchoscope can be therapeutic and even life saving. For safety, this should usually be performed with the rigid bronchoscope [chapter 8, this vol., pp. 83–94].

Other bronchoscopic interventions for treatment of persistent atelectasis such as instillation of acetylcysteine, antibiotics, dornase alfa, surfactant preparations and sodium bicarbonate [chapter 5, this vol., pp. 54–63] have also been reported but for the most part, results are poor or inconclusive [1, 2]. In a recent study [12] of 35 paediatric intensive-care patients with 51 episodes of atelectasis who received intratracheal dornase α, 67% of patients showed radiological signs of improvement after 24 h; however, there was no control group. In another paper [13], 5 children (7 months to 15 years of age) with heterogeneous lung diseases requiring mechanical ventilation were treated with a diluted surfactant preparation (Curosurf^{TM}) in a concentration of 5–10 mg/ml (total dose 120–240 mg) which was instilled into the atelectatic segments. All mechanically ventilated patients were extubated within 24 h following the intervention, and partial or complete resolution of atelectasis without recurrence was reported. This is consistent with a clinical trial showing that surfactant aerosol augments airway mucus clearance in patients with chronic obstructive pulmonary disease [14]. Interventional bronchoscopic techniques can provide treatment of various endobronchial lesions such as tumours or mucus plugging [15; chapter 6, this vol., pp. 64–74].

Middle Lobe Syndrome

MLS in children is a distinct clinical and radiographic entity [16]. It may be symptomatic or asymptomatic, and cause persistent or recurrent atelectasis primarily of the ML and/or the lingula. The anatomical characteristics of the ML bronchus such as narrow diameter of the lobar orifice, acute angle of the lobar bronchus and surrounding lymphoid tissue create conditions for poor secretion drainage, resulting in impaired ventilation and eventually alveolar collapse. Poor collateral ventilation decreases the chance of re-inflation once atelectasis has occurred.

There are many causes of MLS involving intrinsic and extrinsic bronchial obstruction. Many of these conditions are considered to be due to asthma and may resolve spontaneously [17]. However, patient recovery after an asthma attack may not be accompanied by a concomitant re-expansion of the atelectatic lobe. Therefore, atelectasis of the ML may persist for a prolonged period of time, and repeated episodes of infection, inflammation and obstruction may eventually lead to bronchiectasis. Three recent studies evaluated the lung disease in children with primary ciliary dyskinesia using high-resolution computed tomography and found that ML and lingula were the most common areas to manifest bronchiectasis [18–20]. Apparently, in these patients an increase in the usually protective mucus secretory response to inflammation is also present, called secretory hyperresponsiveness [21].

The Role of Bronchoscopy in MLS
The value of bronchoscopy in MLS may be diagnostic and therapeutic. Bronchoscopy allows visualization of the airway and offers the ability to determine whether intrabronchial obstruction is the cause of MLS. It can be immediately therapeutic in removing mucus and clearing the airway, and can be curative in some cases (fig. 4–6; online suppl. video 2). BAL fluid can be obtained to determine cellular

elements and to assess the presence of infection by culturing and staining for pathogens.

In a case series of 55 children with MLS [16, 22], we initially treated all patients with antibiotics, inhaled bronchodilators, inhaled corticosteroids and physiotherapy for 4–6 weeks. When MLS did not resolve, the patients were re-evaluated by high-resolution computed tomography, FB and BAL. Complete obstruction of the ML bronchus was found in only 3 cases: due to a tumour, a foreign body and external compression by enlarged lymph nodes. In the remaining 52 patients, FB revealed secondary disorders, such as bronchial mucosal oedema, scarring, secretions or, less commonly, mucus plugging. Thus, even if MLS is primarily the result of a non-obstructive process, this may lead to the development of secondary obstruction.

Positive findings in BAL fluid culture were detected in 49.1% of patients, although none had clinically diagnosed infection, most frequently *Haemophilus influenzae*, followed by *Streptococcus pneumoniae* and *Staphylococcus aureus*. There was an association between culture positivity and the duration or worsening of symptoms suggesting that infection may hold a pathogenic role in the perpetuation of atelectasis. Bronchiectasis was documented by high-resolution computed tomography scans in 15 patients (27.3%). The duration of symptoms before diagnosis positively correlated with the development of bronchiectasis and an unfavourable clinical outcome (worsening or no change).

The cytology of BAL fluid showed an increased number of eosinophils in 58.2% of the patients. The positive association between an increased number of eosinophils in BAL fluid and a favourable clinical outcome is in agreement with the concept that certain cases of MLS are of 'asthmatic' origin and therefore MLS is expected to recover spontaneously or to respond to appropriate anti-asthma treatment [22].

Plastic Bronchitis

Plastic bronchitis is a rare disease characterized by the formation of branching airway casts that are more cohesive than those seen in ordinary mucus plugging [21]. The casts can be spontaneously expectorated and patients will sometimes expectorate large casts of their tracheobronchial tree (fig. 7). Patients may require bronchoscopy for cast removal [23], and death due to airway obstruction from a cast is not uncommon. Chest radiographs often show collapse of the involved segment or lobe, with compensatory hyperinflation of adjacent lung regions, although there are reports of patients with bilateral patchy consolidations without

Video

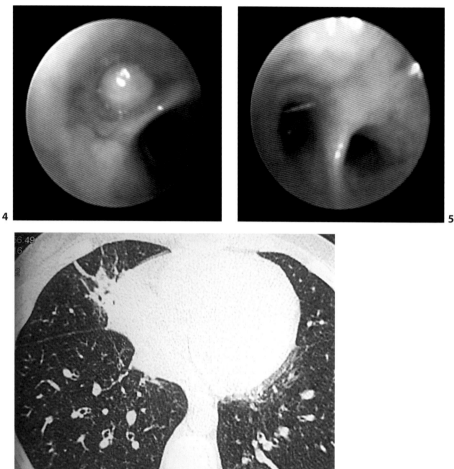

Fig. 4–6. Orifice of the ML bronchus before and after removal of a purulent mucus plug in an 11-year-old girl with 'recurrent pneumonias', and the high-resolution computed tomography scan showing atelectasis and bronchiectasis in the medial segment of the ML of the same patient (online suppl. video 2).

evidence of volume loss [24, 25]. The diagnosis is confirmed by bronchoscopy demonstrating airway obstruction with thick casts or by expectoration of casts.

The prevalence of plastic bronchitis is unknown. It is likely that many patients with plastic bronchitis are not diagnosed. This diagnosis may also overlap with diseases such as asthma and the severe mucus plugging sometimes seen in bronchopulmonary aspergillosis or MLS. Differentiating between severe asthma with mucus plugging and plastic bronchitis can be difficult; plastic bronchitis can present with acute respiratory failure, wheezing and thoracic air leakage refractory to standard asthma therapy [26] or 'bronchial casts' in gastric washings [27]. A case of a cystic fibrosis patient with recurrent airway obstruction caused by plastic bronchitis was also recently reported [28].

The natural history of plastic bronchitis depends on the associated disease and cast type (table 1). Patients with CHD are at the greatest risk for death; the mean reported mortality in these patients is 33% (14–50%). However, death due

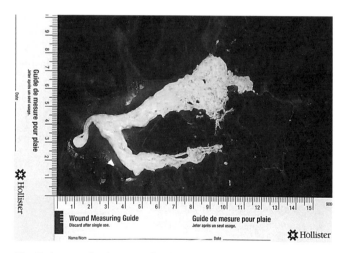

Fig. 7. Large cohesive cast of major airways.

Table 1. Summary of descriptive statistics for published cases of plastic bronchitis, 1965 to the present, where age and cast type are known [24]

Plastic bronchitis classification	Sample size	Male:female ratio	Mean age years	Standard deviation	Mortality ratio
Structural CHD	24	1.7:1	6.2	3.6	0.33
Mucinous casts	13	1.6:1	6.1	2.9	0.38
Inflammatory casts	7	2.5:1	7.4	5.3	0.14
Chylous casts	4	1:1	4	1.4	0.50
Non-structural heart disease	32	1.3:1	12.8	17.6	0.10
Lymphatic diseases or chylous casts[1]	5	1:0	43.8[2]	17.0	0
Atopy or eosinophilic casts	22	0.8:1	6.0	8.75	0.14
SCACS or fibrinous casts[3]	5	0.8:1[4] (n = 26)	11.8	15.9	0

F = Female; M = male; SCACS = sickle cell acute chest syndrome. All cases lost to follow-up or unknown were assumed to be alive for the purposes of data analysis.
[1] Two cases reported in table 1 were not analysed as clinical details were not available to the authors.
[2] The only mean age that significantly differs from all other groups, using one-way ANOVA with Scheffé's method for multiple comparisons.
[3] The paper by Moser et al. [25] was not included in mean age analysis as individual clinical details of patients were not available. In this series of 21 patients with plastic bronchitis associated with acute chest syndrome, the mean age was 8 years (range 3–18), and there were no deaths.
[4] The paper by Moser et al. [25] was included because it offers information on gender distribution.

to obstructing casts is extremely rare in patients with plastic bronchitis due to acute chest syndrome in sickle cell disease [29]. Patients who die usually succumb to respiratory failure related to central airway obstruction [30–34].

Treatment for plastic bronchitis has included bronchodilators, inhaled and oral corticosteroids, mucolytics, airway clearance therapy and antibiotics. Other therapies reported include inhaled heparin [31], urokinase [35], tissue plasminogen activator [36], dornase alfa [24], and oral macrolide antibiotics as mucoregulatory therapy [37]. There is only anecdotal evidence that any of these therapies are beneficial, and this evidence has been generally provided only by single case reports.

Treatment for children with cyanotic CHD and plastic bronchitis should include a careful evaluation of the cardiovascular system, looking for evidence of stenosis or thrombosis [33, 35] and optimizing cardiac rhythm [27, 38] and cardiac output [39]. If there are chylous casts present, dietary modification [24] or thoracic duct ligation, when appropriate [40], may help. Removal of central casts should be attempted before medical therapy to mobilize the casts, as propagation to the trachea is the primary reported cause of death. In patients with CHD, bronchoscopy can be life saving, and many patients require more than one bronchoscopy when cough is ineffective.

References

1 Duggan, M, Kavanagh MB: Atelectasis; in Chernick V, Boat TF, Willmott RW, Bush A (eds): Kendig's Disorders of the Respiratory Tract in Children, ed 7. Philadelphia, Saunders, 2006, pp 616–621.
2 Peroni DG, Boner AL: Atelectasis: mechanisms, diagnosis and management. Paediatr Respir Rev 2000;1:274–278.

3 Gross T, Zmora E, Levi-Kalisman Y, Regev O, Berman A: Lung-surfactant-meconium interaction: in vitro study in bulk and at the air-solution interface. Langmuir 2006;22:3243–3250.
4 Midulla F, Guidi R, Barbato A, Capocaccia P, Forenza N, Marseglia G, Pifferi M, Moretti C, Bonci E, De Benedictis FM: Foreign body aspiration in children. Pediatr Int 2005;47:663–668.

5 Ibrahim Sersar S, Hamza UA, Abdel Hameed WA, Abul Maaty RA, Gowaeli NN, Moussa SA, Al Morsi SM, Hafez MM: Inhaled foreign bodies: management according to early or late presentation. Eur J Cardiothorac Surg 2005;28:369–374.

6   Fauroux B, Aynie V, Larroquet M, Boccon-Gibod
    L, Ducou le Pointe H, Tamalet A, Clément A: Car-
    cinoid and mucoepidermoid bronchial tumours
    in children. Eur J Pediatr 2005;164:748–752.

7   Boogaard R, Huijsmans SH, Pijnenburg MW,
    Tiddens HA, de Jongste JC, Merkus PJ: Trache-
    omalacia and bronchomalacia in children: inci-
    dence and patient characteristics. Chest 2005;
    128:3391–3397.

8   Cerda J, Chacón J, Reichhard C, Bertrand P, Hol-
    mgren NL, Clavería C, Sánchez I: Flexible fi-
    beroptic bronchoscopy in children with heart
    disease: a twelve years experience. Pediatr Pul-
    monol 2007;42:319–324.

9   Lee SL, Cheung YF, Leung MP, Ng YK, Tsoi NS:
    Airway obstruction in children with congenital
    heart disease: assessment by flexible bronchos-
    copy. Pediatr Pulmonol 2002;34:304–311.

10 Weber MD, Thammasitboon S: A critical ap-
    praisal of 'Blind and bronchoscopic sampling
    methods in suspected ventilator-associated
    pneumonia: a multicentre prospective study' by
    Mentec et al (Intensive Care Med 2004;30:1319–
    1326). Pediatr Crit Care Med 2007;8:272–275.

11 Wu KH, Lin CF, Huang CJ, Chen CC: Rigid venti-
    lation bronchoscopy under general anesthesia for
    treatment of pediatric pulmonary atelectasis
    caused by pneumonia: a review of 33 cases. Int
    Surg 2006;91:291–294.

12 Riethmueller J, Kumpf M, Borth-Bruhns T, Bre-
    hm W, Wiskirchen J, Sieverding L, Ankele C,
    Hofbeck M, Baden W: Clinical and in vitro effect
    of dornase alfa in mechanically ventilated pedi-
    atric non-cystic fibrosis patients with atelectases.
    Cell Physiol Biochem 2009;23:205–210.

13 Krause MF, von Bismarck P, Oppermann HC,
    Ankermann T: Bronchoscopic surfactant admin-
    istration in pediatric patients with persistent
    lobar atelectasis. Respiration 2008;75:100–104.

14 Anzueto A, Jubran A, Ohar JA, Piquette CA, Ren-
    nard SI, Colice G, Pattishall EN, Barrett J, Engle
    M, Perret KA, Rubin BK: Effects of aerosolized
    surfactant in patients with stable chronic bron-
    chitis: a prospective randomized controlled trial.
    JAMA 1997;278:1426–1431.

15 Breen DP, Dubus JC, Chetaille B, Payan MJ, Du-
    tau H: A rare cause of an endobronchial tumour
    in children: the role of interventional bronchos-
    copy in the diagnosis and treatment of tumours
    while preserving anatomy and lung function.
    Respiration 2008;76:444–448.

16 Priftis KN, Mermiri D, Papadopoulou A, Anthra-
    copoulos M, Vaos G, Nicolaidou P: The role of
    timely intervention in middle lobe syndrome in
    children. Chest 2005;128:2504–2510.

17 Sekerel BE, Nakipoglu F: Middle lobe syndrome
    in children with asthma: review of 56 cases. J
    Asthma 2004;41:411–417.

18 Santamaria F, Montella S, Tiddens HA, Guidi G,
    Casotti V, Maglione M, de Jong PA: Structural
    and functional lung disease in primary ciliary
    dyskinesia. Chest 2008;134:351–357.

19 Kennedy MP, Noone PG, Leigh MW, Zariwala MA,
    Minnix SL, Knowles MR, Molina PL: High-resolu-
    tion CT of patients with primary ciliary dyskine-
    sia. AJR Am J Roentgenol 2007;188:1232–1238.

20 Jain K, Padley SP, Goldstraw EJ, Kidd SJ, Hogg C,
    Biggart E, Bush A: Primary ciliary dyskinesia in
    the paediatric population: range and severity of
    radiological findings in a cohort of patients receiv-
    ing tertiary care. Clin Radiol 2007;62:986–993.

21 Okamoto K, Kim JS, Rubin BK: Secretory phos-
    pholipases A_2 stimulate mucus secretion, induce
    airway inflammation, and produce secretory
    hyperresponsiveness to neutrophil elastase in
    ferret trachea. Am J Physiol Lung Cell Mol
    Physiol 2007;292:L62–L67.

22 Priftis KN, Anthracopoulos M, Mermiri D, Papa-
    dopoulou A, Xepapadaki P, Tsakanika C, Nico-
    laidou P: Bronchial hyperresponsiveness in per-
    sistent middle lobe syndrome in children.
    Pediatr Pulmonol 2006;41:805–811.

23 Manna SS, Shaw J, Tibby SM, Durward A: Treat-
    ment of plastic bronchitis in acute chest syn-
    drome of sickle cell disease with intratracheal
    rhDNase. Arch Dis Child 2003;88:626–627.

24 Madsen P, Shah SA, Rubin BK: Plastic bronchitis:
    new insights and a classification scheme.
    Paediatr Respir Rev 2005;6:292–300.

25 Moser C, Nussbaum E, Cooper DM: Plastic bron-
    chitis and the role of bronchoscopy in the acute
    chest syndrome of sickle cell disease. Chest
    2001;120:608–613.

26 Kruger J, Springer C, Picard E, Kerem E: Thorac-
    ic air leakage in the presentation of cast bronchi-
    tis. Chest 2009;136:615–617.

27 Brogan TV, Finn LS, Pyskaty DJ, Redding GJ,
    Ricker D, Inglis A, Gibson RL: Plastic bronchitis
    in children: a case series and review of the medi-
    cal literature. Pediatr Pulmonol 2002;34:482–
    487.

28 Mateos-Corral D, Cutz E, Solomon M, Ratjen F:
    Plastic bronchitis as an unusual cause of mucus
    plugging in cystic fibrosis. Pediatr Pulmonol
    2009;44:939–940.

29 Cajaiba MM, Borralho P, Reyes-Múgica M: The
    potentially lethal nature of bronchial casts: plas-
    tic bronchitis. Int J Surg Pathol 2008;16:230–232.

30 Hug MI, Ersch J, Moenkhoff M, Burger R, Fan-
    coni S, Bauersfeld U: Chylous bronchial casts
    after Fontan operation. Circulation 2001;103:
    1031–1033.

31 Schmitz J, Schatz J, Kirsten D: Plastic bronchitis.
    Pneumologie 2004;58:443–448.

32 Le Pimpec-Barthes F, Badia A, Febvre M, Leg-
    man P, Riquet M: Chylous reflux into localized
    pulmonary lymphangiectasis. Ann Thorac Surg
    2002;74:575–578.

33 Nair LG, Kurtz CP: Lymphangiomatosis present-
    ing with bronchial cast formation. Thorax 1996;
    51:765–766.

34 Liu DB, Zeng QY, Zhong JW, Huang ZY, Zhou LF:
    Perioperative management of plastic bronchitis
    in children. Int J Pediatr Otorhinolaryngol 2010;
    74:15–21.

35 Quasney M, Orman K, Thompson J, Ring JC,
    Salim M, Schoumacker RA, Watson D, Novick
    W, Deitcher SR, Joyner R: Plastic bronchitis oc-
    curring late after the Fontan procedure: treat-
    ment with aerosolized urokinase. Crit Care Med
    2000;28:2107–2111.

36 Do TB, Chu JM, Berdjis F, Anas NG: Fontan pa-
    tient with plastic bronchitis treated successfully
    using aerosolized tissue plasminogen activator: a
    case report and review of the literature. Pediatr
    Cardiol 2009;30:352–355.

37 Shinkai M, Rubin BK: Macrolides and airway
    inflammation in children. Paediatr Respir Rev
    2005;6:227–235.

38 Di Cindio S, Theroux M, Costarino AT Jr, Cook
    S, O'Reilly R: Plastic bronchitis: a case report.
    Paediatr Anaesth 2004;14:520–523.

39 Chaudhari M, Stumper O: Plastic bronchitis after
    Fontan operation: treatment with stent fenestra-
    tion of the Fontan circuit. Heart 2004;90:801.

40 Shah SS, Drinkwater DC, Christian KG: Plastic
    bronchitis: is thoracic duct ligation a real surgi-
    cal option? Ann Thorac Surg 2006;81:2281–2283.

Kostas N. Priftis
Allergy-Pneumonology Department, Penteli Children's Hospital
GR–152 36 P. Penteli, Athens (Greece)
Tel. +30 210 8036484, Fax +30 210 6131173
E-Mail kpriftis@otenet.gr

Chapter 15

Priftis KN, Anthracopoulos MB, Eber E, Koumbourlis AC, Wood RE (eds): Paediatric Bronchoscopy.
Prog Respir Res. Basel, Karger 2010, vol 38, pp 156–172

Lung Infection in Cystic Fibrosis and Other Chronic Suppurative Lung Diseases

Jane C. Davies · Andrew Bush · Claire L. Hogg

Royal Brompton Hospital, London, and Imperial College London, London, UK

Abstract

Many conditions cause chronic infection and inflammation within the paediatric airway, including cystic fibrosis, primary ciliary dyskinesia and a host of other conditions all leading to bronchiectasis. Here we describe the background to each of these conditions, what is known about persistent infection, the nature of the inflammatory response and factors which might explain differences in severity of these conditions. We focus on the roles of bronchoscopy in diagnosis and management. Finally, we outline some of the ways in which bronchoscopic research has increased our understanding of these diseases and highlight the areas in which further research is required.   Copyright © 2010 S. Karger AG, Basel

Causes of Chronic Suppurative Lung Diseases in Childhood

Cystic Fibrosis

Cystic fibrosis (CF) is the commonest single cause of suppurative airway disease in childhood, with an incidence varying from 1:1,500 to 1:6,500 in various populations. The phenotype is complex, with involvement of multiple organs; chronic infection and inflammation of the respiratory tract, exocrine pancreatic insufficiency, male infertility and elevated sweat electrolytes are among the typical features of the disease. However, most morbidity and mortality are caused by progressive lung failure. Abnormal transport of chloride and sodium ions across the respiratory epithelium is central to the basic defect in CF and is caused by mutations in the CF transmembrane conductance regulator (CFTR) gene, which was cloned in 1989.

CFTR protein is expressed in the apical membrane of epithelial cells, including airway and intestinal epithelium. Many studies have indicated its role as a cyclic-adenosine-monophosphate-regulated chloride channel. In addition, it is becoming increasingly appreciated that CFTR has a growing number of other functions, including regulation of other ion channels such as the epithelial sodium channel and calcium-activated chloride channels and the transport of glutathione. The relative importance of each of these functions as well as others is yet to be determined.

The link between ion transport defects and the pathogenesis of CF lung disease most likely involves dysregulated airway surface liquid volume and deficient mucus clearance (the 'low-volume hypothesis'; fig. 1) [1, 2]. In addition, there is good evidence that CF airway epithelia possess an intrinsically enhanced pro-inflammatory response; however, whether that occurs only in the presence of infection or can be triggered by non-microbial substances such as obstructed mucus or pollutants remains uncertain.

Patients with CF can present at any age [3]: antenatally, diagnosis may result from screening due to a family history or because of associated problems detected on scanning, most commonly hyperechogenic bowel. Newborn screening is undertaken in many countries, but otherwise, most patients present as infants or children with either respiratory or gastrointestinal problems, or both. Respiratory symptoms include recurrent cough, chest infections, wheeze and respiratory distress. Older children may present with finger clubbing. Chest X-ray may be normal, or show hyperinflation or areas of consolidation. Later in the course of the disease, widespread bronchiectasis with cyst formation and fibrosis may be visible. Bacterial infection should be sought (see later), although viruses likely play an important role.

A proportion (10–15%) of children with CF present in the neonatal period with meconium ileus, and most (>90%) patients have exocrine pancreatic insufficiency,

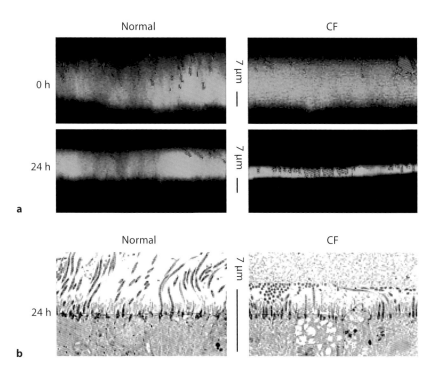

Fig. 1. The low-volume hypothesis of disease pathogenesis in the CF airway. **a** Wild-type (normal) and CF cell monolayers were exposed to a fixed volume of surface liquid (green); 24 h later, the volume was well maintained in the wild-type cultures but significantly decreased in the CF cultures; importantly any particulate matter, like micro-organisms etc. (represented here by red fluorescent beads) present on the liquid surface, was now in direct contact with the cell glycocalyx, a mechanism known to trigger inflammatory responses. **b** Transmission electron micrographs demonstrate the effect of this surface liquid depletion on ciliary position; whilst wild-type cilia were seen extending from the cell surface, the CF cilia were compressed and bent. Indeed, in contrast to ciliary movement visible on the wild-type cultures, complete stasis had occurred in the CF cultures after 24 h. With permission from Matsui et al. [1].

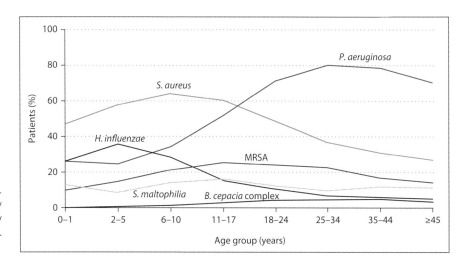

Fig. 2. The age-related prevalence of bacterial infection in CF. Adapted from http://www.cff.org/UploadedFiles/research/ClinicalResearch/2007-Patient-Registry-Report.pdf.

which may lead to failure to thrive if undiagnosed. Other modes of presentation include: nasal polyps, rectal prolapse, fat-soluble vitamin deficiency, peripheral oedema, hypo-albuminaemia and anaemia, neonatal obstructive jaundice (rare) and pseudo-Bartter syndrome (hypochloraemic, hypokalaemic alkalosis). Older males may present with infertility due to congenital bilateral absence of the vas deferens. With the advent of genetic testing, it has become clear that milder forms of CF exist, which have been termed 'atypical' or 'variant' disease. Diagnosis can

be challenging in these individuals, many of whom present later in life.

Almost all patients with CF have bacteria identified from airway secretions at some point in their lives [4]. For the majority, such an infection occurs first in childhood and is chronic by early adulthood (fig. 2). In infants and small children, the commonest infecting bacteria are *Staphylococcus aureus*, *Haemophilus influenzae* and then *Pseudomonas aeruginosa*. Later, organisms including *Stenotrophomonas maltophilia*, *Alcaligenes xylosoxidans* and bacteria from the *Burkholderia cepacia* complex may be acquired. Non-tuberculous mycobacteria are also more common than in the general population; *Mycobacterium abscessus* can be particularly problematic.

Non-CF Bronchiectasis

Non-CF bronchiectasis is a well-recognized condition in children in developing countries, in particular in some indigenous populations [5], although it has received little attention in the developing world. This likely relates to the relatively fewer cases, underrecognition and lack of research in this area but also the increased focus on asthma, which may be a coexisting morbidity, in these countries. Non-CF bronchiectasis in children may represent around 10% of all referrals to a paediatric respiratory service, although the delay in referral and diagnosis may be as long as 7 years from the onset of symptoms [6]. In this group, 75% had a previous diagnosis of asthma reversed.

In many cases, impaired mucociliary clearance (MCC), which may be primary (see next section) or acquired, is likely to contribute to endobronchial infection by facilitating bacterial colonization of the lower airway [7]. An underlying aetiology remains elusive in around 20% but identified causes include: previous infection, immunodeficiency, obliterative bronchiolitis, congenital thoracic malformations, chronic aspiration, eosinophilic oesophagitis, familial bronchiectasis, primary ciliary dyskinesia (PCD) and middle lobe syndrome. Around 8% of children may have two co-morbidities such as obliterative bronchiolitis and bronchiectasis, both of which commonly result from previous infection such as adenovirus.

High-resolution computed tomography is the current gold standard for diagnosis; there is a very poor correlation with plain chest radiographs, highlighting the gross insensitivity of the latter. Following treatment of childhood bronchiectasis, some cases may be seen to resolve on repeat high-resolution computed tomography [8], and in some centres this may affect the terminology used to address cases where the pathology may represent bronchial wall thickening rather than established bronchiectasis. Terms such as prebronchiectasis are now common and may overlap with the increasingly recognized phenomenon of persistent or chronic bacterial bronchitis (see below).

Primary Ciliary Dyskinesia

PCD, although rare, is one of the well-defined causes of non-CF bronchiectasis and as such merits further detail here. Like CF, it is an autosomal recessive disease characterized by impaired MCC, in this case due to abnormalities of ciliary structure and function. The reported incidence of

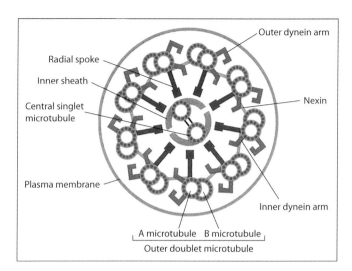

Fig. 3. Diagram of normal ciliary ultrastructure. With permission from Alberts et al. [10].

1:15,000–30,000 is likely to be an underestimate as improved screening and diagnostics become available. Furthermore, in certain isolated or consanguineous communities, the incidence may be significantly higher.

The abnormalities of ciliary function result in a multisystem disease with a wide spectrum of disease severity. Cilia are complex and highly specialized organelles made up of over 360 proteins [9]. Each respiratory cilium is composed of microtubules arranged with 9 peripheral pairs surrounding a central pair, the 9 + 2 formation, known as the axoneme (fig. 3). The peripheral microtubular pairs have a complete A and partial B microtubule, which are connected to the other pairs by nexin links and anchored centrally by radial spokes. Dynein arms, the ATPase motor unit of the cilium, are connected to the A microtubule and effect the motion of the cilium, resulting in the ciliary beat. The basal body anchors the cilium into the apical epithelium of the cell; however, much less is known about this part of the axoneme, which has no central pair, but 9 triplet microtubular sets peripherally. Abnormalities of the basal body relating to PCD have not yet been determined, but within the typical phenotype a significant minority of patients has no known ultrastructural anomaly [11].

Several ultrastructural defects have been identified in PCD, the most common being those affecting the dynein arms, but abnormalities can occur in almost any part of the axonemal structure. The type and frequency of the ultrastructural defects are listed in table 1 [11–13], and the electron micrographs in figure 4 demonstrate these findings.

Table 1. Ultrastructural defects in PCD listed in order of reported frequency

Ultrastructural defects at electron microscopy	Reported frequencies %
Outer dynein arm defect	30–43
Inner dynein arm defect	11–30
Inner and outer dynein arm defect	9–36
Normal ultrastructure	25
Radial spoke defect	7
Transposition defect	14
Ciliary aplasia	6
Central pair defect	9
Disorders of ciliary disorientation	not reported
Nexin link defect	not reported

Disruption of the mucociliary escalator leads to persistent infection in both upper and lower respiratory tracts resulting in the classical symptoms of chronic productive cough, persistent rhinitis and nasal congestion, chronic serous otitis media and hearing impairment. Older children and adults may suffer recurrent sinusitis.

The average age of diagnosis at 4 years belies the fact that the majority of cases will have symptoms or signs present from the time of birth. More than 50% of patients will have situs anomalies (approx. 50% situs inversus totalis; 6% heterotaxy; fig. 5), 75% suffer neonatal respiratory distress at term and nearly all patients have experienced troublesome rhinitis from birth. As recurrent respiratory infections are so prevalent in the normal population, distinguishing the clues that might warrant specialist investigation can be a challenge. Early diagnosis is likely to have significant benefit in terms of both short-term symptom control and prevention of lung disease progression, thereby reducing long-term morbidity [13].

Chronic Bacterial Bronchitis
Over the last decade, there has been an increase in reports of persistent bacterial infection in the lower airways by respiratory paediatricians. This is possibly due to a reduction in antibiotics prescribed for presumed viral infections [14], but also the increasing use of fibre-optic bronchoscopy for investigating children with chronic wet cough. Within this group, persistent bacterial infection may be the commonest cause identified, as well as being a significant co-morbidity factor in patients with difficult asthma.

The importance of chronic bacterial infection of the lower airways in both CF and non-CF bronchiectasis is well established, and our management approach is mainly focused on this issue. More controversial is the debate around when bacterial infection of the lower airways in patients without significant underlying airway disease becomes chronic and potentially pathological. The 'vicious cycle' hypothesis [15] proposes that chronic infection may exist for a prolonged period and lead to the development of bronchiectasis. This hypothesis is that infection results in impaired mucociliary transport, allowing infection to become chronic and persistent with the formation of biofilms, resulting in inflammation and mucosal damage with more damage to the ciliated epithelium further impairing the clearance of bacteria.

The organisms most commonly isolated from children with chronic wet cough without an underlying diagnosis are non-typable *H. influenzae*, *Streptococcus pneumoniae* and *Moraxella catarrhalis*. They may be cultured from both the lower and upper airways, including the sinuses and middle ear, where they are ideally suited to take advantage of reduced MCC mechanisms. It is likely, therefore, that chronic bacterial bronchitis is the mildest end of a spectrum that eventually may lead to end-stage bronchiectasis. This process can be reversed if treated early. It is important to identify and investigate the child with chronic wet cough to prevent the development of bronchiectasis, which may not be easy. The clinical picture is highly variable: at one end of the spectrum, cough may be intermittent and not too troublesome, whilst at the other, the child may have a persistent wet cough and be productive of copious amounts of sputum. Systemic symptoms may be non-existent, mild or severe, but often have little correlation with disease severity.

Taking a 'cough history' is the best initial step to determine which children to investigate further. Those with persistent bacterial bronchitis or more advanced chronic suppurative lung disease typically describe a wet cough although expectoration is rare in children. The presence of a wet cough correlates with intraluminal secretions seen at bronchoscopy. Symptoms are often worst in the morning and patients may suffer prolonged bouts of severe coughing with exertion. It is important to distinguish whether it is the cough that leaves the child feeling breathless or true chest tightness and wheeze. The rattle associated with a wet cough may also be described as wheeze by parents, and further questioning may be necessary to elucidate the exact nature and cause of airway noises. Finally it is important to establish whether the patient has the symptom-free periods more characteristic of episodic viral infections.

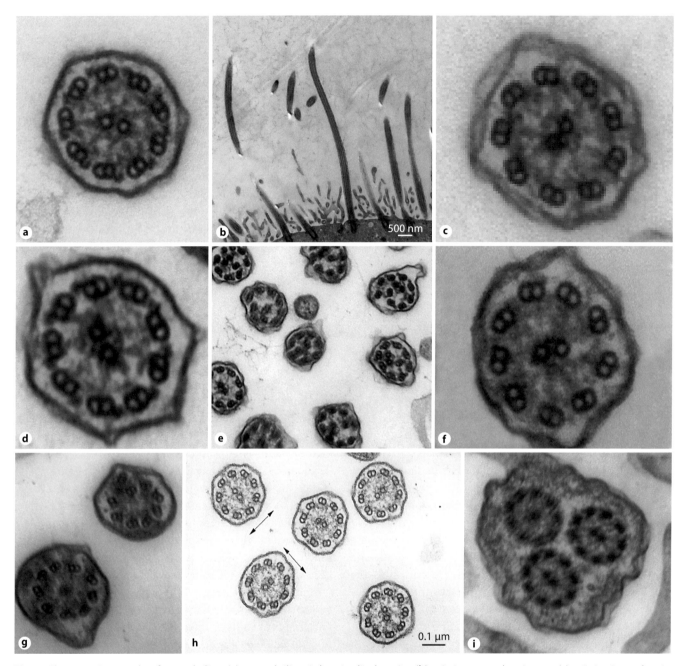

Fig. 4. Electron micrographs of normal cilium (**a**), normal cilium in longitudinal section (**b**), missing outer dynein arms (**c**), missing inner dynein arms (**d**), inner arm and radial spoke defect (**e**), absence of both arms (**f**), transposition defect (**g**), ciliary disorientation (double arrows; **h**) and compound cilium (**i**).

Aspiration Syndromes

Aspiration into the lung is a significant cause of chronic suppurative airway disease. In normal subjects, sophisticated protective mechanisms exist which either prevent aspiration completely or respond to small amounts of aspiration which may occur. These include anatomical features (a close-fitting epiglottis and adduction of the true and false vocal cords), physiological responses to foreign material in the airway (cough, bronchospasm and occasionally apnoea) and innate immunological mechanisms (the mucociliary escalator and pulmonary macrophages).

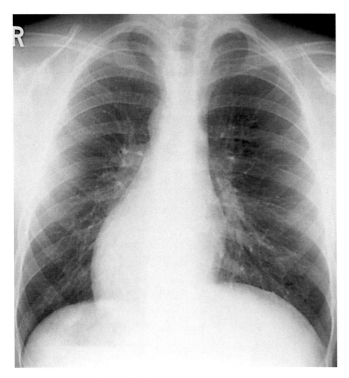

Fig. 5. Chest radiograph from a patient with PCD showing situs inversus.

Despite these mechanisms, pathological aspiration does occur in a minority of patients. Anatomical or mechanical problems should be sought and excluded throughout the upper gastrointestinal tract: from the swallow mechanism, through the oesophagus and into the stomach. Problems may coexist but for clarity it is easiest to consider the causes using mechanistic categories: abnormal swallow, direct tracheo-oesophageal communication and gastro-oesophageal reflux. Table 2 lists possible causes in these categories.

Abnormal Swallow
The act of swallowing is a complex mechanism that involves 3 stages: the oral, the pharyngeal and the oesophageal, using both skeletal muscle (tongue) and smooth muscles of the pharynx and oesophagus. The autonomic nervous system coordinates this process in the pharyngeal and oesophageal phases. As can be seen in table 2, many congenital and acquired causes for an abnormal swallow exist, but it may occur in patients with no detectable underlying cause. Intercurrent illness resulting in tachypnoea or weakness may influence coordination of breathing and swallowing in small infants [16].

Oesophageal Defects
Tracheo-oesophageal fistula is most commonly a congenital defect but, more rarely, may occur secondary to trauma such as tracheostomy [17] or ingestion of caustic materials. Tracheo-oesophageal fistula may be associated with other local anatomical defects as in oesophageal atresia or with a more global set of congenital malformation. The communication allows free flow of swallowed substances and refluxed gastric contents from below into the respiratory tract, and may result in chronic and severe lung disease.

Gastro-Oesophageal Reflux
Gastro-oesophageal reflux is possibly universal in infants and remains very common in older children. However, the relationship between gastro-oesophageal reflux and lung disease is poorly understood, and respiratory illness is not always a consequence even in severe cases [18]. Patients with chronic respiratory disease have an increased risk of gastro-oesophageal reflux, due to cough-associated increases in abdominopleural pressure gradients and increased work of breathing. Factors such as the pH [19], volume, content [20] and presence of bacteria in the aspirated material, the frequency of events and the presence of underlying airway pathology influence the severity of the effects on the lungs. These effects include: spasm of vocal cords and/or lower airways, airway inflammation and airway hyperreactivity, infection such as tracheitis, pneumonia and lung abscesses and, ultimately, bronchiectasis. Laryngospasm may result in apnoea in younger children and is an important aspect of the diagnostic workup in infants presenting with this symptom [21].

Chronic Bacterial Infection: Common Themes

Much is now understood about the steps involved in the chronic, biofilm mode of bacterial growth common to these conditions. The first step in establishing infection is for the organism to acquire a niche, most commonly adhering to surface mucus or to cell surfaces. In CF and PCD, impaired MCC is thought to facilitate this process, although mechanisms in the other conditions are less well understood. In addition, in CF, several other hypotheses have been proposed, including the increased availability of cell surface receptors for *S. aureus* and *P. aeruginosa* [22], impaired ingestion of bacteria by epithelial cells [23], low levels of nasal and exhaled nitric oxide and low concentrations of the host defence molecule glutathione (fig. 6). *P. aeruginosa*, one of the commonest organisms chronically infecting these diseased airways, has developed a huge armamentarium of strategies by which it evades host

Table 2. Causes of aspiration

Aspiration from the top	Aspiration via oesophagus	Aspiration from below
Abnormal swallow	*Breech of oesophageal integrity*	*Gastro-oesophageal reflux*
Congenital	Congenital	Primary
Anatomical	H-type TOF	Idiopathic
Cleft palate	Oesophageal atresia with TOF	Hiatus hernia
Laryngeal cleft	VACTERL association	
Micrognathia	Broncho-oesophageal fistula	Secondary
Macroglossia		Respiratory disease
Cysts/tumours		Medication (xanthines, caffeine)
Vascular rings/slings		Obesity
Choanal atresia		Reduced lower oesophageal sphincter pressure/hypotonia
Neuromuscular/autonomic		
Cerebral palsy		*Oesophageal dysmotility*
Myasthenia gravis and other myopathies		Primary
Hypotonia of any cause		Achalasia
Spinal muscular atrophy		Diffuse oesophageal spasm
Familial dysautonomia		
Acquired	Acquired	Secondary
Anatomical	Traumatic TOF	Cerebral palsy
Tracheostomy	After tracheostomy	Neuromuscular disorders
After intubation	Ingestion of caustics	Hirschsprung disease
Respiratory distress/cough	Abrasive foodstuffs	Post-TOF repair
Acute bronchiolitis	Acquired broncho-oesophageal fistula	
Bronchopulmonary dysplasia	Crohn disease	
Asthma		
CF/non-CF bronchiectasis		
Accidental		
Foreign-body aspiration		

TOF = Tracheo-oesophageal fistula; VACTERL = vertebral anomalies, anal atresia, cardiovascular anomalies, tracheo-oesophageal fistula, oesophageal atresia, renal anomalies, limb anomalies.

defences and ensures its survival. These include exoproducts such as elastase and alkaline protease (which cleave immunoglobulins, complement components and cytokines), exotoxin A (which inhibits phagocytosis and suppresses the cell-mediated immune response) and pyocyanin (which breaks down intercellular tight junctions, slows ciliary beat frequency and thereby may impair MCC). This organism and many of the other bacteria associated with chronic respiratory tract infections either possess or develop antibiotic resistance strategies related to poorly permeable outer membranes, efficient multidrug efflux pumps and β-lactamases.

In the CF airway at least, hypoxic conditions have been described within mucus plugs [24], which attract motile organisms capable of anaerobic survival, such as *P. aeruginosa*. This is now understood to be one of the triggers causing bacteria to switch from their usual, 'planktonic' mode of growth to a chronic, biofilm-based system. Bacteria regulate gene expression in response to population density through a

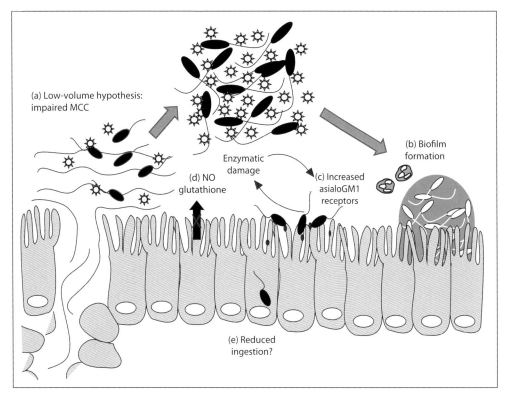

Fig. 6. Hypothesized mechanisms of bacterial infection in the CF airway: (a) bacteria become trapped in viscous mucus, which is not cleared by the usual mucociliary clearance mechanisms; freely diffusible signalling molecules (symbolized as yellow stars) allow a mechanism of 'quorum sensing' and once critical concentrations are reached, bacteria form into biofilms (b), protected from host defence cells and antibiotic agents by a thick matrix. Alternative suggestions for early acquisition include: (c) the presence of increased bacterial receptors on the CF epithelial cell surface, which can be further increased by neuraminidase-mediated cleavage of sialic acid from cell surface glycolipids, (d) decreased secretion of antibacterial agents such as nitric oxide (NO) and glutathione, and (e) the possibility that ingestion of bacteria by epithelial cells is reduced in the presence of defective CFTR.

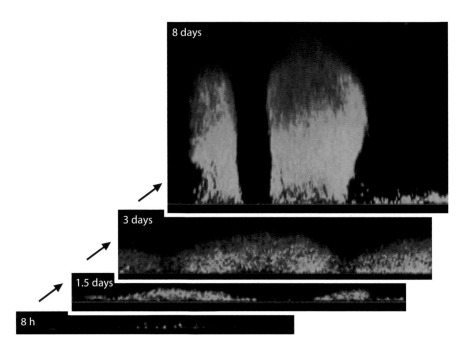

Fig. 7. The evolution of a biofilm in culture over time. Adapted with permission from Fuqua and Greenberg [25].

mechanism termed 'quorum sensing'. Cell-to-cell communication via auto-inducers allows bacteria to coordinate gene expression and therefore the behaviour of the entire colony. This not only occurs within a single bacterial species, but may also serve to communicate between species [25]. This process allows bacteria to use a diverse array of physiological activities, including symbiosis, virulence, biofilm formation and conjugation [26]. Organisms growing within a biofilm (fig. 6, 7) are protected by a thick matrix from host defences and are, unsurprisingly, less susceptible than their planktonic counterparts to antibiotic agents. Several new therapeutic approaches based on our increased understanding of this mechanism are currently being explored; there is some evidence that the macrolide group of antibiotics, associated with significant clinical improvement in diffuse panbronchiolitis and more recently studied in CF, may possess antibiofilm properties.

Bronchoscopy in Chronic Suppurative Lung Disease

In this section, we will consider the role of bronchoscopy in these diseases as a group, highlighting any areas which may be of specific relevance to one disease.

Indications for and Benefits of Bronchoscopy

Microbiological Diagnosis
Across all the conditions described here, making an accurate microbiological diagnosis is probably the commonest reason for bronchoscopy. Many patients fail to expectorate sputum, most particularly children and adults with mild disease. Alternative techniques directed at lower airway secretions include cough swabs, cough plates and sputum induction. The sensitivity and specificity of these techniques have mostly been addressed in patients with CF, and experience differs between centres. Bronchoscopy with bronchoalveolar lavage (BAL) is considered the 'gold standard' for obtaining reliable lower airway cultures.

There are, however, technical considerations. At least in CF, different quantities of bacteria (and even different organisms) have been cultured from geographically distinct lung areas [27]. This is also possible in other suppurative airway diseases, so samples should most usefully be obtained from more than one site. Avoidance of contamination of the bronchoscope by the upper airway is important, as is meticulous cleaning of equipment between patients; reports exist in the literature of 'pseudo-epidemics' and even genuine cross-infection from poorly cleaned bronchoscopes.

When should BAL be considered for microbiological diagnosis?
- Around the time of diagnosis of CF; at our centre, we have a programme of early BAL after diagnosis; we have previously reported high rates of otherwise undetected bacterial infection [28] and are observing similar rates of positive culture in infants diagnosed on newborn screening
- Non-expectorating children with suboptimal clinical status
- Children failing to respond to conventional antimicrobial agents
- Opportunistically, when children with these disease groups are undergoing general anaesthesia for another procedure

Removal of Mucus Plugs
Localized areas of collapse can occur secondary to mucus plugging; the thick, viscous secretions produced by CF patients make them a group particularly at risk of this complication. Standard treatment including chest physiotherapy and mucolytics (recombinant human DNAse, hypertonic saline) may succeed, but if not, the blood supply will be irreversibly shunted away from the area of collapsed, non-ventilated lung parenchyma, and long-term damage will ensue [chapter 14, this vol., pp. 149–155]. Bronchoscopic attempts at removing plugs are therefore worthwhile, although this may be technically challenging (fig. 8); in unsuccessful cases, there may be a place for rigid bronchoscopy [chapter 8, this vol., pp. 83–94]. There have been some reports of success with the targeted instillation of the mucolytic agent recombinant human DNAse [29, 30].

Assessment of Disease Severity
Although rarely the sole indication for a bronchoscopy in these disease groups, macroscopic examination of the airways can be a useful guide for both physician and patient. If the airway disease is much worse than expected, with large amounts of thick sticky secretions/mucus (fig. 9; online suppl. videos 1 and 2), plugging, hyperaemia and friability of the airways, the demonstration of this may lead to increased adherence to treatment by the child and family, and intensification of therapy by the medical team.

Assessment of Posttransplantation Status
Lung transplantation in these diseases is mainly limited to CF, and even in this group, it is uncommon in children. Full details are outside the scope of this chapter, but this is likely

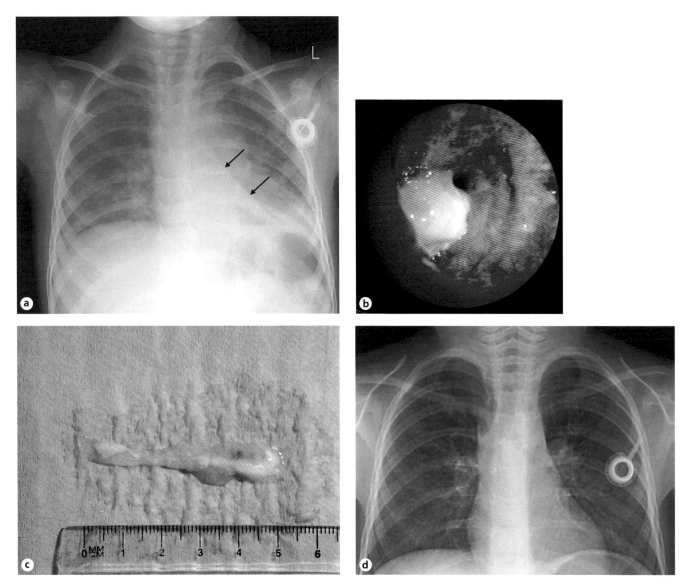

Fig. 8. a Chest radiograph showing left lower lobe collapse (arrows) in a patient with CF; a Portacath® is also visible on the left anterior chest wall. **b** Bronchoscopic findings in the same patient showing mucosal inflammation and a large mucopurulent plug in the left main bronchus. **c** The mucus plug has been removed from the left main bronchus of the same patient. **d** Resolution of the left lower lobe collapse after bronchoscopic plug removal.

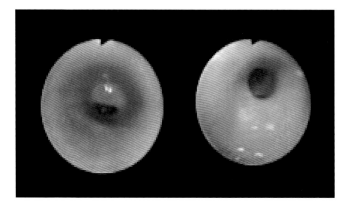

Fig. 9. Typical bronchoscopic findings in a patient with PCD with pooling of secretions; in general, these are easier to aspirate than the typically thick, viscous secretions found in the CF airway.

to be the only indication for transbronchial biopsy, within which rejection will be apparent. The technique is discussed in detail in chapter 19 [this vol., pp. 200–204].

The Search for Associated Conditions

As discussed above, any form of respiratory disease increases the likelihood of gastro-oesophageal reflux, which in some cases may lead to aspiration. The presence of large numbers of lipid-laden macrophages in BAL fluid (BALF) may be supportive, although it is important to remember that these are not specific; as bacterial membranes are composed of fat, these can also be seen in the presence of significant bacterial infection; however, the complete absence of such cells makes significant aspiration unlikely [chapter 3, this vol., pp. 30–41]. Areas of airway malacia or compression can be identified using both rigid and flexible bronchoscopic techniques [chapter 12, this vol., pp. 130–140]. The rigid bronchoscope offers the advantage of being able to ventilate throughout the procedure and maintain the airway safely, but it may obscure dynamic changes by splinting of the malacic airway and result in a false-negative examination. The flexible bronchoscope, whilst not allowing ventilation, affords a dynamic view of the large conducting airways throughout the respiratory cycle. When utilizing a flexible bronchoscope alone for this investigation, the smallest instrument possible should be employed to avoid airway trauma and potential oedema which may compromise the already reduced airway calibre. If significant airway obstruction is suspected or present prior to the procedure, it is prudent to have a rigid bronchoscopist present to assist with the procedure.

What Have We Learned about Disease Mechanisms from Bronchoscopic Samples and Techniques?

The Airway Lumen

BALF studies have largely focused on CF, data from which have resulted in our recognizing several unusual features of the neutrophilic inflammatory response in this disease: it occurs very early in life; for a given trigger, it appears exaggerated; it is prolonged, and it is incompletely effective, failing to eradicate the organisms which may have triggered it. Several studies have reported raised levels of neutrophils and the major neutrophil chemoattractant interleukin 8 in CF BALF. Few studies have included patients with other suppurative airway diseases, but we have found similar levels of these mediators in PCD, suggesting that this may not be disease specific. One vexing issue in CF is whether inflammation occurs only in response to a trigger (most likely infective) or can be a primary abnormality. Results from cell culture [31] and xenograft [32] experiments have lent some support to the latter. However, a series of excellent BAL-based studies would strongly support the former, reporting repeatedly that levels of inflammatory mediators and cells are normal in the non-infected CF airway (fig. 10) [33, 34]. We have reported that this neutrophilic inflammation correlated with raised levels of matrix degradation products such as glycosaminoglycans in CF BALF, perhaps reflecting tissue breakdown and therefore potentially representing a step in the process towards airway remodelling [35]; levels also correlated with forced expiratory volume in 1 s. However, this was not disease specific and was also seen in samples from patients with PCD. Muhlebach et al. [36] studied the degree of the inflammatory response, adjusted for the colony count of infecting bacteria, in CF children compared with non-CF children with acute bacterial infections. They discovered a 10-fold increase in both BAL neutrophil count and interleukin 8 level in CF samples, suggesting an abnormally exaggerated response (fig. 11). However, this has not been compared with children with chronic disorders such as PCD and other causes of non-CF bronchiectasis. Cleavage of CXCR1, a molecule required for the internalization of pathogens, from the surface of BAL neutrophils in the presence of high levels of neutrophil elastase, is thought to account for the relative inefficiency of these cells in the CF airway lumen [37]. A significant relative deficiency of lipoxins, molecules which terminate the inflammatory response, was discovered in BALF from CF patients, which may explain the prolonged nature of the inflammatory response in this disease [38]. Intriguingly, recent studies on both BALF and sputum are beginning to reveal the fact that we significantly underestimate the bacterial burden in the diseased airway using standard, culture-based techniques. Anaerobic culture [39] and molecular tools being used on BAL and sputum have unexpectedly detected multiple bacterial species within airway samples [40, 41]. Further studies of these and other mechanisms in non-CF bronchiectasis may begin to shed some light on the pathogenic mechanisms underlying these conditions and potentially could highlight therapeutic targets for these orphan diseases.

The Airway Wall

Early reports in the CF literature focused on end-stage airway samples, usually obtained from explanted or post-mortem lung tissue. We have recently reported on the safety [42], the utility [43] and the time required to perform endobronchial

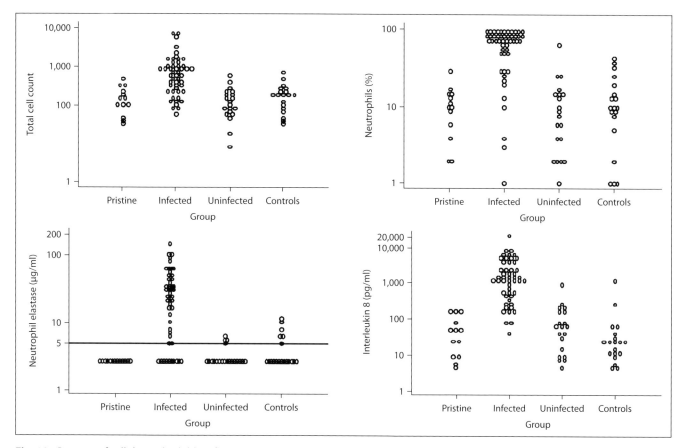

Fig. 10. Patterns of cellular and soluble inflammatory markers in the BALF of infants with a diagnosis of CF on newborn screening. The 'pristine' group (<6 months of age, never infected or symptomatic, no antibiotic treatment and negative culture on BALF) were not different from the group of non-CF controls. The highest levels of inflammation were seen in the group with infection at the time of bronchoscopy. With permission from Armstrong et al. [33].

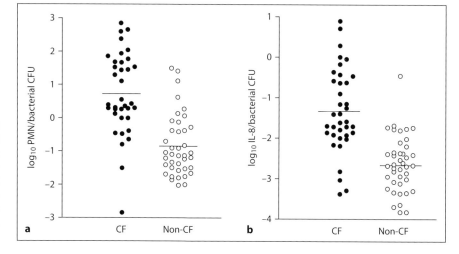

Fig. 11. Children with CF had significantly (p < 0.01) greater numbers of neutrophils (PMN; **a**) and levels of interleukin 8 (IL-8; **b**), when corrected for the number of bacteria cultured per millilitre of BALF, than did infected children without CF. With permission from Muhlebach et al. [36]. Reprinted with permission of the American Thoracic Society. Copyright© American Thoracic Society.

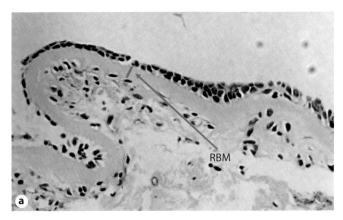

Fig. 12. a Haematoxylin-eosin stain of an endobronchial biopsy showing the RBM, which in this sample is thickened. **b** RBM thickness was increased in CF compared with non-CF patients, although not to the levels reported in asthma (up to 14 μm). CRS = Non-specific chronic respiratory symptoms. **c** RBM thickness did not correlate with any inflammatory markers but was positively related to BALF levels of the profibrotic growth factor transforming growth factor β₁ (TGF-β₁). With permission from Hilliard et al. [35]).

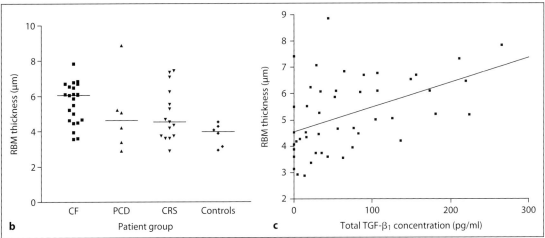

biopsy [44] as part of a clinically indicated bronchoscopy. Data from our studies and those of other groups are helping to increase our understanding of changes in the airway wall and appreciate that these may not reflect those in the lumen. The following features of remodelling and inflammation have been described:

Obstruction of Submucosal Glands, Goblet and Mucus Cell Hyperplasia/Hypertrophy

This was one of the first features described in association with CF and was seen both in advanced disease and in some postmortem specimens from children several decades ago [45]. The composition of CF mucus is abnormal; there is reduced hydration and bicarbonate level, and it is oversulphated. The resultant increased viscosity leads to obstruction of the narrow submucosal gland ducts. The inflammatory response in chronic bronchitis results in bronchial gland hyperplasia and goblet cell metaplasia leading to mucus hypersecretion and persistent cough. Increased staining of mucus and

goblet cells has been described in CF, although whether this is hypertrophy, hyperplasia or both, remains uncertain.

Thickening of the Reticular Basement Membrane

The reticular basement membrane (RBM) lies just below the epithelial layer separating it from the submucosa. In normal healthy people it is very thin, around 3 μm in depth. Increased RBM thickness was first reported in asthma, although interestingly it appears not to be related directly to the characteristic inflammation seen in this condition [46; chapter 13, this vol., pp. 142–148]. Based on observations that lung function was already abnormal in newly diagnosed CF infants [47], we examined biopsies from children with a variety of lung diseases for RBM thickening. We found increased thickness of RBM in children with CF, although not to the levels reported in asthmatics [35] (fig. 12). Measurements correlated positively with BAL levels of the profibrotic, pro-inflammatory cytokine transforming growth factor β₁, although not with other markers of luminal inflammation,

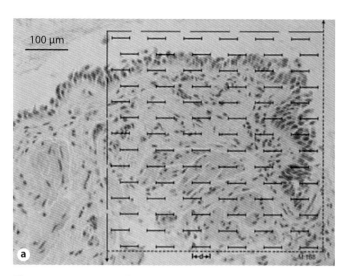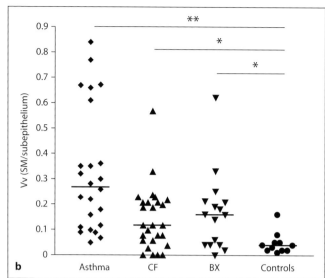

Fig. 13. a Airway smooth muscle can be reliably quantified using stereological analysis and point counting. **b** With this technique, our group reported increased amounts of smooth muscle (SM; both number and size of cells) in children with asthma, CF and non-CF bronchiectasis (BX); in the asthmatic group, where data on bronchodilator responsiveness were available, there was a significant correlation between these two measures. Vv (SM/subepithelium) = Volume fraction of ASM indexed to volume of airway subepithelial tissue. Horizontal bars represent medians. * $p < 0.01$; ** $p < 0.001$. With permission from Regamey et al. [49]. Reprinted with permission of the American Thoracic Society. Copyright© American Thoracic Society.

suggesting two separate mechanisms of remodelling: one associated with and another independent of inflammation. A small group of patients with PCD appeared to have less RBM thickening, although we were underpowered to reach firm conclusions. The significance of RBM thickness has not been established for any disease. Whilst initially considered to be a marker of severity, an alternative proposal is that the thickened RBM in asthma protects the airway from excessive constriction. Further studies are needed in this area, which remains incompletely understood.

Increased Smooth Muscle Mass

Patients with asthma have an increased amount of smooth muscle in their airway wall, which has been shown by some to correlate with severity. Woodruff et al. [48] reported increased smooth muscle in the airway wall of a small group of adults with CF. We have recently examined this feature in the biopsies of children with both CF and non-CF bronchiectasis (including PCD) and compared them to children with asthma and with no lower airway disease (fig. 13) [49]. The greatest amount of muscle was seen in the asthmatic group, where it was found to relate to bronchodilator responsiveness. However, both the CF and non-CF bronchiectasis groups also had significantly more muscle than

the healthy controls, reflecting an increase in both myocyte number and size. There was no clear relationship with lung function or any parameter of airway inflammation in these groups, although there were no data available on bronchial responsiveness; further work is planned in this area.

Submucosal Inflammatory Infiltrate

Airway inflammation is most commonly assessed in sputum or BALF, both of which reflect the milieu of the airway lumen. Recently, we have questioned whether findings in this compartment reflect those in the airway wall itself; the latter is the site of the destructive processes of tissue breakdown leading to bronchiectasis, and mechanisms here may be of more direct pathophysiological relevance. Preliminary data from CF suggest that the airway wall inflammatory infiltrate is composed of lymphocytes, in contrast to the typical neutrophil-dominated inflammation in the lumen. Further work is ongoing both to characterize these lymphocytes and to explore these findings in other non-CF bronchiectatic diseases, including PCD.

Local Airway Physiology

In addition to the data provided by biopsy studies, much has been gained from studying physiological processes occurring in the airway wall. Electrophysiological studies measuring potential differences have confirmed the basic ion transport defect in the lower airways of patients with CF and have demonstrated a degree of improvement following *CFTR* gene therapy [50, 51]. Direct pH measurements have also shown the CF airway to be more acidic than the healthy airway [52], which could have host defence implications. However, studies on exhaled breath condensate suggest that this may reflect chronic inflammation as opposed to a specific, CFTR-related acid-base disturbance [53].

Ex vivo Culture Techniques

Investigators have used lower airway brush biopsy samples to culture epithelial monolayers; there are significant technical challenges to such attempts although success has been reported by some groups. In many cases, cells were obtained by a non-bronchoscopic technique in an endotracheally intubated child [54, 55], although these techniques are equally suited for use down a bronchoscope, which would have the added benefit of allowing targeted sampling under direct vision.

Future Directions and Outstanding Questions

We have learned much from research in this area of childhood airway diseases, but there is still much to understand; we strongly encourage the opportunistic approach to further our knowledge of these diseases. Below we highlight some areas of particular interest, some of which are being studied by other groups worldwide, others of which appear, to date, relatively neglected:

1 *Is there any benefit to regular bronchoscopy and BAL in patients with chronic suppurative lung diseases?* A large Australasian study will seek to address this issue on young children with CF (ACTRN 012605000665639; http://www.anzctr.org.au/). Although the results may not be directly transferable to those with other chronic, suppurative airway diseases, the results may encourage other groups to conduct similar trials targeting these conditions.

2 *Why does CF have a much worse prognosis than PCD?* Most investigators support the low-volume hypothesis which places impaired MCC at the centre of CF pathophysiology. However, MCC is markedly impaired in PCD, a disease with a much better prognosis. Children acquire bacterial infection, on average, at a later age and lung function declines less rapidly; it is rarely severe enough to be life-threatening. There is

some suggestion that this prognostic gap may reflect preserved cough clearance in PCD, although other possibilities, including the potentially detrimental inflammatory response to infection, may play important roles. Our group has a strong interest in this area and is attempting to define some factors which may explain these differences; such understanding has the potential to highlight new therapeutic targets for these diseases.

3 *Which inflammatory mechanisms are occurring in the submucosa, and are they driving luminal inflammation?* We now know that the two compartments of the lumen and the airway wall appear to reflect different types of inflammation. Studies and interventional trials have largely focused on BAL or sputum assays, whereas the irreversible changes of bronchiectasis occur in the airway wall itself. Are the two compartments linked? Do cells in the submucosa direct the luminal inflammatory responses or vice versa? In the absence, to date, of a good animal model of CF lung disease, these sorts of questions are ideally suited to bronchoscopic sampling. The limitations of repeated bronchoscopy can be overcome in some part by including patients at every stage of disease, from asymptomatic newborns to older children and adults with established bronchiectasis.

4 *Can we more accurately identify lower airway pathogens and determine their relevance?* Clinical microbiological techniques rely on culture and identification of organisms. The use of molecular tools in recent years has allowed a greater insight into the presence of many more organisms than we have previously appreciated. These may not be best detected by conventional culture (e.g. strict anaerobes) or may grow so slowly that they are masked by more rapidly growing and higher-density pathogens. However, in addition to detecting these, we need to establish their clinical relevance; certain studies have reported high levels of such organisms also in the apparently healthy lower respiratory tract.

In summary, therefore, bronchoscopy in children with CF and other forms of chronic suppurative airway disease has many clinical applications. It is increasing in popularity and acceptability, and it is likely that this has, in part, led to the recognition of a relatively new condition, chronic bacterial bronchitis. Bronchoscopic research in children has to be opportunistic, but we have learned much from the groups who have taken such opportunities and there is very much hope that this will be a field that will continue to grow and bear fruit over future years.

References

1 Matsui H, Grubb BR, Tarran R, Randell SH, Gatzy JT, Davis CW, Boucher RC: Evidence for periciliary liquid layer depletion, not abnormal ion composition, in the pathogenesis of cystic fibrosis airways disease. Cell 1998;95:1005–1015.

2 Boucher RC: Cystic fibrosis: a disease of vulnerability to airway surface dehydration. Trends Mol Med 2007;13:231–240.

3 Davies JC, Alton EW, Bush A: Cystic fibrosis. BMJ 2007;335:1255–1259.

4 Davies JC, Bilton D: Bugs, biofilms, and resistance in cystic fibrosis. Respir Care 2009;54:628–640.

5 Chang AB, Masel JP, Boyce NC, Wheaton G, Torzillo PJ: Non-CF bronchiectasis: clinical and HRCT evaluation. Pediatr Pulmonol 2003;35:477–483.

6 Eastham KM, Fall AJ, Mitchell L, Spencer, DA: The need to redefine non-cystic fibrosis bronchiectasis in childhood. Thorax 2004;59:324–327.

7 Chang AB, Redding GJ, Everard ML: Chronic wet cough: protracted bronchitis, chronic suppurative lung disease and bronchiectasis. Pediatr Pulmonol 2008;43:519–531.

8 Gaillard EA, Carty H, Heaf D, Smyth RL: Reversible bronchial dilatation in children: comparison of serial high-resolution computer tomography scans of the lungs. Eur J Radiol 2003;47:215–220.

9 Pazour GJ, Agrin N, Leszyk J, Witman GB: Proteomic analysis of a eukaryotic cilium. J Cell Biol 2005;170:103–113.

10 Alberts B, Johnson A, Lewis J, Raff M, Roberts K, Walter P (eds): Molecular Biology of the Cell. London, Garland Science/Taylor & Francis, 2008.

11 Jorissen M, Willems T, De Boeck K: Diagnostic evaluation of mucociliary transport: from symptoms to coordinated ciliary activity after ciliogenesis in culture. Am J Rhinol 2000;14:345–352.

12 Chilvers MA, Rutman A, O'Callaghan C: Ciliary beat pattern is associated with specific ultrastructural defects in primary ciliary dyskinesia. J Allergy Clin Immunol 2003;112:518–524.

13 Noone PG, Leigh MW, Sannuti A, Minnix SL, Carson JL, Hazucha M, Zariwala MA, Knowles MR: Primary ciliary dyskinesia: diagnostic and phenotypic features. Am J Respir Crit Care Med 2004;169:459–467.

14 Arnold SR, Bush AJ: Decline in inappropriate antibiotic use over a decade by pediatricians in a Tennessee community. Ambul Pediatr 2006;6:225–229.

15 Cole P: The damaging role of bacteria in chronic lung infection. J Antimicrob Chemother 1997;40(suppl A):5–10.

16 Hernandez E, Khoshoo V, Thoppil D, Edell D, Ross G: Aspiration: a factor in rapidly deteriorating bronchiolitis in previously healthy infants? Pediatr Pulmonol 2002;33:30–31.

17 Birman C, Beckenham E: Acquired tracheoesophageal fistula in the pediatric population. Int J Pediatr Otorhinolaryngol 1998;44:109–113.

18 Orenstein SR, Orenstein DM: Gastroesophageal reflux and respiratory disease in children. J Pediatr 1988;112:847–858.

19 Marik PE: Aspiration pneumonitis and aspiration pneumonia. N Engl J Med 2001;344:665–671.

20 Wolach B, Raz A, Weinberg J, Mikulski Y, Ben AJ, Sadan N: Aspirated foreign bodies in the respiratory tract of children: eleven years experience with 127 patients. Int J Pediatr Otorhinolaryngol 1994;30:1–10.

21 Orenstein SR: An overview of reflux-associated disorders in infants: apnea, laryngospasm, and aspiration. Am J Med 2001;111(suppl 8A):S60–S63.

22 Saiman L, Prince A: *Pseudomonas aeruginosa* pili bind to asialoGM1 which is increased on the surface of cystic fibrosis epithelial cells. J Clin Invest 1993;92:1875–1880.

23 Pier GB, Grout M, Zaidi TS, Olsen JC, Johnson LG, Yankaskas JR, Goldberg JB: Role of mutant CFTR in hypersusceptibility of cystic fibrosis patients to lung infections. Science 1996;271:64–67.

24 Worlitzsch D, Tarran R, Ulrich M, Schwab U, Cekici A, Meyer KC, Birrer P, Bellon G, Berger J, Weiss T, Botzenhart K, Yankaskas JR, Randell S, Boucher RC, Doring G: Effects of reduced mucus oxygen concentration in airway *Pseudomonas* infections of cystic fibrosis patients. J Clin Invest 2002;109:317–325.

25 Fuqua C, Greenberg EP: Listening in on bacteria: acyl-homoserine lactone signalling. Nat Rev Mol Cell Biol 2002;3:685–695.

26 Miller MB, Bassler BL: Quorum sensing in bacteria. Annu Rev Microbiol 2001;55:165–199.

27 Gutierrez JP, Grimwood K, Armstrong DS, Carlin JB, Carzino R, Olinsky A, Robertson CF, Phelan PD: Interlobar differences in bronchoalveolar lavage fluid from children with cystic fibrosis. Eur Respir J 2001;17:281–286.

28 Hilliard TN, Sukhani S, Francis J, Madden N, Rosenthal M, Balfour-Lynn I, Bush A, Davies JC: Bronchoscopy following diagnosis with cystic fibrosis. Arch Dis Child 2007;92:898–899.

29 Kamin W, Klar-Hlawatsch B, Truebel H: Easy removal of a large mucus plug with a flexible paediatric bronchoscope after administration of rhDNAse (Pulmozyme). Klin Paediatr 2006;218:88–91.

30 Slattery DM, Waltz DA, Denham B, O'Mahony M, Greally P: Bronchoscopically administered recombinant human DNAse for lobar atelectasis in cystic fibrosis. Pediatr Pulmonol 2001;31:383–388.

31 Bonfield TL, Konstan MW, Berger M: Altered respiratory epithelial cell cytokine production in cystic fibrosis. J Allergy Clin Immunol 1999;104:72–78.

32 Tirouvanziam R, de Bentzmann S, Hubeau C, Hinnrasky J, Jacquot J, Peault B, Puchelle E: Inflammation and infection in naive human cystic fibrosis airway grafts. Am J Respir Cell Mol Biol 2000;23:121–127.

33 Armstrong DS, Hook SM, Jamsen KM, Nixon GM, Carzino R, Carlin JB, Robertson CF, Grimwood K: Lower airway inflammation in infants with cystic fibrosis detected by newborn screening. Pediatr Pulmonol 2005;40:500–510.

34 Armstrong DS, Grimwood K, Carlin JB, Carzino R, Gutierrez JP, Hull J, Olinsky A, Phelan EM, Robertson CF, Phelan PD: Lower airway inflammation in infants and young children with cystic fibrosis. Am J Respir Crit Care Med 1997;156:1197–1204.

35 Hilliard TN, Regamey N, Shute JK, Nicholson AG, Alton EW, Bush A, Davies JC: Airway remodelling in children with cystic fibrosis. Thorax 2007;62:1074–1080.

36 Muhlebach MS, Stewart PW, Leigh MW, Noah TL: Quantitation of inflammatory responses to bacteria in young cystic fibrosis and control patients. Am J Respir Crit Care Med 1999;160:186–191.

37 Hartl D, Latzin P, Hordijk P, Marcos V, Rudolph C, Woischnik M, Krauss-Etschmann S, Koller, B, Reinhardt D, Roscher AA, Roos D, Griese M: Cleavage of CXCR1 on neutrophils disables bacterial killing in cystic fibrosis lung disease. Nat Med 2007;13:1423–1430.

38 Karp CL, Flick LM, Park KW, Softic S, Greer TM, Keledjian R, Yang R, Uddin J, Guggino WB, Atabani SF, Belkaid Y, Xu Y, Whitsett JA, Accurso FJ, Wills-Karp M, Petasis NA: Defective lipoxin-mediated anti-inflammatory activity in the cystic fibrosis airway. Nat Immunol 2004;5:388–392.

39 Tunney MM, Field TR, Moriarty TF, Patrick S, Doering G, Muhlebach MS, Wolfgang MC, Boucher R, Gilpin DF, McDowell A, Elborn JS: Detection of anaerobic bacteria in high numbers in sputum from patients with cystic fibrosis. Am J Respir Crit Care Med 2008;177:995–1001.

40 van Belkum A, Renders NH, Smith S, Overbeek SE, Verbrugh HA: Comparison of conventional and molecular methods for the detection of bacterial pathogens in sputum samples from cystic fibrosis patients. FEMS Immunol Med Microbiol 2000;27:51–57.

41 Bittar F, Richet H, Dubus JC, Reynaud-Gaubert M, Stremler N, Sarles J, Raoult D, Rolain JM: Molecular detection of multiple emerging pathogens in sputa from cystic fibrosis patients. PLoS One 2008;3:e2908.

42 Molina-Teran A, Hilliard TN, Saglani S, Haxby E, Scallan M, Bush A, Davies JC: Safety of endobronchial biopsy in children with cystic fibrosis. Pediatr Pulmonol 2006;41:1021–1024.

43 Regamey N, Hilliard TN, Saglani S, Zhu J, Scallan M, Balfour-Lynn IM, Rosenthal M, Jeffery PK, Alton EW, Bush A, Davies JC: Quality, size, and composition of pediatric endobronchial biopsies in cystic fibrosis. Chest 2007;131:1710–1717.

44 Regamey N, Balfour-Lynn I, Rosenthal M, Hogg C, Bush A, Davies JC: Time required to obtain endobronchial biopsies in children during fiberoptic bronchoscopy. Pediatr Pulmonol 2009;44:76–79.

45 Sturgess J, Imrie J: Quantitative evaluation of the development of tracheal submucosal glands in infants with cystic fibrosis and control infants. Am J Pathol 1982;106:303–311.

46 Payne DN, Rogers AV, Adelroth E, Bandi V, Guntupalli KK, Bush A, Jeffery PK: Early thickening of the reticular basement membrane in children with difficult asthma. Am J Respir Crit Care Med 2003;167:78–82.

47 Ranganathan SC, Stocks J, Dezateux C, Bush A, Wade A, Carr S, Castle R, Dinwiddie R, Hoo AF, Lum S, Price J, Stroobant J, Wallis C: The evolution of airway function in early childhood following clinical diagnosis of cystic fibrosis. Am J Respir Crit Care Med 2004;169:928–933.

48 Woodruff PG, Dolganov GM, Ferrando RE, Donnelly S, Hays SR, Solberg OD, Carter R, Wong HH, Cadbury PS, Fahy J: Hyperplasia of smooth muscle in mild to moderate asthma without changes in cell size or gene expression. Am J Respir Crit Care Med 2004;169:1001–1006.

49 Regamey N, Ochs M, Hilliard TN, Muhlfeld C, Cornish N, Fleming L, Saglani S, Alton EW, Bush A, Jeffery PK, Davies JC: Increased airway smooth muscle mass in children with asthma, cystic fibrosis, and non-cystic fibrosis bronchiectasis. Am J Respir Crit Care Med 2008;177:837–843.

50 Alton EW, Stern M, Farley R, Jaffe A, Chadwick SL, Phillips J, Davies J, Smith SN, Browning J, Davies MG, Hodson ME, Durham SR, Li D, Jeffery PK, Scallan M, Balfour R, Eastman SJ, Cheng SH, Smith AE, Meeker D, Geddes DM: Cationic lipid-mediated CFTR gene transfer to the lungs and nose of patients with cystic fibrosis: a double-blind placebo-controlled trial. Lancet 1999;353:947–954.

51 Davies JC, Davies M, McShane D, Smith S, Chadwick S, Jaffe A, Farley R, Collins L, Bush A, Scallon M, Pepper J, Geddes DM, Alton EW: Potential difference measurements in the lower airway of children with and without cystic fibrosis. Am J Respir Crit Care Med 2005;171:1015–1019.

52 McShane D, Davies JC, Davies MG, Bush A, Geddes DM, Alton EW: Airway surface pH in subjects with cystic fibrosis. Eur Respir J 2003;21:37–42.

53 Tate S, MacGregor G, Davis M, Innes JA, Greening AP: Airways in cystic fibrosis are acidified: detection by exhaled breath condensate. Thorax 2002;57:926–929.

54 Doherty GM, Christie SN, Skibinski G, Puddicombe SM, Warke TJ, de Courcey F, Cross AL, Lyons JD, Ennis M, Shields MD, Heaney LG: Non-bronchoscopic sampling and culture of bronchial epithelial cells in children. Clin Exp Allergy 2003;33:1221–1225.

55 McNamara PS, Kicic A, Sutanto EN, Stevens PT, Stick SM: Comparison of techniques for obtaining lower airway epithelial cells from children. Eur Respir J 2008;32:763–768.

J.C. Davies
Consultant in Paediatric Respiratory Medicine
Royal Brompton Hospital, Sydney Street
London SW3 6NP (UK)
Tel. +44 207 352 8121, Fax +44 207 351 8340, E-Mail j.c.davies@imperial.ac.uk

Priftis KN, Anthracopoulos MB, Eber E, Koumbourlis AC, Wood RE (eds): Paediatric Bronchoscopy.
Prog Respir Res. Basel, Karger 2010, vol 38, pp 173–181

Endobronchial Tuberculosis

Elif Dagli[a] · Robert P. Gie[b] · Zeynep Seda Uyan[a] · Pierre Goussard[b]

[a]Division of Paediatric Pulmonology, Marmara University, Istanbul, Turkey; [b]Desmond Tutu Tuberculosis Center, Department of Paediatrics and Child Health, Faculty of Health Sciences, Stellenbosch University, Stellenbosch, South Africa

Abstract

Childhood tuberculosis (TB) is characterized by enlarged mediastinal lymph nodes which compress and infiltrate the airways resulting in endobronchial tuberculosis (ETB). ETB has been reported in 41–63% of children suspected of pulmonary TB. In children the disease is typically pausibacillary, which hinders the microbiological confirmation of the diagnosis. Flexible bronchoscopy (FB) is a useful tool for the confirmation of paediatric ETB. Indications for performing FB in children suspected of having TB include: confirmation of the diagnosis, determination of the degree of airway compression in children with radiological evidence of airway obstruction, management of life-threatening airway obstruction and evaluation of the response to treatment. Common bronchoscopic presentations of ETB are airway compression (42–59%) and TB lymph node ulceration into the airway (18–29%). The most commonly involved site is the right main bronchus. The bronchoscopic presentation of ETB in HIV-positive and HIV-negative children does not differ. The diagnostic yield of the microbiological analysis of bronchoalveolar lavage fluid in childhood pulmonary TB is greatly enhanced when taking into account the endobronchial abnormalities that are detected by endoscopy. The diagnostic value of endobronchial and/or transbronchial biopsy has not been reported.

Childhood tuberculosis (TB) is a common disease that affects approximately 1 million children annually around the world and contributes by approximately 10–15% to the global TB case load. It is estimated that 75% of the affected children live in the 22 countries that have the highest burden of TB disease [1]. It should be noted that the technology required to make the diagnosis is quite limited in these countries. Unfortunately, the epidemiological data required to estimate the proportion of children with severe disease who would benefit from bronchoscopic intervention at a global level is lacking; therefore, the true extent to which airway endoscopy can benefit the management of pulmonary TB in children is unclear.

Pathogenesis of Childhood Tuberculosis

After inhalation, *Mycobacterium tuberculosis* causes a localized alveolitis, termed the Ghon focus, from which the bacilli spread to the hilar and mediastinal lymph nodes. The localized alveolitis and the enlarged mediastinal glands form the primary complex (Ghon complex). In children, when the infection is not contained, the lymph nodes enlarge and involve the central airways (fig. 1). The airway can be narrowed either by external compression from the enlarged lymph node(s) or by tuberculous infiltration of the airway due to this compression [2]. In case of tuberculous infiltration, the airway lumen is narrowed by the inflammatory reaction or by the intraluminal caseating material, granulation tissue or polyps that may follow the ulceration of the lymph node into the airway. The caseating material may cause airway obstruction or may be inhaled into a lung segment or lobe, thus resulting in a hypersensitivity pneumonia, which clinically presents as expansile pneumonia. The enlarged lymph nodes may not infiltrate only the airway, but also other intrathoracic structures such as the oesophagus, the phrenic nerve, the ductus thoracicus and various blood vessels, thus resulting in diverse clinical presentations; the common feature of these presentations is the airway involvement due to the tuberculous nodes.

The degree of airway obstruction is influenced by the severity of the disease and the age of the child. Indeed, younger children suffer more extended airway obstruction as compared to older ones; this is ascribed to the smaller airways and the more pliable cartilage rings at a young age. Infants with culture-proven pulmonary TB presented with airway compression diagnosed by chest radiography in 56% of cases [3]. The extrathoracic airway is rarely involved in childhood TB [4, 5].

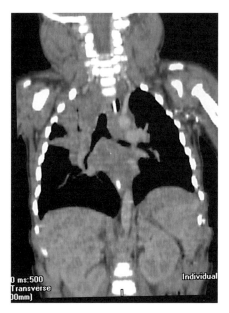

Fig. 1. Coronal reconstruction of a CT scan of the chest demonstrating compression of the left and right main bronchi by enlarged tuberculous lymph nodes. The importance of the enlarged subcarinal nodes in the airway compression is clearly demonstrated.

The diagnosis of TB in children can be quite challenging as it is extremely difficult to demonstrate acid-fast bacilli. Symptoms and signs of *M. tuberculosis* infection in children are often non-specific and can be misdiagnosed as other diseases such as HIV-related lung disease, intrathoracic lymphoma and fungal infections [6, 7]. For the diagnosis of TB, isolation of *M. tuberculosis* from culture is important. However, adequate diagnostic specimens are often difficult to obtain in children younger than 8 years of age due to lack of sputum production. In the majority of cases, the diagnosis is established using a combination of indirect evidence such as history of exposure to an adult with active TB, positive tuberculin skin test, positive chest radiograph and physical examination findings that are consistent with TB [8].

Definition of Endobronchial Tuberculosis

Endobronchial TB (ETB) is most often a complication of primary pulmonary TB. Since bronchoscopy is not routinely performed in all patients with TB, the exact incidence of ETB is unknown [9–11]. However, studies that investigated the results of flexible fibre-optic bronchoscopy (FB) in children with suspected TB have shown bronchial involvement in 41–63% of patients [11–13]. The

pathogenesis of ETB is not yet fully understood. Sources of ETB may include: direct implantation of bacilli into a bronchus from an adjacent pulmonary parenchymal lesion, direct airway infiltration from an adjacent tuberculous mediastinal lymph node, erosion and protrusion of an intrathoracic tuberculous lymph node into the bronchus, haematogenous spread and extension to the peribronchial region by lymphatic drainage [9]. ETB has been classified according to the bronchoscopic findings as: extrinsic bronchial compression, actively caseating lesion, granuloma formation, polypoid mass lesion, lymph node protrusion, and mucosal erosion with ulceration [10, 11]. Early detection and effective treatment of ETB are important to decrease disease complications such as bronchiectasis and bronchial stenosis [13].

Unlike adults, the most common form of ETB in children is airway compression by enlarged lymph nodes. As a result, the term lymphobronchial tuberculosis has been suggested for childhood ETB as it describes more accurately the relevant pathology and thus helps to differentiate childhood from adult disease; this discrimination allows for better targeting of treatment and accuracy in prognosis.

Bronchoscopy in Suspected Pulmonary Tuberculosis

Indications

The role of FB in the investigation of paediatric airway disease continues to expand [7, 14]; it is most often used to investigate children with airway obstruction [introduction and chapter 1, this vol., pp. 12–21]. The use of FB in ETB has advantages such that smaller divisions of the airways can be reached and airway obstruction can be bypassed enabling the evaluation of the distal airway [15]. Therefore, FB offers a safe and rapid means of confirming the cause of obstruction by directly visualizing the airway abnormality [7, 14, 16–19].

Nevertheless, the use of bronchoscopy in the diagnosis and management of childhood TB remains controversial [20]. Most authors agree that the role of bronchoscopy is to exclude other possible causes of airway obstruction and coexistent opportunistic infections, especially in immunocompromised children. There are no officially endorsed indications for performing bronchoscopy in children with ETB, but the following propositions are generally agreed upon [15]:

1 in children suspected of having TB to confirm the diagnosis when this is not possible by other non-invasive techniques;

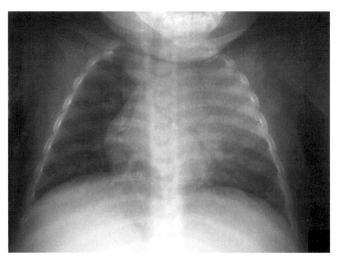

Fig. 2. Chest radiograph demonstrating the compression of the left main bronchus by enlarged tuberculous lymph nodes. Alveolar consolidation is visible in the left upper lobe.

2 in cases of airway obstruction that is visible on chest radiography to determine the degree, the cause and ultimately the management of the obstruction;

3 in children with life-threatening airway obstruction to determine the cause, the degree and the treatment of the obstruction;

4 in children being treated for ETB to determine the response to treatment.

Endoscopic Evaluation of Endobronchial Tuberculosis
The prevalence of ETB in children remains uncertain. In the prechemotherapeutic era, the incidence was stated to be 86%, with 28% of cases suffering bronchial perforation [2]. In more recent studies, the incidence of complicated lymph node disease varies from 8 to 38% (fig. 2); the low percentage was found in the community, while the high percentage was reported, not surprisingly, among hospitalized patients [21]. In paediatric studies, where FB was used to determine the presence of airway involvement, such involvement was found in 41–63% of patients [11–13]. The reported difference is not surprising as the degree of airway obstruction is underestimated when evaluated by chest radiography. There is a positive correlation between the frequency of airway involvement and the severity of the disease. In industrialized countries, where the majority of cases are diagnosed early in the course of the disease, the clinical presentation of TB and the airway compression are less severe. Conversely, in countries where children usually present with symptomatic disease, they are more likely to have more advanced

disease, and a larger proportion is diagnosed with airway compression.

FB has been found to be useful not only in providing rapid confirmation of ETB, but also in excluding other causes of bronchial obstruction; indeed, ETB cases can be misdiagnosed as pneumonia, asthma or foreign-body aspiration [22–28]. Moreover, FB helped to diagnose ETB in patients in whom it was not suspected on the basis of their clinical findings and chest radiography [13].

FB has been proven to be valuable when making a decision between the conservative and the surgical approach to treat ETB. Corticosteroids are recommended in children with airway compression caused by mediastinal lymph node enlargement [15]. Although their role in the prevention of bronchial obstruction is controversial [29–32], there are studies that demonstrate the efficacy of adding corticosteroids to the routine anti-TB therapy in ETB [33–35]. The degree and the duration of the obstruction (as assessed by FB) are important factors in deciding which children would require surgical intervention [11].

FB is also used in children with TB to assess the response to treatment [13, 15]. The improvement, or the worsening, of the lymphobronchial lesion can be followed by repeat bronchoscopies [36]. It has been reported that some children with ETB have experienced initial worsening of airway compression and an increase in the size of granulation tissue when starting anti-TB treatment [13, 28]. This response is considered to be the result of a hypersensitivity reaction. Therefore, serial FBs have been suggested in order to assess the patient's response to therapy and to decide whether to continue anti-TB chemotherapy or resort to surgical treatment [36, 37].

The treatment of ETB remains uncertain, and there are many unanswered questions. The role of adjuvant corticosteroids, endobronchial or transthoracic enucleation of the lymph nodes eroding into or compressing the bronchus is not yet clear. In most cases, ETB is treated by 3 or 4 first-line anti-TB drugs, to which methylprednisolone (2 mg/kg/day) is added for the first month of treatment. The mean time to regression after initiation of treatment, as determined by FB, has been found to be 5.5 ± 2.7 months, while radiological improvement was observed in 5.3 ± 2.7 months [11]. The rate of regression is dependent on the grade of the bronchoscopic classification of the lymphobronchial lesions and the severity of the airway compression [10]. In cases with airway compression, resolution occurs in 9–90 days, while in 80% of cases with endoluminal granulation, tissue resolution was observed in 3–10 weeks [11]. Among children, in whom the airway compression is estimated to be greater than 75%, approximately 33% fail to respond to medical therapy [P. Goussard, pers. observation]. Of 31 reported cases, 4 (12%) developed stenosis of the bronchi, with 1 requiring surgical intervention. This is considerably less than the reported frequency of 41% in adult patients who develop stenosis [38].

Bronchoalveolar Lavage and Endobronchial Biopsy
It has been argued that bronchoscopy is of limited value in the diagnosis of childhood TB due to the low diagnostic yield of cultured *M. tuberculosis* from bronchoalveolar lavage fluid (BALF). Numerous studies have demonstrated that the diagnostic yield of BALF is lower than that of gastric aspirate for *M. tuberculosis* culture [7, 39]. These results, however, do not take into account the lymphobronchial airway involvement, which can be visualized by the bronchoscope during the procedure.

In adults with pulmonary TB, the BALF culture has been reported to yield a higher recovery rate for *M. tuberculosis* than sputum cultures, especially in sputum-smear-negative patients [40]. In a study of children with suspected pulmonary TB, designed to investigate whether BALF is superior to gastric lavage for the isolation of *M. tuberculosis*, gastric lavage was found to perform better than BALF in the bacteriological confirmation of pulmonary TB [41]. However, in another study, Brown et al. [42] showed that the use of induced sputum samples was more sensitive than the use of gastric lavage or BALF samples for the diagnosis of TB in patients who could not expectorate spontaneously.

In their study of paediatric patients, Cakir et al. [11] demonstrated that the isolation rate of *M. tuberculosis* was 10% from gastric lavage, 12.8% from BALF, while it increased to 20% when both procedures were performed. When the authors reviewed the results of previous reports on the isolation rate of *M. tuberculosis* from samples obtained from different sites, they found that *M. tuberculosis* was isolated from gastric lavage in 14–47% of cases, and from BALF in 10–43% of cases [11]. Taking into account the available information, every effort, including BALF culture, should be made to recover the mycobacterium in order to perform anti-TB drug susceptibility testing, especially in regions where the prevalence of resistant *M. tuberculosis* is high. It is worth noting that in the study of Cakir et al. [11], while the total positive culture yield for *M. tuberculosis* was 20%, the frequency with which abnormalities due to ETB were visualized bronchoscopically reached 47%. Hence, when BALF culture of *M. tuberculosis* is the only means utilized to diagnose childhood TB, the diagnostic value of FB is grossly underestimated.

It is possible to perform endobronchial biopsy [chapter 4, this vol., pp. 42–53] of the airway sites affected by ETB.

The size of the working channel is the limiting factor for the size of the biopsy that can be obtained, thus making the diagnosis more challenging. We routinely remove caseating material that herniates into the airway, and process it for culture and pathology. No study to date has systematically evaluated the diagnostic yield of endobronchial biopsy in children with ETB.

Use of Rigid versus Flexible Bronchoscopy
Since the working channel of the 2.8-mm flexible bronchoscope used in young children is small [chapter 1, this vol., pp. 12–21], interventional bronchoscopy using this instrument is quite limited. In cases where transbronchial enucleation of tuberculous lymph nodes ulcerating into the airways is required, the rigid bronchoscope can be very useful. This instrument has the added advantage that the patient can be ventilated throughout the procedure, thus giving more time to perform the procedure [chapters 2 and 8, this vol., pp. 22–29 and 83–94].

Bronchoscopy versus Computed Tomography
The modern multidetector computed tomography (CT) scanners make multiplanar reconstruction of the chest possible, thus allowing for accurate demonstration of airway narrowing in children [43; chapter 9, this vol., pp. 95–112]. In a study, in which 3-dimensional volume-rendered CT scans were used to determine airway narrowing caused by TB lymph node enlargement in children, the sensitivity of the examination was 92% and the specificity 85% when FB was used as the gold standard [44]. The 3-dimensional multidetector CT scan could not determine the tissue characteristics of the airway involvement and was less accurate when the airway compression was less than 50%. Where severe compression was present, its length could not be measured by FB, while it could be estimated from the CT scan images. These and other relevant data illustrate that the comprehensive management of patients suspected of having ETB should include both bronchoscopy and chest CT scan. Based on the above data, it is also evident that bronchoscopy should precede CT scan as the presence of less than 50% compression of the airway, as witnessed during FB, would indicate that the CT scan of the chest will most likely not contribute to the further management of the child, except in cases where the cause of the external compression is uncertain.

Studies Evaluating Flexible Bronchoscopy
There are three large series that have evaluated the role of FB in the diagnosis and treatment of ETB in children:

Chan et al. [13] investigated the usefulness of FB in the diagnosis and management of 36 children younger than 16 years of age with active pulmonary TB. ETB was detected in 41.7% of the patients, while one third of children thought to have primary uncomplicated TB, which was diagnosed by conventional means (i.e. history, physical examination and plain chest radiography), were found to have ETB by FB. *M. tuberculosis* was isolated from the gastric washing in 47.2% and from the BALF in 10.8% of the patients. None of the children had a major complication during or after the procedure.

De Blic et al. [12] evaluated 121 FB procedures in 54 children aged 3 months to 14 years who were suspected of having pulmonary TB. ETB was detected in 57% of the patients. FB helped to guide the use of oral corticosteroid therapy. It proved to be particularly useful in children with chest radiographs that were not suggestive of bronchial involvement, it indicated the need for resection of granulation tissue by rigid bronchoscopy in 3 cases, and its findings were crucial in the decision to proceed to surgical intervention in 2 children with persistent bronchial obstruction.

In their study, Cakir et al. [11] evaluated 70 TB patients aged 5 months to 15 years with suspected TB and an inadequate response to more than 8 weeks of anti-TB treatment. In patients with endobronchial lesions and extrinsic bronchial compression that obstructed the airway by more than 50% of the original lumen, methylprednisolone at a dose of 2 mg/kg/day was added to the standard anti-TB chemotherapy (20 patients), and FB was repeated every 2 months until resolution of the lesion. ETB was more common in children less than 3 years of age, in those with a history of contact with TB, and those with lymphadenopathy detected by chest CT scan. All of the patients in this series were treated without any complications, but 1 patient required surgical resection.

A separate evaluation of 193 FB procedures was carried out in 122 children, younger than 16 years of age with suspected pulmonary TB, at the paediatric pulmonary clinic of Marmara University Hospital. ETB was detected in 47.6% of the patients. In those with endobronchial lesions and/or extrinsic bronchial compression obstructing the airway by more than 50% of its original lumen, systemic corticosteroid treatment at a dose of 2 mg/kg/day was added to standard anti-TB chemotherapy, and serial FBs were performed every 2 months until resolution of the lesion. Among patients with ETB, 41.3% were found to have extrinsic bronchial compression, 31% actively caseating lesions (online suppl. videos 1 and 2), 13.7% granuloma formation (online suppl. videos 3 and 4), 3.4% protrusion

of an enlarged lymph node (online suppl. video 5), 8.6% polypoid mass lesion (online suppl. videos 6 and 7), 1.7% mucosal erosion with ulceration and 13.7% more than one type of endobronchial lesion. During the follow-up, only a 1-year-old girl with a polypoid mass in the right main bronchus required surgical intervention to remove the endobronchial lesion and dilate the bronchial stenosis that complicated the surgical intervention (online suppl. videos 8–11).

Common Bronchoscopic Presentations of Endobronchial Tuberculosis

The most common lesion of ETB seen on bronchoscopy is compression of the airways (42–59%) [11, 12] (fig. 3). The few studies that have systematically investigated the compression of the airways by enlarged tuberculous lymph node(s) in children have found that the most common site of obstruction is the right main bronchus (58%), followed by the left main bronchus (21%) [11]. The degree of obstruction varies, but in most cases (79%) it is estimated to be less than 50% of the original airway lumen [11]. The next two most common lesions are granulation tissue at the site of lymph node ulceration into the airway (18–29%) and caseating material, which originates from the lymph node and protrudes into the airway (12–39%) [11, 12]. The least common lesion in children is polyp formation (6%) [11].

Another feature of childhood ETB is that airway involvement is multifocal (41%) [12] and commonly involves both the left and right bronchial trees (12%) [11].

These findings are similar to airway involvement as reported by chest CT scan in children with TB. The most common site of airway compression demonstrated by this modality was the left main bronchus (21%), followed by the right main bronchus (14%) and the bronchus intermedius (8%) [45].

Endobronchial Involvement in Children Infected with Human Immunodeficiency Virus

In children with severe immunosuppression, the deferential diagnosis of lymph node enlargement that involves the airway is expanded. Bronchoscopy in HIV-infected children is valuable for collecting specimens for culture, cytology and histopathology [chapters 3 and 4, this vol., pp. 30–41 and 42–53]. The bronchoscopic images of tuberculous

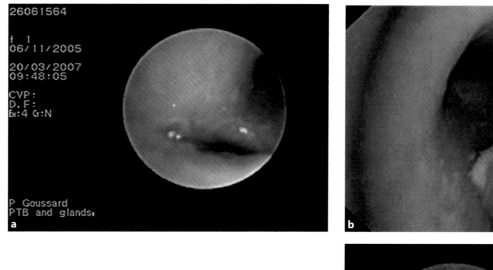

Fig. 3. a. Medial and lateral compression of the bronchus intermedius by adjacent lymph nodes in a child with proven tuberculosis as seen at FB. PTB = Pulmonary TB. **b** Tuberculous node ulcerating into the airway with caseating material visible. **c** Tuberculous node ulcerating into the airway with granuloma tissue visible.

lymphobronchial involvement in children have not been reported in the literature but in our experience it does not differ from that seen in children who are HIV negative. *Cryptococcus neoformans,* Karposi sarcoma and lymphoma cause lymph node enlargement, which can be confused with that of tuberculous aetiology.

The role of FB in the evaluation of immune reconstitution inflammatory syndrome has not been determined yet but it will most likely become an important additional investigation.

Unusual Cases of Endobronchial Tuberculosis

Expansile Pneumonia Caused by M. tuberculosis
Expansile pneumonia in children due to *M. tuberculosis* commonly presents with the clinical picture of a pneumonia that is not responding to treatment. The chest radiograph reveals a dense opacification, especially of the upper lobes (75%), with displacement of the fissures indicating an increase in volume of the involved lobe (fig. 4). The left (42%) and right (33%) upper lobes are the most commonly involved lobes [46]. The severity of this form of the disease is reflected by the fact that 88% of patients are culture positive for *M. tuberculosis*.

On FB, airway compression was present in 95% of patients, with the obstruction estimated to be more than 75% of the original airway lumen in 83% of the cases. In 21% of the children, the lumen occlusion was complete. Accompanying the airway compression were lymph nodes ulcerating into the airways in 21% of the patients, while tracheal compression was present in 63% of the cases [46].

The severity of the disease positively correlates with the degree of airway obstruction. In cases where the obstruction was greater than 75%, there was evidence of necrotic liquefaction of the affected lobe while this was not present in those where the airway obstruction was less than 75%.

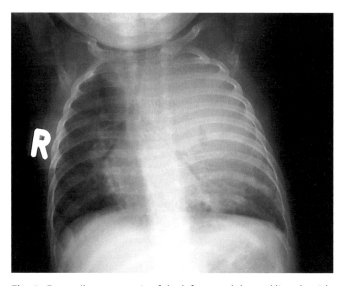

Fig. 4. Expansile pneumonia of the left upper lobe and lingula with compression of the left main bronchus and the trachea.

Often, the compression was so severe that 42% of children required enucleation of the tuberculous lymph node(s). Of the 10 cases that required nodular enucleation, this was achieved bronchoscopically in 3 cases [46].

Bronchoscopy is essential for the follow-up of children treated for expansile pneumonia due to *M. tuberculosis*. Transthoracic enucleation of the mediastinal lymph nodes should be carried out in those patients who, after 1 month of anti-TB therapy (to which oral steroids have been added), show no improvement of a bronchoscopically estimated airway obstruction which remains greater than 75%.

Broncho-Oesophageal Fistula Caused by M. tuberculosis
Tuberculous lymph nodes that involve the bronchi and the oesophagus can rupture into both structures, thus causing an acquired broncho-oesophageal fistula. Children with this form of fistula present clinically in one of two ways [5]:

The first clinical presentation is that of acute respiratory failure requiring assisted ventilation. When initiating mechanical ventilation, it becomes apparent that there is air leak into the gastrointestinal system. The presence of the suspected broncho-oesophageal fistula is best determined by FB. The fistula is visualized in the majority of cases in the medial wall of the left main bronchus. It needs to be blocked to ensure adequate ventilation. This is best achieved by placing a stent in the oesophagus at the level of the fistula [47].

The second is one of a child who coughs when fed, either prior to or after initiating anti-TB therapy. In these cases, FB demonstrates the fistula in the medial wall of the left main bronchus. Proving the patency of the fistula may present a challenge. However, the fistula can be demonstrated by injecting a dye (we use rifampicin) into the oesophagus and observe the dye enter from the oesophagus into the airway, through the fistula, during spontaneous ventilation.

Repeated bronchoscopy is useful in following the clinical course of these children. Although we have reported in the past that fistulas caused by *M. tuberculosis* in children do not resolve after 6 or more months of medical treatment, we have subsequently observed this to actually occur in children.

Laryngeal Tuberculosis
Laryngeal TB used to be common in adult patients with severe TB, especially prior to the modern chemotherapy era. In children this lesion is rare. We recently reported 2 cases of laryngeal TB with severe upper airway obstruction during sleep. When bronchoscoped, both children had severe supraglottic swelling with nodular compression of the proximal trachea [4]. The pathogenesis of these lesions is unclear. Both children had a miliary picture on a chest radiograph that was consistent with haematogenous spread, but the accompanying nodular compression of the trachea suggests that lymphatic spread may also have contributed to the pathogenesis.

Accompanying Intrathoracic Chest Disease
Tracheal compression, ball valve obstruction of the main bronchi [5], phrenic nerve palsy [48], chylothorax [49] and cold abscess of the thorax [5] have been associated with ETB. Bronchoscopy plays an important role in the diagnosis and management of such cases. In life-threatening airway obstruction, relief can be provided by endoscopically removing part of the lymph node ulcerating into the airway and the caseating material obstructing its lumen.

Future Trends

There is considerable debate regarding the value of FB in the investigation of a child suspected of pulmonary TB. Most studies have been performed in regions of the world where there is a low prevalence of disease. In reports originating from regions with a high prevalence of TB, FB plays an important role in the diagnosis and management of these children [11]. The exact role of endoscopy in high-burden countries needs to be explored.

With the continuous improvements in the image quality of FB and the potential increase in the size of the working channel, it may become possible to perform more invasive diagnostic procedures through this instrument. In adult patients transbronchial aspiration biopsies are feasible [50]. Children with nodal compression of the airways are probably ideal candidates for this procedure. Nevertheless, the precise role of FB in the diagnosis and management of pulmonary TB in children still needs to be determined.

References

1 Nelson LJ, Wells CD: Global epidemiology of childhood tuberculosis. Int J Tuberc Lung Dis 2004;8:363–647.
2 Marais BJ, Gie RP, Schaaf HS, Hesseling AC, Obihara CC, Enarson DA, Donald PR, Beyers N: The natural history of childhood intrathoracic tuberculosis: a critical review of the literature from the pre-chemotherapy era. Int J Tuberc Lung Dis 2004;8:392–402.
3 Schaaf HS, Gie RP, Beyers N, Smuts N, Donald PR: Tuberculosis in infants less than 3 months of age. Arch Dis Child 1993;69:371–374.
4 Gregg KK, Detjen AK, Goussard P, Gie RP: Laryngeal involvement in two severe cases of childhood tuberculosis. Pediatr Infect Dis J 2009;28: 1136–1138.
5 Gie RP, Goussard P, Kling S, Schaaf HS, Beyers N: Unusual forms of intrathoracic tuberculosis in childhood and their management. Pediatr Respir Rev 2004;5:S139–S141.
6 Starke JR, Taylor Watts KT: Tuberculosis in the pediatric population of Houston, Texas. Pediatrics 1989;84:28–35.
7 Bibi H, Mosheyev A, Shoseyov D, Feigenbaum D, Kurzbart E, Weiller Z: Should bronchoscopy be performed in the evaluation of suspected pediatric pulmonary tuberculosis? Chest 2002;122: 1604–1608.
8 Karadağ B: Pulmoner tüberkülozun klinik bulguları ve tanısı; in Dagli E, Karakoc F, (eds): Çocuk Göğüs Hastalıkları. Istanbul, Nobel Tıp Kitabevleri, 2007, pp 187–192.
9 Chung HS, Lee JH: Bronchoscopic assessment of the evolution of endobronchial tuberculosis. Chest 2000;117:385–392.
10 Lee JH, Park SS, Lee DH, Shin DH, Yang SC, Yoo BM: Endobronchial tuberculosis: clinical and bronchoscopic features in 121 cases. Chest 1992; 102:990–994.
11 Cakir E, Uyan ZS, Oktem S, Karakoc F, Ersu R, Karadag B, Dagli E: Flexible bronchoscopy for diagnosis and follow-up of childhood endobronchial tuberculosis. Pediatr Infect Dis J 2008;27: 783–787.
12 De Blic J, Azevedo I, Burren CP, Le Bourgeois M, Lallemand D, Scheinmann P: The value of flexible bronchoscopy in childhood pulmonary tuberculosis. Chest 1991;100:688–692.
13 Chan S, Abadco DL, Steiner P: Role of flexible fiberoptic bronchoscopy in the diagnosis of childhood endobronchial tuberculosis. Pediatr Infect Dis J 1994;13:506–509.
14 Wood RE: The emerging role of flexible bronchoscopy in pediatrics. Clin Chest Med 2001;2:311–317.

15 Goussard P, Gie R: Airway involvement in pulmonary tuberculosis. Pediatr Respir Rev 2007;8: 118–123.
16 Joos L, Patuto N, Chhajed PN, Tamm M: Diagnostic yield of flexible bronchoscopy in current clinical practice. Swiss Med Wkly 2006;136:155–159.
17 De Charnace G, de Lacourt C: Diagnostic techniques in paediatric tuberculosis. Paediatr Respir Rev 2001;2:120–126.
18 Donato L, Helms P, Barats A, Lebris V: Bronchoscopy in childhood pulmonary tuberculosis. Arch Pediatr 2005;12(suppl 2):S127–S131.
19 Charnace G, Delacourt C: Diagnostic techniques in paediatric tuberculosis. Paediatr Respir Rev 2001;2:120–125.
20 Shingadia D, Novelli V: Diagnosis and treatment of tuberculosis in children. Lancet Infect Dis 2003;3:624–632.
21 Marais BJ, Gie RP, Schaaf HS, Enarson D, Beyers N: The spectrum of disease in children treated for tuberculosis is a high endemic area. Int J Tubercl Lung Dis 2006;10:732–738.
22 Wood GS, Gonzalez C, Done S, Albus RA: Endobronchial tuberculosis in children: a case report and review. Int J Pediatr Otorhinolaryngol 1990;20:241–245.
23 Abdulla F, Dietrich KA: Endobronchial tuberculosis manifested as obstructive airway disease in a 4-month-old infant. South Med J 1990;83:715–717.
24 Uzuner N, Anal O, Karaman O, Sevinç C, Türkmen M, Canda T, Kazan E. Endobronchial tuberculosis complicated with Staphylococcus aureus pneumonia and empyema in a child. Turk J Pediatr 2003;45:254–257.
25 Park AH, Fowler SS, Challapalli M: Suspected foreign body aspiration in a child with endobronchial tuberculosis. Int J Pediatr Otorhinolaryngol 2000;53:67–71.
26 Caglayan S, Coteli I, Acar U, Erkin S: Endobronchial tuberculosis simulating foreign body aspiration. Chest 1989;95:1164.
27 Weiner GM, Batch AJ: Endobronchial tuberculosis masquerading as foreign body aspiration. J Laryngol Otol 1995;109:1192–1194.
28 Williams D, York E, Nobert E, Sproule B: Endobronchial tuberculosis presenting as asthma. Chest 1988;93:836–837.
29 Alzeer AH, FitzGerald JM: Corticosteroids and tuberculosis: risks and use as adjunct therapy. Tuber Lung Dis 1993;74:6–11.

30 Dooley DP, Carpenter JL, Rademacher S: Adjunctive corticosteroid therapy for tuberculosis: a critical reappraisal of the literature. Clin Infect Dis 1997;25:872–887.
31 Senderovitz T, Viskum K: Corticosteroids and tuberculosis. Respir Med 1994;88:561–565.
32 Rikimaru T: Therapeutic management of endobronchial tuberculosis. Expert Opin Pharmacother 2004;5:1463–1470.
33 Chan HS, Pang JA: Effect of corticosteroids on deterioration of endobronchial tuberculosis during chemotherapy. Chest 1989;96:1195–1196.
34 Chan HS, Sun A, Hoheisel GB: Endobronchial tuberculosis: is corticosteroid treatment useful? A report of 8 cases and review of the literature. Postgrad Med J 1990;66:822–826.
35 Toppet M, Malfroot A, Derbe MB, Toppet V, Spehl M, Dab I: Corticosteroids in primary tuberculosis with bronchial obstruction. Arch Dis Child 1990;65:1222–1226.
36 De Blic J: The value of flexible bronchoscopy in childhood pulmonary tuberculosis. Pediatr Pulmonol 1995;11(suppl):24–25.
37 Hsu HS, Hsu WH, Huang BS, Huang MH: Surgical treatment of endobronchial tuberculosis. Scand Cardiovasc J 1997;31:79–82.
38 Um SM, Yoon YS, Lee SM, Yim JJ, Yoo CG, Chung HS, Kim YW, Han SK, Shim YS, Kim DK: Predictors of airway stenosis in patients with endobronchial tuberculosis. Int J Tuberc Lung Dis 2007;12:57–62.
39 Abadaco D, Steiner P: Gastric lavage is better than bronchoalveolar lavage for isolation of Mycobacterium tuberculosis in childhood pulmonary tuberculosis. Pediatr Infect Dis J 1993;11: 735–738.
40 Norman E, Keistinen T, Uddenfeldt M, Perolof Rydstrom P, Lundgren R: Bronchoalveolar lavage is better than gastric lavage in the diagnosis of pulmonary tuberculosis. Scand J Infect Dis 1988;20:77–80.
41 Somu N, Swaminathan S, Paramasivan CN, Vijayasekaran D, Chandrabhooshanam A, Vijayan VK, Prabhakar R: Value of bronchoalveolar lavage and gastric lavage in the diagnosis of pulmonary tuberculosis in children. Tuber Lung Dis 1995;76:295–299.
42 Brown M, Varia H, Bassett P, Davidson RN, Wall R, Pasvol G: Prospective study of sputum induction, gastric washing and bronchoalveolar lavage for the diagnosis of pulmonary tuberculosis in patients who are unable to expectorate. Clin Infect Dis 2007;44:1415–1420.

43 Andronikou S, Wieselhaler N: Modern imaging of tuberculosis in children: thoracic, central nervous system and abdominal tuberculosis. Pediatr Radiol 2004;34:861–875.

44 Du Plessis J, Goussard P, Andronikou S, Gie R, George R: Comparing three-dimensional volume-rendered CT images with fibre-optic tracheobronchoscopy in the evaluation of airway compression caused by tuberculous lymphadenopathy. Pediatr Radiol 2009;39:694–702.

45 Andronikou S, Joseph E, Lucas S, Brachmeyer S, du Toit G, Zar H, Swingler G: CT scanning for the detection of TB mediastinal and hilar lymphadenopathy in children. Pediatr Radiol 2004;34:232–234.

46 Goussard P, Gie RP, Kling S, Beyers N: Expansile pneumonia in children caused by *Mycobacterium tuberculosis:* clinical, radiological and bronchoscopic appearances. Pediatr Pulmonol 2004;38:451–455.

47 Goussard P, Sidler D, Kling S, Andronikou S, Rossouw G, Gie R: Esophageal stent improves the ventilation in a child with broncho-esophageal fistula caused by *Mycobacterium tuberculosis.* Pediatr Pulmonol 2007;42:93–97.

48 Goussard P, Gie RP, Kling S, Andronikou S, Jansen J, Rossouw G: Phrenic nerve palsy in children associated with confirmed intrathoracic tuberculosis: diagnosis and clinical course. Pediatr Pulmonol 2008:44:345–350.

49 Cakir E, Gocmen B, Uyan ZS, Oktem S, Kiyau G, Karadoc F, Ersu R, Karadag B, Dagli T, Dagli E: An unusual case of chylothorax complicating childhood tuberculosis. Pediatr Pulmonol 2008; 43:611–614.

50 Cetinkaya E, Yildiz P, Kadakal F, Tekin A, Soysal T, Elibol S, Yilman V: Transbronchial needle aspiration in the diagnosis of intrathoracic lymphadenopathy. Respiration 2002;69:335–338.

Dr. Elif Dagli
Division of Paediatric Pulmonology, Marmara University
Istanbul (Turkey)
E-Mail esezginer@gmail.com

Priftis KN, Anthracopoulos MB, Eber E, Koumbourlis AC, Wood RE (eds): Paediatric Bronchoscopy.
Prog Respir Res. Basel, Karger 2010, vol 38, pp 182–190

Chronic Cough

I. Brent Masters[a] · Anne B. Chang[a,b]

[a]Queensland Children's Respiratory Centre, Royal Children's Hospital, Brisbane, Qld., and [b]Child Health Division, Menzies
School of Health Research, Darwin, N.T., Australia

Abstract

Cough occurs as a result of a complex of neurophysiological and mechanical interactions within the respiratory system, and as such its efficiency is vital to human homeostasis and well-being. However, it may also be an indicator of many respiratory illnesses. Cough characteristics vary with illnesses but some disorders such as structural airway disorders/malacia have very characteristic brassy cough qualities and bronchoscopic findings. In chronic wet cough and other forms of cough without defining audible properties, the bronchoscopic visual appearance of the airways and bronchoalveolar lavage (BAL) cytological and culture assessments allow for identification and confirmation of specific conditions and organisms. Bronchoscopy is not indicated in all chronic coughs but is necessary where the chronic cough is unresolving and wet, has otherwise atypical features, associated with radiological or underlying congenital or acquired immunodeficiency, or suggests aspiration disorders or a foreign body. In these circumstances, consideration should be given to performing a flexible fibre-optic bronchoscopy and BAL even when the levels of physiological dysfunction appear minor. In the research context, bronchoscopy and BAL for chronic cough are providing considerable insight into diagnoses, overlapping and concomitant diagnoses and disease mechanisms but the role of brush and tissue biopsy is yet to be fully elucidated. Research dealing with the interface between cough and bronchoscopically derived data needs to be extended in the paediatric setting as it potentially offers enhanced understanding and treatment options for many conditions.

Copyright © 2010 S. Karger AG, Basel

Cough, the most common symptom of respiratory disease, is also the commonest acute reason for presentation to doctors. Cough has an important defensive role in health and disease. Inefficient cough is associated with acute and respiratory morbidity such as aspiration pneumonia and bronchiectasis. However, chronic cough can be troublesome; it impairs the quality of life of children and their parents. For the clinician, defining who should investigate and the type

of investigation (if any), to delineate an underlying aetiology, is a key management decision. This chapter reviews the utility of flexible fibre-optic bronchoscopy (FFB) and bronchoalveolar lavage (BAL) in children with chronic cough. As chronic cough encompasses the entirety of respiratory illness in children, this chapter is limited to cough with specific bronchoscopic characteristics and to cough when the diagnosis is uncertain.

Cough: Mechanism and Receptors

With the increased interest in cough, understanding of cough mechanisms has substantially improved in the last 10 years. Many reviews are available [1–4], and readers are referred to these for further in-depth study of physiological mechanisms. We limit this abbreviated physiology section to the relevance to clinicians.

Cough comprises 3 phases (inspiratory, compressive, expiratory) and serves as a vital defensive mechanism for lung health. Unlike other reflexes, cough is one that is both voluntarily and involuntarily regulated. While physiologists argue about what constitutes a cough (e.g. expiratory or laryngeal reflex, single bouts or epochs), clinicians are certain that cough refers to a distinct expiratory sound. The involuntary laryngeal reflex component of cough prevents pulmonary aspiration and the tracheobronchial component (which is both voluntary and involuntary) promotes ciliary activity and clears airway debris. The importance of an intact cough mechanism is reflected in the occurrence of pulmonary problems when cough is inefficient. Cough efficiency is dependent on physical/mechanical aspects (respiratory muscles, mucous, airway calibre, larynx) and integrity of the neurophysiology

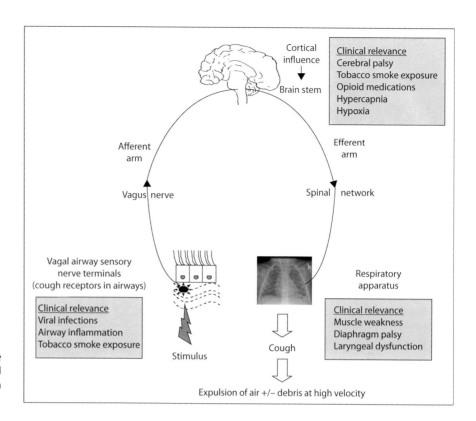

Fig. 1. Schematic representation of the cough pathway, with examples of clinical relevance affecting the cough pathway in grey boxes.

pathway of cough [3, 5]. When the neurophysiology pathway of cough is dysfunctional, for example in children with neurological impairment, cough may be absent during airway aspiration [6].

Neurophysiological Aspects of the Cough Pathway
The understanding of this aspect of cough (simplified in fig. 1) has significantly progressed (albeit mostly in animals) with the characterization of airway afferent nerve subtypes implicated in coughing (cough receptors: bronchopulmonary C fibres, rapidly adapting airway mechanoreceptors and Aδ sensory nerve fibres) and discovery of how they function. The latter occurs via the transient receptor potential family of ion channels that can be stimulated by tussogenics or vanniloid receptors (and subtypes) [1, 2, 4]. The relative contributions of these airway afferents/receptors to cough (especially in disease) are however still disputed [2]. All these cough receptors are terminal endings of vagal sensory nerves that project into the epithelial layer of the extra- and intrapulmonary airways. Thus, cough receptors are absent in mucosal areas that are not innervated by the vagus nerve, a fact that has been poorly appreciated by some clinical reviews describing the cough reflex. Vagal afferents are more mechanosensitive in the extrapulmonary airways and

more chemosensitive in the intrapulmonary airways [2]. As prevention of airway aspiration involves stimulation of the low-threshold mechanosensitive receptors to activate the cough laryngeal reflex, it makes biological sense that extrapulmonary airways are more mechanosensitive than intrapulmonary airways.

Activation of sensory nerve terminals forms a generator potential (membrane depolarization) arising from opening of non-selective cation channels in a graded manner. If sufficiently activated and if the threshold is achieved, voltage-gated sodium channels are opened and action potentials initiated. These action potentials spread along the nerve fibre travelling to the brain stem (nucleus tractus solitarii, NTS) where synaptic vesicles release their neurotransmitters (mainly glutamate or neuropeptides) into multiple relay neurons that then activate other action potentials in the brain stem, resulting in respiratory reflexes. The quantity of released neurotransmitters depends on the frequency of action potential formation (impulses per second), duration of activation and number of neurons activated [1, 2]. Local anaesthetics used during FFB for inhibiting cough block the action potentials (formation, peak and/or frequency) evoked by the tussive mechanical stimuli of the FFB. The 'urge to cough'

Table 1. Clinical indications for FFB in a child with chronic cough to identify the aetiology and/or for therapeutic purposes

Indication	Examples of aetiologies of chronic cough identified or treated using FFB
BAL for microbiology, airway cellularity	protracted bacterial bronchitis, atypical infections, eosinophilia, tuberculosis, *Mycobacterium* and other pathogens
Localized changes on radiology of the chest	mucous plug, localized airway obstruction or compression
Suspicion of inhaled foreign body	diagnosis and/or retrieval of foreign body
Evaluation of aspiration lung disease	laryngeal cleft, vocal cord palsy, tracheo-oesophageal fistula, BAL findings
Suspicion of airway abnormality	tracheobronchomalacia, localized bronchial stenosis, airway obstruction or compression
Unexplained persistent cough	airway eosinophilia, Mounier-Kuhn syndrome, tracheopathia osteoplastica

sensation which may or may not precede a cough may be related to subthreshold action potential levels or a different afferent pathway [2].

Sensory afferent terminals have their cell bodies in the jugular and nodose ganglia. The first synapse of these primary cough-related sensory inputs is the second-order neurons in the brain stem, primarily the NTS. Nerve projections to and from the NTS that can enhance or inhibit cough link with other brain stem functions and from there the efferent arm of the cough pathway emerges [1, 2]. The efferent arm involves the nerve supply to the larynx, respiratory muscles and pelvic sphincters (fig. 1) [5]. The latter – if not fully functioning (muscle or nerve) – can clinically manifest as incontinence as a complication of cough.

Up- and down-regulation (plasticity) of the cough reflex have been described and likely related to changes in nerve excitability and brain stem synaptic activity. Plasticity of peripheral and central afferent cough pathways is important in pathological states associated with increased cough. Centrally, the NTS exhibits most plasticity with its many neuronal relays [7, 8]. Less is known about peripheral plasticity and even less about the developmental aspects of the cough mechanism and neurophysiology in humans. Animal studies suggest that very early exposure in the developing human can alter airway innervations and expression of cough [8].

Thus, while the cough reflex arc that consists of vagal afferents, brain stem, respiratory motor nerve and muscles is a simple arc, its complexity when examined at the system, synaptic, cellular and molecular levels is yet to be fully determined. Furthermore, the non-reflexic component of the cough can be influenced by higher cortical function that influences clinical manifestations.

Indications to Perform Flexible Bronchoscopy in the Evaluation of Chronic Cough and Its Clinical Advantages

The indications for FFB in children with chronic cough can be formulated for diagnostic and therapeutic reasons. These diagnostic indications are embedded in the importance of diagnostic accuracy and the pathophysiology of particular conditions to medical management balanced against the likelihood of the potential risks of the procedure. Cough disrupts sleep and daily function, and the associated anxieties of children and families surrounding the lack of a specific diagnosis [9] need to be considered in this milieu of factors important to decision-making. Safety issues must be considered in defining indications to perform a bronchoscopy, with or without BAL and/or brush and tissue biopsies.

Specific indications for a bronchoscopy in a child with chronic cough include (a) visual inspection of the airways, (b) obtaining a BAL, brush biopsy or tissue biopsy for microbiology and airway cellularity, (c) localized changes on radiology of the chest, (d) suspicion of inhaled foreign body, (e) evaluation of aspiration lung disease, (f) suspicion of airway abnormality and (g) unexplained cough. Table 1 provides examples of what may be found for the indications above. However, the evidence for its yield in the different clinical situations is limited. Indeed, the utility and yield of FFB are dependent on the child's medical history and the available expertise. Furthermore, in some situations (e.g. suspicion of an aspirated or inhaled foreign body), a negative finding may be equally important.

In one of the earliest published series of paediatric FFB, Wood [10] described that the diagnostic efficiency of FFB for the primary indication of chronic cough (n = 12 of 695)

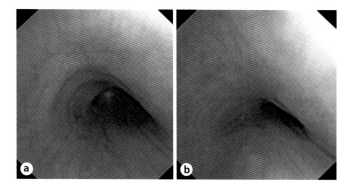

Fig. 2. Tracheomalacia in inspiration (**a**) and expiration (**b**). Note the significantly reduced area of the lumen during inspiration but the near-complete closure of the lumen during the expiratory phase.

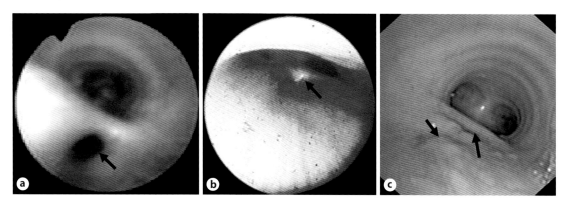

Fig. 3. Tracheo-oesophageal fistula of the H type (arrows). **a** An H-type fistula may present as an open or mucus-filled orifice with a bar/ridge distal to the orifice in the left image. **b** The fistula is a pinhole at the top of a bulging pars membranacea. Tracheomalacia is also present here. **c** Two fistulae were present: H shaped at the proximal end of the posterior groove and just proximal to the bar across the distal pars.

Fig. 4. **a** The fistula was at the mid tracheal level visible as an S-shaped opening with a distal bar or linear tissue ridge. Horseshoe-shaped ridging may also occur. Fistulae may present at any site and even involve the proximal main stem bronchus and carina itself. **b** A residual diverticulum following repair of the fistula: the diverticulum was 1.2 cm in depth. These children had chronic cough.

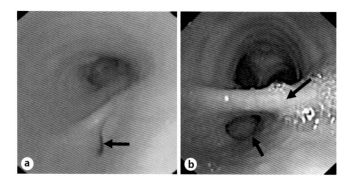

was 55%. In a tertiary-centre-based study, bronchoscopically defined airway abnormalities (mainly tracheobronchomalacia) were present in 46% of the 49 children with chronic cough [11]. In a European series, chronic cough was the indication in 11.6% of the 1,233 paediatric bronchoscopies performed but the yield was not described [12]. In Callahan's [13] series of 95 children with chronic cough (>3 weeks), bronchoscopy assisted in the diagnosis in only 5 (5.3%) children. Thus, the yield of FFB in children with

chronic cough with an unknown aetiology is likely dependent on the local expertise and sampling frame.

Endoscopic Findings in Different Types of Cough
Bronchoscopic airway inspection provides for the confirmation of diagnosis for visually diagnosed conditions such as tracheobronchomalacia (fig. 2), tracheo-oesophageal fistula (fig. 3 and 4), stenosis or endobronchial foreign bodies (fig. 5) and allows biopsy of visually obvious granuloma

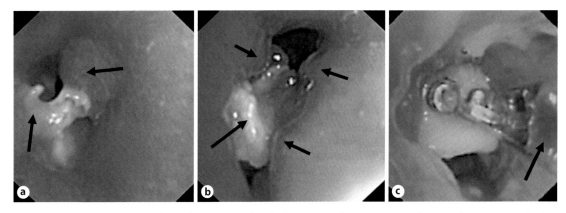

Fig. 5. Foreign bodies in 3 children who presented with chronic cough. **a** Large granuloma with mucus attached to an ulcer all hiding a foreign body. **b** Foreign body sandwiched between granulation tissues. **c** Use of biopsy forceps to remove a small piece of impacted peanut.

Fig. 6. a, b Micronodular mucosal appearance (arrows) involving the trachea and various segmental orifices in 2 different children with protracted bacterial bronchitis and chronic moist cough.

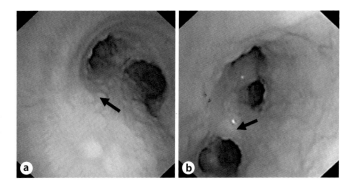

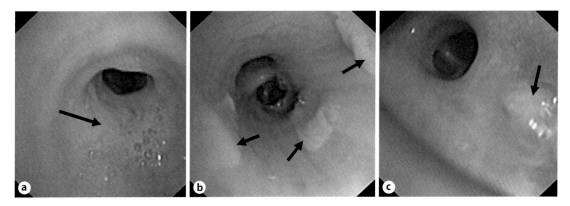

Fig. 7. Endotracheal and endobronchial mucus (arrows) presenting as a sleeve, plaques and endobronchial plug in 3 children (**a–c**) with chronic cough from protracted bronchitis or suppurative lung disease.

and other endobronchial abnormalities (fig. 6). Airway inspection also provides for an accurate description of the anatomical site, estimates of the degree of cross-sectional area loss and length of specific lesions [14], the colour and nature of secretions (fig. 7) and the colour of mucosal surfaces, textural appearance, anatomical changes (fig. 8) and

depth of mucosal surfaces pending the appearance or non-appearance of cartilage rings, and, when blood is present, the potential site of bleeding or its persistence with BAL during suctioning.

Some specific chronic cough qualities are known to be associated with characteristic bronchoscopic findings.

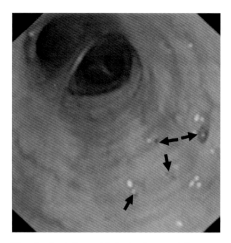

Fig. 8. Endobronchial pits (arrows) from mucus glands presenting as open or glistening (mucus-filled) spots on the lateral wall of the middle lobe bronchus and 'circumferential ribbing' seen in a child with chronic cough related to bronchiectasis after removal of endobronchial mucus.

Tracheomalacia is a common lesion associated with specific cough qualities of a brassy cough [15]. The sensitivity and specificity for brassy cough (for tracheomalacia diagnosed on FFB) were 0.57 and 0.81, respectively. Intra- and interobserver clinician agreement for brassy cough was excellent (for both κ = 0.79, 95% confidence interval = 0.73–0.86) [15]. However, there are numerous bronchoscopic appearances attributed to malacia disorders, and there is also overlap with malacia and some stenotic appearances where mixtures of cough, stridor and wheeze occur. These disorders and their pathophysiological effects may be complicated or altered by infective states, aspiration or coexistent illness such as cardiovascular disorders or syndrome effects. Appearances associated with the malacia disorders can be triangular, oval and circumferential shapes [14]. Examples of malacia associated with tracheo-oesophageal fistula of various types, primary malacia and secondary malacia are shown in figures 2–4.

Children with wet cough have airway secretions seen bronchoscopically [15]. However, children with dry cough may have minimal to mild airway secretions [15]. Bronchitic disorders such as protracted bronchitis, chronic suppurative lung disease and bronchiectasis are associated with chronic wet cough [16]. They may be entities in their own right or complicate structural lesions (e.g. malacia disorders, fig. 2–4). Protracted bacterial bronchitis (fig. 6, 7; online suppl. video 1) is a common cause of wet cough in children, and their BAL displays airway neutrophilia and has significant growths of common respiratory bacteria (*Streptococcus*

pneumoniae, Haemophilus influenzae and/or *Moraxella catarrhalis*) [17]. In young children with wet cough undergoing FFB, a bronchoscopic secretion scoring system for quantifying airway secretions has been validated [15, 18]. This scoring system (range from bronchoscopic grade 1 to 6) takes into account the amount of secretions seen (relative to airway size) and the number of bronchi involved. It is freely available in the article online [15]. The scoring system also related well to airway cellularity and neutrophilia, as well as to an airway infective state. However, the scoring system is only complementary to cell counts and cultures and cannot replace these laboratory quantification techniques [18].

FFB is not indicated in all children with chronic cough. However, for selected children, normal FFB findings may be equally important for the exclusion of severe conditions such as presence of an airway foreign body. In children without lung disease, the common coexistence of cough with symptoms of gastro-oesophageal reflux is independent of the occurrence of oesophagitis. As airway neutrophilia is absent in these children (when endobronchial airway bacterial infection is absent) [19], no macroscopic abnormality is seen bronchoscopically. Likewise FFB appearances in children with psychogenic cough are usually macroscopically normal. However, there are minor levels of change in the form of laryngeal oedema where flattening of mucosal surfaces over the arytenoids may be seen. While psychogenic cough may have unusual tracheal and vibratory qualities, habitual cough is usually single and dry.

BAL Findings in Children with Chronic Cough
Cough may coexist with conditions discussed in other chapters (e.g. asthma, atelectasis). In situations when the diagnosis is uncertain and/or the chronic cough is non-resolving or worse than expected, FFB and BAL are also indicated. For example in children with asthma, the unresolved chronic cough may be related to coexistent bacterial bronchitis that requires antimicrobial therapy to achieve a cough-free clinical endpoint [16]. Chronic cough is a common symptom in children with tracheobronchomalacia, and these children have an increased likelihood of respiratory illness frequency, severity, significant cough and a tendency for delayed recovery. However, neither site nor severity of malacia exhibited any significant dose effect on respiratory illness profiles [20]. It is highly likely that the chronic cough in children with airway lesions relates to reduced cough efficiency and an increased likelihood of bacterial bronchitis. Indeed, the BAL in these children when coughing is often culture

positive with significant ($\geq 10^5$ CFU/ml) growth of respiratory pathogens [17].

Several groups have examined BAL fluid cellular and inflammatory indices in children with unexplained chronic cough. Fitch et al. [21] examined the BAL in children with untreated unexplained persistent cough and showed that only a minority (3 of 23) of children had asthma-type airway inflammation. Zimmerman et al. [22] studied children with postinfectious cough as well as treated and untreated children with asthma and concluded that postinfectious cough in children has different pathophysiological features than allergic asthma and represents a different disease. Although 6 of the 11 children with postinfectious cough had airway hyperresponsiveness, airway eosinophils and eosinophilic cationic protein were normal [22]. In 150 children without lung disease, we described that the common coexistence of cough with symptoms of reflux oesophagitis is independent of the occurrence of oesophagitis [19]. Unlike adults, airway neutrophilia was not found in children with reflux oesophagitis, and when present is more likely to be related to airway bacterial infection and not to oesophagitis [19]. Also abnormal microbiology of the airways, when present, is not related to reflux oesophagitis and does not reflect that of gastric juices [23]. In a small study of 12 children with chronic cough, Marguet et al. [24] described that the BAL cell profiles of children with chronic cough were similar to those of controls and dissimilar to those of children with asthma.

An increased lipid-laden macrophage index, which represents increased lipid numbers and/or content in alveolar macrophages, was thought to be a useful indicator for recurrent small-volume pulmonary aspiration as a cause of chronic cough. However, significant counts of lipid-laden macrophages can be found in lung diseases from other causes in the absence of aspiration [25]. Indeed Colombo reported that the lipid-laden macrophage index was highest in patients undergoing chemotherapy and suffering from graft-versus-host disease [25]. Thus, the utility of the lipid-laden macrophage index as a sensitive and specific marker of aspiration in children has been questioned. Currently, lipid-laden macrophages as a marker of aspiration are utilized as supportive but not diagnostic evidence.

Thus, other than assessment of airway specimens for microbiological purposes, the use of airway cellular and inflammatory profiles in children with chronic cough is currently limited to supportive diagnosis and research rather than definitive diagnosis. This is in contrast to that in adults with chronic cough where some have suggested to use an airway inflammatory profile (airway eosinophilia in eosinophilic bronchitis) to direct therapy.

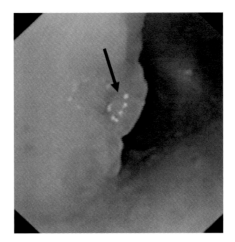

Fig. 9. Foreign body granuloma (arrow) in the right main bronchus in a young infant.

Indications for Bronchial Brushing and Bronchial Biopsy in Chronic Cough

In children with chronic cough, the indications for bronchial brushing and bronchial biopsy are generally related to the macroscopic appearances like a mass lesion such as an endobronchial mass, granulations of uncertain origin or granuloma after foreign body (fig. 9). A biopsy is also indicated in the context of a child with chronic cough and an underlying malignancy or after transplantation. Under such circumstances adequate caution must be taken to ensure adequate samples (size and number) and optimal control of bleeding and/or airway compromise. Outside the situations mentioned above, there is currently insufficient data to advocate a biopsy or bronchial brushing on clinical grounds. This is in contrast to adults in whom subtle changes in airway mucosa may be representative of an airway carcinoma.

Current Unmet Needs and Research Trends

The many large gaps in our knowledge of most clinical aspects of paediatric cough include:

(a) Aspects relevant to FFB and BAL
- The yield of FFB and BAL in defining the aetiology of chronic cough, following specific criteria and management steps
- The role and timing of FFB in different types of cough (e.g. wet, dry, brassy) and clinical settings

(b) Generic aspects

- The criteria for children requiring further investigations based on large cohort studies inclusive of primary care setting
- Understanding how cough and markers of cough severity relate (or otherwise) with other conditions (e.g. a marker of, association with and/or chance occurrence)
- When and which (clinical features and timing) antibiotics should be used in children with chronic moist cough and children with chronic cough after viral infection
- Determination of the optimal definition of acute, subacute and chronic cough based on diagnosis, treatment and outcome criteria
- Natural history and outcomes of children with non-specific cough
- High-quality randomized controlled trials specifically relating to cough as highlighted in many Cochrane reviews on common medication used for cough where no studies were found [26]

Future Research Trends

- *Understanding pathophysiology:* use of bronchial biopsies with staining and examination of sensory nerves, neuropeptides and their precursors

- *Measurement of cough outcomes:* development and use of validated outcomes specific for children in clinical care and research, including patient-important outcomes, objective measures
- *Evidence-based medicine:* improvements in evidence-based recommendations for cough management specific to children and increasing acceptability that children with chronic cough should not be managed like adults with chronic cough
- *Development of cough-specific medications:* medications that can enhance the cough reflex (for conditions where the cough reflex is down-regulated such as in neurological abnormalities) as well as those that can suppress cough when cough is troublesome as opposed to beneficial in airway clearance (e.g. in prolonged postviral dry cough)

Acknowledgements

We thank Barry Dean for obtaining all the images for this chapter.

A.C. is supported by the Australian NHMRC, Queensland Smart State Fund and the Royal Children's Hospital Foundation.

References

1 Canning BJ: The cough reflex in animals: relevance to human cough research. Lung 2008;186(suppl 1):S23–S28.

2 Lee MG, Undem BJ. Basic mechanisms of cough: current understanding and remaining questions. Lung 2008;186(suppl 1):S10–S16.

3 McCool FD: Global physiology and pathophysiology of cough: ACCP evidence-based clinical practice guidelines. Chest 2006;129:48–53.

4 Mazzone SB, Undem BJ: Cough sensors. V. Pharmacological modulation of cough sensors. Handb Exp Pharmacol 2009;187:99–127.

5 Chang AB: The physiology of cough. Paediatr Respir Rev 2006;7:2–8.

6 Weir K, McMahon S, Barry L, Masters IB, Chang AB: Clinical signs and symptoms of oropharyngeal aspiration and dysphagia in children. Eur Respir J 2009;33:604–611.

7 Sekizawa S, Chen CY, Bechtold AG, Tabor JM, Bric JM, Pinkerton KE, Joad JP, Bonham AC: Extended secondhand tobacco smoke exposure induces plasticity in nucleus tractus solitarius second-order lung afferent neurons in young guinea pigs. Eur J Neurosci 2008;28:771–781.

8 Yu M, Zheng X, Peake J, Joad JP, Pinkerton KE: Perinatal environmental tobacco smoke exposure alters the immune response and airway innervation in infant primates. J Allergy Clin Immunol 2008;122:640–647.

9 Newcombe PA, Sheffield JK, Juniper EF, Halstead RA, Masters IB, Chang AB: Development of a parent-proxy quality-of-life chronic cough-specific questionnaire: clinical impact vs psychometric evaluations. Chest 2008;133:386–395.

10 Wood RE: The diagnostic effectiveness of the flexible bronchoscope in children. Pediatr Pulmonol 1985;1:188–192.

11 Thomson F, Masters IB, Chang AB: Persistent cough in children – overuse of medications. J Paediatr Child Health 2002;38:578–581.

12 De Blic J, Marchac V, Scheinmann P: Complications of flexible bronchoscopy in children: prospective study of 1,328 procedures. Eur Respir J 2002;20:1271–1276.

13 Callahan CW: Etiology of chronic cough in a population of children referred to a pediatric pulmonologist. J Am Board Fam Pract 1996;9:324–327.

14 Masters IB: Congenital airway lesions and lung disease. Pediatr Clin North Am 2009;56:227–242.

15 Chang AB, Eastburn MM, Gaffney J, Faoagali J, Cox NC, Masters IB: Cough quality in children: a comparison of subjective vs bronchoscopic findings. Respir Res 2005;6:3.

16 Chang AB, Redding GJ, Everard ML: Chronic wet cough: protracted bronchitis, chronic suppurative lung disease and bronchiectasis. Pediatr Pulmonol 2008;43:519–531.

17 Marchant JM, Masters IB, Taylor SM, Cox NC, Seymour GJ, Chang AB: Evaluation and outcome of young children with chronic cough. Chest 2006;129:1132–1141.

18 Chang AB, Faoagali J, Cox NC, Marchant JM, Dean B, Petsky HL, Masters IB: A bronchoscopic scoring system for airway secretions – airway cellularity and microbiological validation. Pediatr Pulmonol 2006;41:887–892.

19 Chang AB, Cox NC, Faoagali J, Cleghorn GJ, Beem C, Ee LC, Withers GD, Patrick MK, Lewindon PJ: Cough and reflux esophagitis in children: their co-existence and airway cellularity. BMC Pediatr 2006;6:4.

20 Masters IB, Zimmerman PV, Pandeya N, Petsky HL, Wilson SB, Chang AB: Quantified tracheobronchomalacia disorders and their clinical profiles in children. Chest 2007;133:461–467.

21 Fitch PS, Brown V, Schock BC, Taylor R, Ennis M, Shields MD: Chronic cough in children: bronchoalveolar lavage findings. Eur Respir J 2000;16:1109–1114.

22 Zimmerman B, Silverman FS, Tarlo SM, Chapman KR, Kubay JM, Urch B: Induced sputum: comparison of postinfectious cough with allergic asthma in children. J Allergy Clin Immunol 2000;105:495–499.

23 Chang AB, Cox NC, Purcell J, Marchant JM, Lewindon PJ, Cleghorn GJ, Ee LC, Withers GD, Patrick MK, Faoagali J: Airway cellularity, lipid laden macrophages and microbiology of gastric juice and airways in children with reflux oesophagitis. Respir Res 2005;6:72.

24 Marguet C, Jouen Boedes F, Dean TP, Warner JO: Bronchoalveolar cell profiles in children with asthma, infantile wheeze, chronic cough, or cystic fibrosis. Am J Respir Crit Care Med 1999;159:1533–1540.

25 Colombo JL: Pulmonary aspiration and lipid-laden macrophages: in search of gold (standards). Pediatr Pulmonol 1999;28:79–82.

26 Chang AB: Cough. Pediatr Clin North Am 2009;56:19–31.

Anne B. Chang
Queensland Children's Respiratory Centre, Royal Children's Hospital
Herston, Brisbane, Qld. 4029 (Australia)
Tel. +61 7 3636 5270, Fax +61 7 3636 1958, E-Mail annechang@ausdoctors.net

Priftis KN, Anthracopoulos MB, Eber E, Koumbourlis AC, Wood RE (eds): Paediatric Bronchoscopy.
Prog Respir Res. Basel, Karger 2010, vol 38, pp 191–197

Lung Transplant Recipients and Other Immunosuppressed Patients

Christian Benden[a] · Paul Aurora[b]

[a]Division of Pulmonary Medicine, University Hospital Zurich, Zurich, Switzerland; [b]Cardiothoracic Transplant Unit and Respiratory Medicine Unit, Great Ormond Street Hospital for Children, London, UK

Abstract

This review examines the utility of flexible bronchoscopy (FB) in paediatric lung transplant recipients and other immunosuppressed children, including indications and contraindications, risk-benefits and potential complications of bronchoalveolar lavage (BAL) and transbronchial biopsy (TBB). FB with BAL/TBB is a valuable tool to establish the presence or absence of acute lung allograft rejection and/or infection that provides a high sensitivity and specificity; however, bronchiolitis obliterans (BO) is less well diagnosed. FB with BAL/TBB can be carried out safely with a good yield. The complication rate of the procedure is low. FB is clinically indicated in every symptomatic paediatric lung transplant recipient. The majority of paediatric centres perform regularly scheduled surveillance bronchoscopies with BAL/TBB, aiming to reduce the incidence of BO by earlier detection of acute rejection or infection and to target therapy; however, it is not clear whether surveillance bronchoscopy improves long-term posttransplantation survival. The role of FB in other immunosuppressed children with pulmonary complications is less well defined, but the technique is valuable in identifying infection and thus guiding treatment. Immunosuppressed patients are often highly symptomatic and sometimes in borderline respiratory failure; therefore, the potential risk-benefit profile of FB has to be assessed first.

Lung transplantation has become an accepted therapy option for end-stage parenchymal and vascular lung disease in children [1]. Sixty to 70 paediatric lung transplantations are performed worldwide each year, mostly in adolescents. Overall, the most common indication for lung transplantation in the paediatric age group is advanced cystic fibrosis lung disease [2].

Besides improvements in short-term survival over the last decade, long-term outcome following lung transplantation remains inferior compared to other solid-organ transplantations [3]. The commonest causes of death in the early posttransplantation period are graft failure and infection, with acute rejection accounting for up to 4% of deaths 1 year after the procedure. Bronchiolitis obliterans (BO) is the major cause (>40%) of morbidity and mortality in paediatric lung recipients in the first 5 years after transplantation [2]. BO has been defined pathologically as the airway response to chronic graft rejection that manifests itself as fibroproliferative obstruction of the airway lumen [3]. Since this condition can only be confirmed by open lung biopsy, a physiological correlate of BO, termed bronchiolitis obliterans syndrome (BOS), has been defined based on the development of permanent airflow obstruction after transplantation [4]. The histological diagnosis of BO is made according to the recently updated recommendations of the International Society for Heart and Lung Transplantation for the standardization of nomenclature for the grading of lung allograft rejection (table 1) [5]. Histological examples of minimal acute cellular allograft rejection (grade A1) and mild acute cellular allograft rejection (A2) are displayed in figures 1 and 2. Likewise, the physiological diagnosis of BOS is made according to the recently updated recommendations [6].

The mechanisms underlying graft deterioration are not entirely understood; however, multiple alloimmunological and non-alloimmunological factors seem to play a role [3]. Acute allograft rejection following lung transplantation is relatively common, with the majority of lung transplant recipients experiencing a minimum of 1 biopsy-proven acute allograft rejection episode during the first 12 months

Table 1. Revised working formulation for classification/grading of pulmonary allograft rejection

Class A: acute rejection
 Grade 0 – none
 Grade 1 – minimal
 Grade 2 – mild
 Grade 3 – moderate
 Grade 4 – severe

Class B: airway inflammation
 Grade 0 – none
 Grade 1 – low grade
 Grade 2 – high grade
 Grade X – ungradeable

Class C: chronic airway rejection – obliterative bronchiolitis
 Grade 0 – absent
 Grade 1 – present

Class D: chronic vascular rejection

Reproduced from Stewart et al. [5], with permission from the publisher.

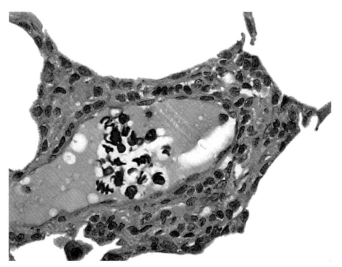

Fig. 1. Minimal acute cellular lung allograft rejection (grade A1) with a characteristic circumferential perivascular interstitial mononuclear cell inflammatory infiltrate (courtesy of Peter Vogt, MD, Institute of Clinical Pathology, University Hospital Zurich, Switzerland). Haematoxylin-eosin staining.

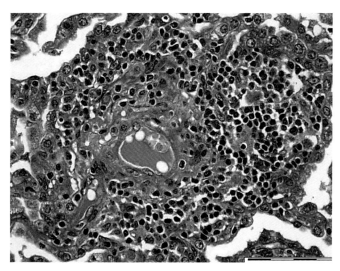

Fig. 2. Mild acute cellular lung allograft rejection (grade A2) with a characteristic circumferential expansion of the perivascular interstitium of small vessels due to a mononuclear cell inflammatory infiltrate (courtesy of Peter Vogt, MD, Institute of Clinical Pathology, University Hospital Zurich, Switzerland). Haematoxylin-eosin staining.

after transplantation [7]. Initially, transbronchial biopsy (TBB) was implemented as the equivalent of endomyocardial biopsy for the diagnosis of acute lung allograft rejection in heart-lung transplant recipients; this provided a high sensitivity and specificity in the detection of acute rejection [8]. However, BO is less efficiently diagnosed by TBB.

Graft function following paediatric lung transplantation can be assessed non-invasively by lung function tests or chest imaging. Unfortunately, none of these investigations can reliably establish the diagnosis of acute graft rejection or distinguish acute rejection from lower airway infection. Plain chest radiography and computed tomography (CT) may be normal in the presence of moderate acute allograft rejection [1]. It should be emphasized that the clinical symptoms of acute allograft rejection can be mild and non-specific, encompassing cough, mild dyspnoea, low-grade pyrexia or just malaise. Bronchoscopy is, therefore, considered to be the gold standard for the diagnosis of acute allograft rejection and for its differentiation from other pathology [1].

It is important to note that the published literature in the field of paediatric lung transplantation consists mostly of single-centre reports that include retrospective studies. There are only a few published articles each year, a situation which is not comparable to the wealth of original literature that is published annually on other respiratory diseases such as childhood asthma. This is rather expected considering the small number of paediatric lung transplantations performed each year. Indeed, there are less than 30 established paediatric lung transplantation programmes worldwide, only 2 of which perform as many as 10–15 transplantations annually;

the vast majority of paediatric centres carry out less than 5 transplantations each year.

Indications for Flexible Bronchoscopy in Lung Transplant Recipients

In the immediate posttransplantation period, flexible bronchoscopy (FB) – including bronchoalveolar lavage (BAL) with or without TBB – is performed to inspect the size of bronchial anastomoses, confirm bronchial healing and assess the appearance of the mucosa. Occasionally, it is necessary to remove mucus plugs or re-inflate atelectatic areas. In the later posttransplantation period, FB with BAL and TBB can be performed to evaluate new-onset clinical symptoms, follow up a confirmed acute rejection episode to ensure successful treatment, or for surveillance purposes.

The first of these indications is uncontroversial, and a low threshold for FB with BAL and TBB is advised in every child who presents with lung function deterioration, worsening respiratory symptoms or unexplained changes on plain chest radiography or CT. Whilst it is sometimes advisable to treat for infection even in the absence of laboratory confirmation, it is rarely acceptable to augment immunosuppression in the absence of histological confirmation of acute graft rejection as the side effects of the treatment are considerable [1].

The necessity for follow-up TBBs after treatment of acute rejection is more controversial [9]. Many centres opt not to perform TBB in children who have shown marked clinical improvement following therapy. However, Aboyoun et al. [10], in a comprehensive study of adult patients, have reported on the results of 173 follow-up TBBs in 99 transplant recipients with acute graft rejection (≥A2); they found that follow-up procedures demonstrated persistent acute rejection (≥A2) in approximately one quarter of the cases, despite corticosteroid therapy. Unfortunately, there are no published data in children, and the protocols of different centres vary on this matter.

Routine surveillance TBB, performed at regular intervals in asymptomatic transplant recipients, aims to detect acute rejection in order to treat patients as early as possible by augmenting immunosuppressive treatment. There is no question that lung transplant recipients can have acute rejection in the absence of symptoms, spirometric deterioration or chest radiographic changes. Faro and Visner [11] summarized the results of 11 recently published studies in adult populations, which demonstrate an incidence of acute rejection (≥A2) of approximately 14%, i.e. treatable

grades of rejection that would have been missed otherwise. There have been 2 studies describing the prevalence of acute rejection in paediatric lung transplant recipients. A North American paediatric study investigated the role of TBB and reported an incidence of acute rejection (≥A2) of 25% among 46 children after lung or heart-lung transplantation [12]; in this study one quarter of TBBs were performed for surveillance purposes. An UK study documented an incidence of acute rejection (≥A2) of 12% in symptomatic as compared to 4% in asymptomatic children during the first year after lung transplantation [13]. The prevalence of silent acute rejection following lung transplantation in both children and adults is therefore well established. It is assumed that detection and prompt treatment of these rejection episodes will result in better outcomes and, more specifically, in a lower incidence of BO/BOS. Unfortunately, there are no specifically designed studies to answer this question even in adult transplant recipients.

According to a recent informal survey of paediatric lung transplantation centres within the International Paediatric Lung Transplant Collaborative, three quarters of paediatric centres currently perform surveillance bronchoscopies with BAL and TBB at least during the first year after transplantation [Faro A., pers. commun.]. In addition, these procedures are performed whenever a paediatric lung transplant recipient presents with symptoms and/or laboratory investigations suggestive of acute rejection and/or infection presenting with cough, sputum production, dyspnoea, malaise, chest radiographic changes or a more than 10% decline in forced expiratory volume in 1 s. Experts in the field recommend routine surveillance bronchoscopy of children with BAL and TBB during the first year after lung transplantation. A minimum of 4 procedures should be undertaken, i.e. at 1 month, and thereafter at 3, 6 and 12 months following transplantation. Nevertheless, it should be noted that the impact of such a protocol of aggressive surveillance and intervention has not been formally evaluated.

Bronchoalveolar Lavage in Lung Transplant Recipients

The main purpose of BAL is the diagnosis of lung graft infection, more particularly of a subclinical one. General instructions regarding the technique of BAL in children are described in chapter 3 of this volume [pp. 30–41]. Details of the volume of BAL fluid (BALF) and the number of aliquots instilled, and details for processing of the recovered BALF are provided in the most recent European Respiratory Society Task Force statement [14].

Briefly, BALF should be examined microscopically as a direct wet preparation and after Gram and Ziehl-Neelsen staining. Additionally, BALF should be cultured semi-quantitatively for bacteria and fungi, including a culture for mycobacteria. Immunofluorescence techniques can be used for detection of cytomegalovirus (CMV), adenovirus, influenza virus types A and B, para-influenza virus types 1–3, respiratory syncytial virus and *Pneumocystis jiroveci*. Supplementary testing for viral DNA is recommended by using the polymerase chain reaction (PCR) technique. CMV detection by PCR in BALF of lung transplant recipients has been proven to be a more sensitive technique as compared to quantitative measurements of viral load in the recipients' plasma for the diagnosis of CMV infection. Moreover, quantification of the CMV load in the BALF seems to correlate with the histological detection of CMV in the lung graft, which probably makes this examination useful for monitoring subclinical CMV replication in the lungs [15]. Michelson et al. [16] have recently published data on quantitative measurements of Epstein-Barr viral load in the BALF of paediatric lung and heart-lung transplant recipients, showing that the Epstein-Barr viral load in the BALF may be a valuable tool to screen for posttransplantation lymphoproliferative disease, possibly superior to peripheral blood assays.

Differential cytology is usually performed on cell preparations after centrifugation [chapter 3, this vol., pp. 30–41]. In the field of lung transplantation, it is vital to take into consideration the natural time course of cellular morphological changes in the BALF of lung transplant recipients. Early posttransplantation (<3 months) BALF total cell counts are elevated, and a neutrophilic alveolitis is common; these findings characterize the cellular response to the lung graft injury. Later in the posttransplantation time course, the CD4:CD8 ratio decreases due to the lower percentage of CD4 cells in the BALF. BALF neutrophilia may even be of prognostic value in the identification of lung transplant recipients at risk for BOS. A recent observational study investigated the potential associations of BALF neutrophilia with lung allograft rejection and BOS in a cohort of stable lung transplant recipients (n = 63). BALF neutrophilia of ≥20% was shown to independently predict BOS ≥1 [17].

Transbronchial Biopsy in Lung Transplant Recipients

The general technique of TBB is described in detail in chapter 4 of this volume [pp. 42–53]. An adult-sized flexible bronchoscope can be used in paediatric lung transplant recipients to perform TBB; however, it may be advantageous to use a laryngeal mask if the external diameter of the flexible bronchoscope is too large to fit through the endotracheal tube. Generally, we recommend that the TBB be performed unilaterally in children following bilateral cadaveric lung (or heart-lung) transplantation to prevent the risk of bilateral pneumothoraces. However, in recipients of living donor transplants, TBB should ideally be carried out bilaterally to sample both lungs, in order to account for the fact that unilateral acute rejection can occur as two different living donors are involved in this type of transplantation procedure. The TBB should be performed in the periphery of the lung, aiming to obtain parenchymal as well as bronchial tissue. Furthermore, we advocate sampling the lower lobes, not only to minimize the risk of pneumothoraces, but also because there is evidence that adequate tissue samples are obtained more reliably from this area of the lung [18].

The main problem with TBB in paediatric lung transplant recipients is the relatively small size of the tissue sample obtained with the small biopsy forceps. In their retrospective study, Visner and Faro [12] showed that adequate tissue specimens were obtained in 85% of TBBs performed in children using a paediatric flexible instrument, while the success rate rose to 97% when using an adult flexible bronchoscope. Therefore, the use of an adult-sized flexible bronchoscope is recommended in older children whenever possible. In smaller children, a paediatric flexible bronchoscope with a smaller instrumentation channel is used. The bronchoscope is positioned above the segment to be sampled, and then the forceps are passed through the instrumentation channel into the lung periphery under fluoroscopic guidance (fig. 3). The biopsy forceps are withdrawn slightly, opened, advanced, then closed and finally pulled back. The tissue specimen is placed in a formalin-filled container, the forceps are cleaned in sterile normal saline, and the procedure is repeated. A minimum of 5 well-sized specimens of tissue should be obtained according to the recently published recommendations [5]. At the end of the procedure, brief visualization of the biopsy site is advisable to exclude prolonged bleeding.

If TBB is unsuccessful in providing an appropriate tissue sample and the establishment of diagnosis is imperative, video-assisted thoracoscopic surgery or open lung biopsy may be required [19].

Complications

Overall, the complication rate of FB in children is low [20]. Details regarding general complications of paediatric FB are described in chapters 2 and 8 of this volume [pp. 22–29

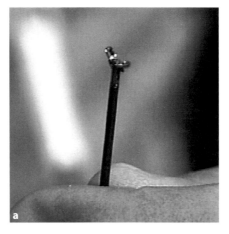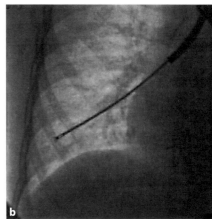

Fig. 3. a A 2.0-mm alligator biopsy forceps (open). **b** Flexible bronchoscope (4.5 mm external diameter) with open alligator biopsy forceps (2.0 mm) positioned in an airway of the right lower lobe.

and pp. 83–94]. The most important specific complications associated with TBB are bleeding and pneumothorax [21]. Chhajed et al. [22] reported that the severity of bleeding was independent of a number of specific risk factors such as gender, type of transplantation, acute rejection, BOS status, number of biopsies per procedure, infections and number of days after transplantation. As is usually the case, data in children are limited. The complication rates quoted in the 2 most recent paediatric studies involving TBB in children after lung transplantation [11, 13] were 1.8 and 3.2%, respectively. Taking the 2 studies together, pneumothoraces occurred in less than 1% of more than 500 procedures performed.

No guidelines exist with regard to the necessary investigations prior to the procedure. Our own practice is to ensure a minimum platelet count of 50,000/mm^3 and a clotting profile within the normal range prior to performing TBB. Minimal bleeding (less than 10 ml) is common. In case of moderate bleeding, the procedure should be interrupted until the bleeding stops. In this situation, the authors recommend to withdraw the bronchoscope, and continue with positive pressure ventilation – ideally with high end-expiratory pressure – for 5–10 min and then re-inspect the bleeding site. Severe bleeding (more than 100 ml) caused by TBB in transplant recipients is very rare. In these circumstances, it may be necessary to wedge the bronchoscope into the relevant segmental bronchus to act as a plug, or to instil iced saline or epinephrine.

The risk of pneumothorax can be reduced by avoiding upper lobe biopsies and by using fluoroscopic guidance. However, it is likely that a regular operator will on occasion encounter this complication; therefore, equipment for pleural drainage should be available in the bronchoscopy suite. Furthermore, we recommend performing a plain chest radiograph 2–4 h after the procedure to detect a slowly developing pneumothorax. However, a chest X-ray is not universally performed after TBB as some centres rely upon clinical deterioration of the patient to detect this complication.

In addition to the risks of bleeding and pneumothorax, a number of other issues need to be considered. In the early posttransplantation period, it is essential to minimize the risk of airway trauma due to instrumentation, particularly at the site of the bronchial anastomosis. If some stenosis at this site is already present, then further trauma may result in critical airway stenosis. Since the use of an adult-sized flexible instrument is required in order to obtain satisfactory biopsy specimens, airway obstruction occurs more frequently in these patients than is generally reported for bronchoscopy.

Transient fever and bacteraemia may occur following BAL. In immunosuppressed children however, transient bacteraemia may set off serious problems and result in septicaemia. The authors recommend a low threshold for the use of antibiotic therapy in this scenario.

Flexible Bronchoscopy in Other Immunosuppressed Children

Children who have received bone marrow transplantation (BMT) or other solid-organ transplants and children who are immunosuppressed due to chemotherapy for malignancy are at risk of lower respiratory tract infections, resulting in substantial morbidity and mortality [chapter 3, this vol., pp. 30–41]. After BMT, 25% of children suffer pulmonary complications [23]. Clinical examination, pulmonary function tests and/or chest imaging (chest X-ray, CT) may assist the diagnosis; however, they are usually unhelpful in providing a definitive diagnosis, identifying possible infectious aetiologies and distinguishing infectious from non-infectious complications. FB with BAL should be considered in immunosuppressed children who develop unexplained pulmonary infiltrates, hypoxaemia or abnormal findings on chest auscultation. This group of immunosuppressed children are often highly symptomatic and sometimes in borderline respiratory failure. Therefore, the physician is obliged to individually assess the potential risk-benefit profile of FB. In selected patients with severe respiratory compromise, non-bronchoscopic BAL may be the preferred diagnostic tool. Non-bronchoscopic BAL is known to have a very good safety profile in children with auto-immune disease or primary immunodeficiency [24].

When bronchoscopy with BAL is undertaken in immunosuppressed children, a good yield is generally reported. *Pneumocystis jiroveci* and CMV are the most commonly isolated pathogens in this group, while bacterial, viral and fungal pathogens are less frequently isolated [25]. McCubbin et al. [26] have reported on the BAL findings of 27 paediatric BMT recipients; an opportunistic pathogen was isolated in more than 50% of cases, most commonly CMV, followed by *P. jiroveci* and other fungi. Furthermore, a recent retrospective North American study in paediatric cancer patients on chemotherapy showed that both positive and negative BAL results contribute to patient care [27]. In this study, diagnosis was established in 30% of 53 paediatric patients in whom BAL was performed, and clinical management was altered in an additional 26%. Moreover, BAL led to a change in the clinical decision-making in one third of ventilated and non-ventilated children after BMT [28]. According to a study from Chicago that included 89 paediatric haematopoietic stem cell transplantation recipients, despite the relatively high diagnostic yield of BAL in children after haematopoietic stem cell transplantation, the procedure is unlikely to provide additional information particularly in recipients with grades II–IV acute graft-versus-host disease (GVHD) and those who are immunosuppressed [29].

Ideally, BAL should be performed prior to the start of antimicrobial therapy. Furthermore, BAL is indicated in children who clinically deteriorate regardless of appropriate antimicrobial therapy. The microbiological results in immunosuppressed children need to be interpreted carefully and, if in doubt, they should be discussed with an infectious disease specialist and/or a microbiologist. BALF results are helpful if pathogenic organisms are isolated to guide antibiotic therapy. BALF neutrophilia suggests bacterial rather

than opportunistic infection such as *P. jiroveci* or CMV. Furthermore, only positive BALF findings for pathogens such as *P. jiroveci* and *Mycobacterium tuberculosis,* which are not part of the normal airway flora, are considered to be diagnostic. Clinical judgement should guide the initiation of antimicrobial therapy despite negative BALF results. In any event, the diagnostic yield of BALF and the sensitivity and specificity of newer molecular techniques such as PCR for the detection of *P. jiroveci* and CMV in the BALF of immunosuppressed children require further research.

To date, there are very few published data on BALF cytology in children following BMT and in paediatric cancer patients. A recently published retrospective study [23] investigated the role of BALF cytology in the diagnosis of pulmonary GVHD by comparing BALF results of children after allogenic BMT to those of paediatric cancer patients undergoing chemotherapy. Both groups presented with rapidly progressing respiratory symptoms and abnormal radiological findings (new or persistent infiltrate on chest radiography and/or CT). Nine BMT patients with respiratory symptoms underwent 17 bronchoscopies that included BAL and were compared to 10 oncological patients who underwent 13 bronchoscopies with BAL. In both groups, the BALF total cell count was increased; however, the BMT BALF samples were characterized by a higher percentage of lymphocytes and a lower percentage of neutrophils. Despite the small cohort size, these data suggest that the presence of BAL lymphocytosis and atypical epithelial cells, concomitantly with respiratory symptoms and GVHD in other organs, may be a useful marker of pulmonary GVHD [23].

The role of TBB in immunosuppressed children is limited, and there is a lack of published data regarding its use in these patients. A recent study of adult haematopoietic stem cell transplant recipients reported that TBB provided additional information to BAL in less than 10% of cases [30]. Tissue diagnosis may be helpful in case of suspected fungal infection (*Aspergillus* or *Candida* spp.), where the specificity of BAL is rather poor [31]. Unfortunately, the small tissue sample size that is obtainable via TBB is often insufficient for pathology. The authors of this chapter consider the use of TBB in immunosuppressed children other than lung transplant recipients of no particular value; therefore, no data are provided on this subject. Video-assisted thoracoscopic surgery or open lung biopsy may be the preferred tool for this application. The role of open lung biopsy for the evaluation of persistent pulmonary infiltrates in immunosuppressed children is beyond the scope of this chapter.

References

1 Benden C, Aurora P: Paediatric aspects of lung transplantation. Eur Respir Mon 2009;45:251–265.

2 Aurora P, Edwards LB, Christie J, Dobbels F, Kirk R, Kucheryavaya AY, Rahmel AO, Taylor DO, Hertz MI: Registry of the International Society for Heart and Lung Transplantation: eleventh official pediatric lung and heart/lung transplantation report – 2008. J Heart Lung Transplant 2008;27:978–983.

3 Belperio JA, Weigt SS, Fishbein MC, Lynch JP 3rd: Chronic lung allograft rejection: mechanisms and therapy. Proc Am Thorac Soc 2009;6:108–121.

4 Hachem RR, Trulock EP: Bronchiolitis obliterans syndrome: pathogenesis and management. Semin Thorac Cardiovasc Surg 2004;16:350–355

5 Stewart S, Fishbein MC, Snell GI, Berry GJ, Boehler A, Burke MM, Glanville A, Gould FK, Magro C, Marboe CC, McNeil KD, Reed EF, Reinsmoen NL, Scott JP, Studer SM, Tazelaar HD, Wallwork JL, Westall G, Zamora MR, Zeevi A, Yousem SA : Revision of the 1996 working formulation for the standardization of nomenclature in the diagnosis of lung rejection. J Heart Lung Transplant 2007;26:1229–1242.

6 Estenne M, Maurer JR, Boehler A, Egan JJ, Frost A, Hertz M, Mallory GB, Snell GI, Yousem S: Bronchiolitis obliterans syndrome 2001: an update of the diagnostic criteria. J Heart Lung Transplant 2002;21:297–310.

7 Knoop C, Estenne M: Acute and chronic rejection after lung transplantation. Semin Respir Crit Care Med 2006;27:512–533.

8 Tazelaar HD, Nilsson FN, Rinaldi M, Murtaugh P, McDouglas JC, McGregor CG: The sensitivity of transbronchial biopsy for the diagnosis of acute lung rejection. J Thorac Cardiovasc Surg 1993;105:761–773.

9 Glanville AR: The role of bronchoscopic surveillance monitoring in the care of lung transplant recipients. Semin Respir Crit Care Med 2006;27:480–491.

10 Aboyoun CL, Tamm M, Chhajed PN, Hopkins P, Malouf MA, Rainer S, Glanville AR: Diagnostic value of follow-up transbronchial lung biopsy after lung rejection. Am J Respir Crit Care Med 2001:164:460–463.

11 Faro A, Visner G: The use of multiple transbronchial biopsies as the standard approach to evaluate lung allograft rejection. Pediatr Transplant 2004;8:322–328.

12 Visner GA, Faro A: Role of transbronchial biopsies in pediatric lung disease. Chest 2004;126:273–280.

13 Benden C, Harpur-Sinclair O, Ranasinghe AS, Hartley JC, Elliott MJ, Aurora P: Surveillance bronchoscopy in children during the first year after lung transplantation – is it worth it? Thorax 2007;62:57–61.

14 De Blic J, Midulla F, Barbato A, Clement A, Dab I, Eber E, Green C, Grigg J, Kotecha S, Kurland G, Pohunek P, Ratjen F, Rossi G: Bronchoalveolar lavage in children. ERS Task Force on bronchoalveolar lavage in children. Eur Respir J 2000;15:217–231.

15 Westall GP, Michaelides A, Williams TJ, Snell GI, Kotsimbos TC: Human cytomegalovirus load in plasma and bronchoalveolar fluid: a longitudinal study of lung transplant recipients. J Infect Dis 2004;190:1076–1083.

16 Michelson P, Watkins B, Webber SA, Wadowsky R, Michaels MG: Screening for PTLD in lung and heart-lung transplant recipients by measuring EBV DNA load in bronchoalveolar lavage fluid using real time PCR. Pediatr Transplant 2008;12:464–468.

17 Neurohr C, Huppmann P, Samweber B, Leuschner S, Zimmermann G, Leuchte H, Baumgartner R, Hatz R, Frey L, Ueberfuhr P, Bittmann I, Behr J, Munich Lung Transplant Group: Prognostic value of bronchoalveolar lavage neutrophilia in stable lung transplant recipients. J Heart Lung Transplant 2009;28:468–474.

18 Hasegawa T, Iacono AT, Yousem SA: The anatomic distribution of acute cellular rejection in the allograft lung. Ann Thorac Surg 2000;69:1529–1531.

19 Choong CK, Haddad FJ, Huddleston CB, Bell J, Guthrie TJ, Mendeloff EN, Schuler P, De la Morena M, Sweet SC: Role of open lung biopsy in lung transplant recipients in a single children's hospital: a 13-year experience. J Thorac Cardiovasc Surg 2006;131:204–208.

20 De Blic J, Marchac V, Scheinmann P: Complications of flexible bronchoscopy in children: prospective study of 1,328 procedures. Eur Respir J 2002;20:1271–1276.

21 Midulla F, de Blic J, Barbato A, Bush A, Eber E, Kotecha S, Haxby E, Moretti C, Pohunek P, Ratjen F, ERS Task Force: Flexible endoscopy of paediatric airways. Eur Respir J 2003;22:698–708.

22 Chhajed PN, Aboyoun C, Malouf MA, Hopkins PM, Plit ML, Glanville AR: Risk factors and management of bleeding associated with transbronchial lung biopsy in lung transplant recipients. J Heart Lung Transplant 2003;22:195–197.

23 Rochat I, Posfay-Barbe KM, Kumar N, Pache JC, Kaiser L, Ozsahin H, Barazzone Argiroffo C, Bongiovanni M: Bronchoalveolar cytology for diagnosing pulmonary GVHD after bone marrow transplant in children. Pediatr Pulmonol 2008;43:697–702.

24 Slatter MA, Rogerson EJ, Taylor CE, Galloway A, Clark JE, Flood TJ, Abinun M, Cant AJ, Gennery AR: Value of bronchoalveolar lavage before haematopoietic stem cell transplantation for primary immunodeficiency or autoimmune diseases. Bone Marrow Transplant 2007;40:529–533.

25 Lanino E, Sacco O, Kotitsa Z, Rabagliati A, Castagnola E, Garaventa A, Dallorso S, Gandolfo A, Manfredini L, Venzano P, Savioli C, Mació L, Dini G, Rossi GA: Fiberoptic bronchoscopy and bronchoalveolar lavage for the evaluation of pulmonary infiltrates after BMT in children. Bone Marrow Transplant 1996;18:117–120.

26 McCubbin MM, Trigg ME, Hendricker CM, Wagener JS: Bronchoscopy with bronchoalveolar lavage in the evaluation of pulmonary complications of bone marrow transplantation in children. Pediatr Pulmonol 1992;12:43–47.

27 Park JR, Fogarty S, Brogan TV: Clinical utility of bronchoalveolar lavage in pediatric cancer patients. Med Pediatr Oncol 2002;39:175–180.

28 Ben-Ari J, Yaniv I, Nahum E, Stein J, Samra Z, Schonfeld T: Yield of bronchoalveolar lavage in ventilated and non-ventilated children after bone marrow transplantation. Bone Marrow Transplant 2001;27:191–194.

29 Kasow KA, King E, Rochester R, Tong X, Srivastava DK, Horwitz EM, Leung W, Woodard P, Handgretinger R, Hale GA: Diagnostic yield of bronchoalveolar lavage is low in allogeneic hematopoietic stem cell recipients receiving immunosuppressive therapy or with acute graft-versus-host disease: the St Jude experience, 1990–2002. Biol Blood Marrow Transplant 2007;13:831–837.

30 Patel NR, Lee PS, Kim JH, Weinhouse GL, Koziel H: The influence of diagnostic bronchoscopy on clinical outcomes comparing adult autologous and allogeneic bone marrow transplant patients. Chest 2005;127:1388–1396.

31 Efrati O, Gonik U, Bielorai B, Modan-Moses D, Neumann Y, Szeinberg A, Vardi A, Barak A, Paret G, Toren A: Fiberoptic bronchoscopy and bronchoalveolar lavage for the evaluation of pulmonary disease in children with primary immunodeficiency and cancer. Pediatr Blood Cancer 2007;48:324–329.

Dr. Christian Benden
Division of Pulmonary Medicine, University Hospital Zurich
Raemistrasse 100
CH–8091 Zurich (Switzerland)
Tel. +41 44 255 2186, Fax +41 44 255 8997, E-Mail Christian_benden@yahoo.de

Epilogue

Priftis KN, Anthracopoulos MB, Eber E, Koumbourlis AC, Wood RE (eds): Paediatric Bronchoscopy.
Prog Respir Res. Basel, Karger 2010, vol 38, pp 200–204

A Four-Decade Perspective on Paediatric Bronchoscopy – Where Have We Come from, and Where Are We Going?

Robert E. Wood

Division of Pulmonary Medicine, Cincinnati Children's Hospital Medical Center, University of Cincinnati College of Medicine, Cincinnati, Ohio, USA

Bronchoscopy is a technique that enables the physician to visualize the interior of the patient's airways – an otherwise dark and mysterious place. During the first 6 or 7 decades after the advent of bronchoscopy, paediatric applications were very limited, and most if not all paediatric procedures were performed for the relief of airway obstruction, primarily by foreign bodies. The first major breakthrough came with the development of the glass rod telescope in the early 1970s, which was also about the same time as the introduction of flexible instruments for adult use. The glass rod telescope remains the gold standard for optical performance, yielding virtually infinite image resolution, but it is of course limited by the inconvenient fact that light travels in straight lines. Rigid instruments simply cannot go into many of the places where flexible instruments will...

While the advent of glass rod telescope technology opened the field of diagnostic paediatric bronchoscopy, the introduction of the flexible bronchoscope (approx. in 1970–1971) opened bronchoscopy to the non-surgical medical specialists. Prior to the 1970s, very few pulmonologists performed (rigid) bronchoscopy. There were, understandably, some issues of role confusion and 'turf' between surgical and non-surgical specialists. Eventually, it became clear that flexible bronchoscopy was a valid, legitimate and extremely useful technique for the pulmonologist treating adult patients, and the surgeons continue to be the predominant users of rigid instruments. The surgeons have since been kept happily occupied dealing with the large influx of patients referred to them by their medical colleagues who have discovered surgical problems in the course of performing flexible bronchoscopies.

It required a decade after the introduction of flexible bronchoscopes to adult practice for the development of a useful paediatric instrument. After appealing to the Olympus Corporation for a paediatric flexible bronchoscope, I was fortunate to have the opportunity to use one of the first, if not the first, such prototype, beginning in 1978. This instrument was 3.5–3.7 mm in diameter and had a suction channel that was only 1.2 mm in diameter. Despite considerable scepticism on the part of the manufacturer, who had difficulty imagining that anyone would ever use such an instrument, it proved to be useful indeed. And predictably, the introduction of this instrument generated considerable controversy among our surgical colleagues. After my first presentation at a national conference, I was publicly accused of 'medical voyeurism' (presumably because it was perceived that a flexible instrument would be useful primarily for visualization, with very limited capability for manipulation such as foreign-body extraction) and 'gross medical malpractice for doing this in children' (I have yet to figure out the basis for *that* concept).

Happily, the climate has changed in paediatrics as well as in medicine for adults. Today, the use of flexible bronchoscopes by paediatric pulmonologists is not only accepted, but expected, at least in most institutions. Even more happily, pulmonologists and surgeons have begun to learn that by working together they can achieve better patient outcomes. Ten years ago, I came to Cincinnati Children's Hospital to work with Dr. Robin Cotton and his colleagues in 'Paediatric Otolaryngology'. This is a programme that draws patients from around the globe and performs hundreds of airway reconstructions annually. Had I not had a close personal relationship with Robin Cotton (and had he perhaps a different personality), I could have literally found myself in a situation like George Bernard Shaw once described as 'a mangy old lion in a den full of Christians'. In the event, as we began to work *together* to evaluate children with complex airway problems, it rapidly became apparent that neither I nor my otorhinolaryngology colleagues fully appreciated either the limitations of our own or the advantages of the other's instruments and techniques! In the first year or two, there were some truly eye-opening experiences on both sides. Now, partly as a result of our enhanced understanding of the advantages of looking at patients from both perspectives (medical/surgical as well as flexible/rigid) and partly as a result of the complex patient population we see, approximately 500 of the 1,200 flexible bronchoscopies I and my pulmonology colleagues perform each year are joint procedures with otorhinolaryngology. As a result, our patients receive, we believe, more accurate diagnoses and more effective care. We believe this to be an effective model for good patient care.

Over the past 40 years, there has been an ongoing development of new instruments for use in the paediatric airways, although flexible instruments have had further to go. It has been difficult to improve on the glass rod telescope, but flexible instruments have become smaller, and their image quality has continued to improve. In flexible bronchoscopes used in adult patients today, the fibre-optic image bundle has been replaced by a video chip at the distal end of the instrument. This has resulted in a significantly improved image resolution and eliminated the problem of broken image fibres with degradation of the image quality. Unfortunately, video chips small enough to be used in paediatric instruments have yet to make their appearance, although this may change in the (hopefully near) future. In the meantime, 'hybrid' instruments, which use a fibre-optic image bundle to deliver the image to a video chip embedded in the proximal end of the instrument, are now available and are quite useful. They are completely compatible with the video instruments used by our colleagues in gastro-enterology and adult pulmonology.

The smallest useful flexible bronchoscope now available is approximately 2 mm in diameter, but such instruments have no suction channel and therefore have very limited utility. They are also more challenging to manipulate than their larger cousins. Nevertheless, they are essential parts of the serious paediatric bronchoscopist's tool chest.

In the search for smaller but useful instruments, we must remain aware of the limits of physics. There are 5 criteria for a useful paediatric flexible bronchoscope: image quality, illumination, manoeuvrability, suction capability and durability. Each of these functions contributes to the diameter of the working part of the instrument. The smallest instrument now available with a useful working channel is 2.8–3.0 mm in diameter. I have thoroughly explored the potential for smaller suction channels and have sadly but firmly concluded that a channel smaller than the current 1.2 mm would not be useful. I believe that the future lies in the production of instruments with improved image quality rather than smaller outer diameters. Improvements could also be made in ergonomic features, but not, realistically, in size. However, with very few exceptions, the 2.8-mm instrument can perform the tasks needed in the diagnosis and management of most paediatric patients. I currently utilize the 2.8-mm 'hybrid' instrument for more than 90% of the procedures I do. While a smaller instrument is occasionally necessary, a smaller instrument would not, in my opinion, be useful for the majority of paediatric procedures.

Prior to the advent of flexible bronchoscopy as a part of paediatric pulmonary practice, issues involving airway structure and dynamics were poorly defined and understood. Over the past 4 decades, much has been learned, and additional new diagnostic tools have been developed, including computed tomography and magnetic resonance imaging. As more paediatric specialists have become comfortable with diagnostic bronchoscopy, barriers to more aggressive and effective diagnosis have fallen. The result has been a dramatic enhancement of our understanding of airway problems in children and improved patient care.

Confucius was right: a picture can be worth many words. The ability to visualize the airways of children can be powerful. Contemporary equipment and techniques for recording video images make it possible for members of the care team as well as parents (and even patients) to see and understand the nature of the child's problems. In my experience, non-medical persons find it much easier to comprehend a video of a bronchoscopy (especially if it has been effectively edited and/or a comparison video of a normal paediatric airway is available) than to understand a chest CT scan. Three-dimensional reconstructions of CT scans can give a dramatic image but do not show dynamics.

My radiology colleagues frequently (teasingly, I think) tell me that they could make bronchoscopy unnecessary for the majority of my patients with 3-dimensional reconstructions and 'virtual bronchoscopy'. 'Fat chance', I retort. 'Show me the dynamics, show me the results of the cytology of the terminal bronchi and alveoli, and define for me the microbial flora of the airways and lungs'. QED. In truth, there are, as with virtually all diagnostic modalities, relative advantages and disadvantages of each technique, and in many cases, *both* bronchoscopy *and* radiological imaging techniques are required to give the whole story.

Not every child who would benefit from diagnostic bronchoscopy has an anatomical airway problem, nor even a problem of airway dynamics (e.g. tracheomalacia). In essence, there is only one indication for diagnostic bronchoscopy: information in the lungs or airways of the patient, necessary for the care of the patient and best obtained by bronchoscopy. One of the issues for the future is to make health care practitioners who are not specialists more aware of the indications for and the utility of bronchoscopic evaluation in their patients. The value of a negative examination, properly conducted, also needs to be appreciated, as it can dramatically reduce anxiety on the part of the patient and family and eliminate or greatly reduce further diagnostic tests or therapeutic trials.

One of the advantages attributed (correctly) to the flexible bronchoscope is its ability to traverse and examine the entire airway, from nostril to bronchus, and the fact that this can be done with minimal mechanical distortion of the airway anatomy and dynamics. Despite the relatively inferior optical performance of flexible instruments, in many paediatric patients, the most critical aspect of bronchoscopy is documentation of the airway dynamics. This can be done more readily with flexible than with rigid instruments, which themselves of necessity distort the anatomy. However, evaluation of some other aspects of the upper airway with flexible instruments is much more difficult than is usually appreciated. Specifically, flexible instruments are seriously limited in their ability to evaluate the structure of the posterior aspect of the larynx. I have been amazed, working with my otorhinolaryngology colleagues in Cincinnati, at how often they are able to demonstrate a laryngo-oesophageal cleft, and how normal the larynx appears to me at the same examination (with a flexible instrument). In our referral population, there are many children who aspirate food or oral secretions; in these children, we have found that examination with both rigid and flexible instruments is needed to gain a full understanding of the anatomy and physiology. The beauty of our cooperative practice model is that both procedures are performed during the same anaesthetic session: both the pulmonologist and the surgeon are present for the examination (and discussion), we approach the patient from different perspectives, and we then speak to the family together. It is clear, to me, at least, that two very strong

indications for rigid instruments are foreign-body removal and the detailed evaluation of the posterior aspect of the larynx.

Therapeutic bronchoscopy involves the restoration of airway patency or stability, or the removal of tissue or substances from the airways or alveolar spaces that interfere with normal function. It is in this arena that the rigid bronchoscope and accessories have a distinct advantage in most circumstances. While it is clearly possible to remove *some* bronchial foreign bodies with a flexible bronchoscope, foreign-body extraction with such instruments is not, and will not become, an easy or preferred technique. There are simply too many limitations, and it makes little sense to me to eschew the advantages of rigid instrumentation for this purpose.

There are some other therapeutic bronchoscopic procedures that can be performed with either rigid or flexible instrumentation. Table 1 shows some of these indications and points out some relative preference. It should be clear that in many cases, *either* rigid or flexible instrumentation can suffice perfectly well. Much depends on the skill and experience of the bronchoscopist. The use of *both* types of equipment should be seriously considered in individual situations.

Early in the history of paediatric flexible bronchoscopy, there was emphasis on the use of intravenous sedation administered by the bronchoscopist and team, rather than 'general anaesthesia' administered by an anaesthesiologist. As we have grown older and gained more experience, most paediatric flexible bronchoscopists today utilize the services of a paediatric anaesthesiologist. The benefit for the bronchoscopist is that someone else takes the responsibility for the primary monitoring of the patient and can use drugs that can get the patient to the precise level of sedation needed for the specific diagnostic or therapeutic purpose (and change that level quickly, as necessary). The benefit for the patient is more rapid induction and emergence, in a safe environment. Bronchoscopy is a serious procedure and should be so treated; patients deserve the benefit of expert care in the most appropriate facilities (i.e. anaesthesiologists and postanaesthesia recovery units). This is not to say that bronchoscopist-administered intravenous sedation is inappropriate, but I, at least, have grown beyond it.

Another issue that continues to evolve is that of training for the performance of bronchoscopy. It is not possible to be a competent bronchoscopist unless one has a good working knowledge of airway anatomy and physiology, and of the many abnormalities one is likely to encounter in paediatric patients. Bronchoscopy is not merely a technical skill but

Table 1. Therapeutic bronchoscopy – rigid versus flexible instrumentation

Indication	Rigid	Flexible
Extraction of mucus plugs[1]	+	+++
Extraction of foreign body[2]	+++	(+)
Haemoptysis – extraction of clots[3]	++	++
Endobronchial mass lesions		
Forceps extraction[4]	+++	+
Endobronchial cauterization[5]	++	+++
Endobronchial laser[6]	++	+++
Dilation of stenosis[7]	++	++
Placement of stent[8] (note: very limited application in paediatrics)	++	++
Therapeutic lung lavage[9]	(+)	+++
Treatment of bronchopleural fistula[10]	(+)	++

[1] Extraction of mucus plugs is in most cases more easily done with flexible instruments, but on occasion, rigid forceps may be useful.
[2] With rare exceptions, the primary utility of a flexible bronchoscope in the management of foreign bodies lies in the initial diagnosis or in the management of very small, peripherally located objects not reachable by rigid forceps.
[3] Large bronchial clots can be difficult to remove with any technique and sometimes require large forceps.
[4] Forceps usable with flexible instruments are very small and, in practice, mostly valuable for diagnostic purposes (if that).
[5] Either instrument can be used to direct a cautery electrode, although I could argue that the ability to direct the electrode precisely (and to go around a corner with the electrode) makes the flexible bronchoscope more useful.
[6] Laser fibres are relatively rigid, but for the treatment of small, benign lesions, a flexible instrument can direct and control the fibre more accurately and easily than a rigid instrument.
[7] The larger the patient, the more useful a flexible instrument can be (i.e. in larger patients, a balloon catheter can be passed via the suction channel of an adult flexible bronchoscope).
[8] Accurate stent placement requires direct observation of the stent; this can be accomplished with either rigid or flexible instruments.
[9] Flexible bronchoscopes are vastly superior at performing bronchoalveolar lavage and/or directing endobronchial catheters or double-lumen endotracheal tubes for large-volume lavages.
[10] Flexible bronchoscopes can deliver glue or direct a Fogarty catheter to the bronchus proximal to the air leak.

involves a large amount of cognitive skill and ability as well. Of all the complications of bronchoscopy, other than death of the patient, I believe that the most serious is to have done the procedure and got the wrong answer. One can get the wrong answer for many reasons, including using the wrong equipment, using the wrong technique for anaesthesia/sedation, not looking in the right place, not taking the right specimen, handling the specimen improperly, by not recognizing the abnormality when it is seen, and others.

Effective bronchoscopy requires considerable training and experience. How does one gain that training and experience? In many paediatric pulmonary training programmes today, fellows in training do not get experience with a large number of procedures. Attempts to define the number of bronchoscopies needed to reach clinical competence naturally fail to account for the quality and intensity of training programmes or the innate skill of the fledgling bronchoscopist. I believe that one of the real challenges in the future will be the development of programmes to adequately train young physicians to safely and effectively perform diagnostic and therapeutic bronchoscopy.

Bronchoscopy is not limited to the purview of surgeons and pulmonologists. In many institutions, specialists in critical care (including neonatology) and anaesthesiology have also expressed interest in learning to perform (flexible) bronchoscopy. While it is critical to have sufficient numbers of skilled practitioners in any given institution to offer the needed patient care and to provide backup coverage, there is a potential danger of having too many bronchoscopists, each with too little skill and experience... This clearly is an issue that will have to be addressed within each institution, with the ultimate goal of providing the best care for patients at the least cost and risk.

In the next several decades, bronchoscopy will become a more substantial part of paediatric pulmonary research. Serious ethical (and other) barriers exist to the use of paediatric subjects in research involving invasive techniques such as bronchoscopy. However, it is clear that bronchoscopy is the only acceptable way to obtain material from the interior of the airways and lungs (other than induced sputum, which has many potential pitfalls…). Flexible bronchoscopes can allow investigators to visualize the airways, obtain specimens (washings, brushings, mucosal biopsies, gas samples, airway surface liquid) and to deposit drugs or materials within the lungs. Research applications of bronchoscopy can involve patients in whom the bronchoscopy is already being performed for clinical reasons, those for whom participation in the research study will bring direct personal benefit and possibly those already undergoing procedures requiring intubation/anaesthesia and from whom small samples can be obtained with very minimal risk. We must and we will find ways to utilize this powerful tool to expand our ability to understand and more effectively treat paediatric pulmonary disease.

What are the challenges for the future? Better instruments – not smaller, but with better optics. Better training – to ensure skilled performance of clinically needed procedures. Better understanding on the part of paediatrics practitioners of the role of bronchoscopy in the diagnosis and management of paediatric patients – to develop more appropriate referral patterns. Better practice models – to improve the multidisciplinary management of difficult diagnostic and therapeutic dilemmas. Better research applications – to improve our understanding of disease and the development of new therapies. There is great potential in all these areas, and I foresee a Golden Age of paediatric bronchoscopy on the horizon.

'We dance around the patient and suppose, but the bronchoscope goes into the patient and knows' (with apologies to Robert Frost).

Robert E. Wood, PhD, MD
Professor of Pediatrics and Otolaryngology
Cincinnati Children's Hospital Medical Center
University of Cincinnati College of Medicine
3333 Burnet Avenue MLC 2021
Cincinnati, OH 45229-3039 (USA)
Tel. +1 513 636 2776, Fax +1 513 636 3845, E-Mail rewood@cchmc.org

Author Index

Subject Index